$53.95
1/21/88

Testicular and Epididymal Pathology

Manuel Nistal
Professor of Histology and Embryology,
Department of Morphology, School of Medicine, Autonomous University of Madrid, Madrid, Spain,
Head of the Section of Pathology, La Paz Hospital, Madrid, Spain

Ricardo Paniagua
Professor of Cytology and Histology,
Faculty of Biology, University of Salamanca, Salamanca, Spain

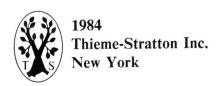

1984
Thieme-Stratton Inc.
New York

Georg Thieme Verlag
Stuttgart • New York

Thieme-Stratton Inc.
381 Park Avenue South
New York, New York 10016

Library of Congress Cataloging in Publication Data

Nistal Martín de Serrano, Manuel.
    Testicular and epididymal pathology.
    Includes bibliographies and index.
    1. Testis—Diseases. 2. Epididymis—Diseases.
I. Paniagua Gómez-Alvarez, Ricardo. II. Title.
[DNLM: 1. Epididymis—abnormalities. 2. Epididymis—
pathology. 3. Testicular Diseases—pathology. 4. Testis
—abnormalities. WJ 830 N727t]

RC898.N57   1984   616.6'8   83-50439
ISBN 0-86577-112-X

Printed in the United States of America

Cover design by Debra Morton

Testicular and Epididymal Pathology
Manuel Nistal and Ricardo Paniagua

TSI ISBN 0-86577-112-X
GTV ISBN 3-13-651701-6

Copyright © 1984 by Thieme-Stratton Inc. All rights reserved. No part of this publication may be reprinted or reused without the express written consent of the publisher.

5 4 3 2 1

To my sons Rodrigo, Gonzalo and Beatriz
(Manuel Nistal)

To Pilar and Alvaro
(Ricardo Paniagua)

ACKNOWLEDGMENTS

Our work could only be fulfilled if the adequate material and installations were available, and with the aid of generous colaborators. We are indebted to Prof. Dr. Felix Contreras, Head of the Department of Pathology of La Paz Hospital, Madrid (Spain), who trained us in the basic histopathologic techniques, introduced us to the study of testicular pathology, supervised our research, and offered us the material from his department for this work. We gratefully acknowledge his cooperation and helpful discussion in the preparation of the manuscript.

We thank Prof. Dr. Fernando Reinoso, Head of the Department of Morphology, School of Medicine, Autonomous University of Madrid, and our colleagues of the Department of Pathology, Drs. M. Patrón, J. Larrauri, M. Gutiérrez, M. Claver, A. Ruiz, M.L. Picazo, C. Gamallo, J. Alba, I. Rodríguez, F. López-Barea, J.M. Viguer, A. Suárez, and C. Morales for their constant support and valuable suggestions during the course of our work.

We are also grateful to Dr. J.J. Vázquez-Rodríguez who wrote chapter 5, Dr. M.A. Abaurrea for her helpful revision of the literature, and Drs. D.B. Krimer and L. Santamaría for contributing excellent illustrations.

Our gratitude goes also to the Departments of Urology, Endocrinology, Sterility, Pediatrics, and Genetics at La Paz Hospital for the contribution of material and studies.

Lastly, the authors wish to thank the technicians and photographer of the department of pathology for their skillful technical assistance.

PREFACE

The purpose of this book is to offer the reader an updated review of the pathology of the testis and epididymis. It summarizes a number of data that have appeared in books and journals devoted to many different medical areas including endocrinology, urology, andrology, radiology, gynecology, and even genetic, pediatric, and basic biomedical sciences.

The basis of the work was to establish a link among the different points of view through which testicular and epididymal pathology has traditionally been focused. A histopathologic prospective was, in our opinion, the best approach for integrating the different approaches to the subject. *Testicular and Epididymal Pathology* is first of all a book of histopathology.

Furthermore we decided to write the book ourselves, preferring the harmony and cohesion of a book with only two authors to an exhaustive opus written by many different authorities. This has enabled us to complete a work in which the available knowledge is adequately distributed in twenty-two chapters, which demonstrate the progressive development of testicular lesion study. This format also facilitates frequent cross references to other chapters.

The work was carried out in the Department of Pathology, in La Paz Hospital, School of Medicine of the Autonomous University of Madrid (Spain). The material used for the compilation of this book includes biopsies, surgical specimens, and autopsies—all of which were collected from November 1966 to December 1983. During this period, the number of testicular biopsies and orchidectomy specimens studied was over 4,000, and from the approximately 6,000 autopsies that were carried out, two-thirds of them were of children.

Although some chapters deal in part with experimental models in order to achieve a better understanding of the lesions, this book is primarily devoted to human pathology.

The book examines the normal testis and epididymis, congenital abnormalities, testicular biopsy interpretation, cryptorchidism, hypogonadisms, vascular pathology of the testis, intersex conditions, inflammatory diseases and testicular and epididymal tumors. Special attention has been devoted to problems that are debated at the moment, such as the fertility prognosis of the early surgically descended cryptorchid testes, the spermatozoon morphological abnormalities having a genetic origin, the causes involved in progressive testicular atrophy in patients with varicocele, and the classification of male pseudohermaphroditism on a histological basis.

Although the focus of the book is mainly histologic, most of the disorders studied include clinical, hormonal, and genetic aspects that facilitate a comprehensive approach to their study. A selected, updated list of references completes each chapter.

Our wish is that the work be useful for our pathologist colleagues as well as for all those who, from different medical specialities, must daily solve problems presented by patients with testicular or epididymal pathology.

The authors
April 1984

CONTENTS

1. Development of the Male Genital Tract ... 1
2. Development of the Testis from Birth to Puberty ... 14
3. Adult Testis ... 26
4. Epididymis and Spermatic Ducts ... 52
5. Hormonal Control of Testicular Function ... 63
   J.J. Vazquez
6. Congenital Anomalies of the Testis and the Epididymis ... 72
7. Testicular Biopsy. Basic Testicular Lesions ... 94
8. Precocious Testicular Maturation (Precocious Puberty) ... 114
9. Cryptorchidism ... 120
10. Retractile Testes ... 140
11. Hypogonadism Due to Primary Testicular Failure ... 145
12. Hypogonadisms Due to Secondary Testicular Failure ... 168
13. Testicular Lesions Secondary to Disorders of Different Endocrine Glands ... 178
14. Testicular Lesions Secondary to Physical-Chemical Agents, Dietary Deficiencies, and Peripheral Nervous System Lesions ... 190
15. Vascular Disorders of the Testis ... 201
16. Morphological Abnormalities in the Spermatozoa ... 227
17. Gonadal Dysgenesis: True Hermaphroditism and Male Pseudohermaphroditism ... 241
18. Inflammatory Diseases of the Epididymis and Testis ... 263
19. Disorders Secondary to Obstruction of the Epididymis and Vas Deferens ... 278
20. Lesions of the Tunica Vaginalis ... 288
21. Testicular Tumors ... 298
22. Tumors of the Epididymis and the Spermatic Cord ... 338
    Index ... 351

1
DEVELOPMENT OF THE MALE GENITAL TRACT

Evolution of the Undifferentiated Gonad

Although genetic sex is established at the time of conception, the development of the genital tract is identical in both sexes until the seventh week of embryonal development (embryos of 17 to 20 mm length). The sequence of events leading to the evolution of the undifferentiated gonad is as follows (Forest, 1982; O'Rahilly, 1983):

1. Primordial germ cells are originally seen toward the third week of gestation in and around the extraembryonal mesoderm lining the posterior wall of the yolk sac near the allantois evagination. The primordial cells are oval shaped, have some cytoplasmic processes and measure 12 to 14 microns. Their nuclei are round and display one or two prominent nucleoli. Their cytoplasm has abundant glycogen and numerous organelles. The latter include mitochondria with tubular cristae, numerous polysomes, rough endoplasmic reticulum displaying short cisternae, scant lipid droplets, lysosomes and bundles of microfilaments. There is marked activity of alkaline phosphatase (Fujimoto and associates, 1977; Fukuda and others, 1975; Ando and Fujimoto, 1983).

2. Development of genital ridge. After 30 or 32 days the embryo shows an area of celomic thickening along the longitudinal axis on either side of the midline between the mesonephros and the root of the dorsal mesentery. This thickening of the celomic epithelium and adjacent loose mesenchyma is designated as genital or gonadal ridges (Fig. 1–1A).

3. Migration of primordial germ cells. Simultaneous to the development of the genital ridges is the incoming migration of primordial germ cells along the dorsal mesentery of the hindgut. The primordial germ cells have reached the genital ridges by the 32nd to 35th day of gestation (Figs. 1–1B and 1–2). This migration is accomplished by ameboid movements probably controlled to some extent by cells of the gonadal blastema. This control does not seem to be androgenic in nature (Jirasek, 1970; Witschi, 1948). The primordial germ cells together with the mesenchymal cells, which both accumulate beneath the coelomic epitheluim, form the gonadal blastema (Wartenberg, 1981).

4. Development of the "indifferent gonad." To most former investigators (Grunwald, 1942), at the time the germinal cells begin to organize in the gonadal blastema the celomic epithelium proliferates inwards resulting in the formation of the primary sex cords in continuity with the celomic epithelium lining the gonad (Figs. 1–1B and 1–3A). These sex cords are made up of irregular cellular nests arranged perpendicularly to the epithelial surface and they become gradually surrounded by primordial germinal cells. At this point, however, the male and female gonads still share common features. Other authors held the view that the male and female inner gonadal structures were derived from the mesenchymal (mesonephric) cells without participation of the superficial epithelium (Gropp and Ohno, 1966). In the last decade a different theory has been developed by Wartenberg (1978 and 1981). He assumes that epithelial and mesonephric cells intermingled to form a common gonadal blastema. The sex cords begin forming by separation of the blastema into a network of plate-like strands (sex cords) and interstitial tissue. The primordial germ cells become enclosed in the sex cords. The germinal cells still retain intense alkaline phosphatase activity and

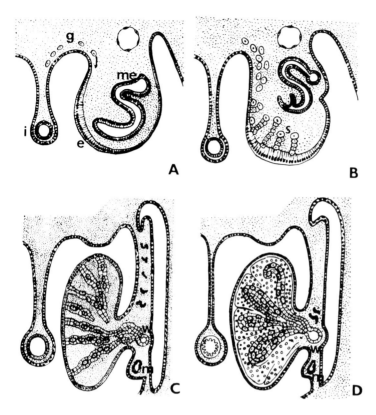

FIGURE 1–1. *Early stages of development of the male gonad. A, Embryo, 4th week. Primordial germ cells migrate from the vitelline sac to the genital ridges. B, Sixth week. Formation of sex cords. C, Seventh week. Development of sex cords and degeneration of mesonephric tubes. D, Eighth week. Sex cords break away from the epithelial surface of the gonad and the tunica albuginea begins to form. g: primordial germ cells; i: intestine; e: surface epithelium of genital ridge; me: mesonephric tube; s: sex cords; w: Wolffian duct; m: Müllerian duct (modified from W. J. Hamilton).*

high glycogen content evidenced by their cytoplasmic PAS positive reaction. After the 37th day both gonads become individualized. A mesonephros, containing blood vessels, and the prolongations of the primitive sexual cords forming the undifferentiated rete testis, are the sole residual structures of the mesonephric mesenchyma. At this time, two folds of the posterior peritoneum appear: the superior fold forms the suspensory ligament; and the inferior fold forms the inguinal ligament.

GENITAL DUCT FORMATION

At the end of the sixth week of embryonal development the undifferentiated gonads have paired genital ducts, the Wolffian (mesonephric) ducts and the Müllerian (paramesonephric) ducts (Figs. 1–1C and 1–4).

The Wolffian ducts originate from the mesonephros thus relating embryologically and anatomically to the excretory system. About the third week of gestation the embryonal mesoderm divides in three parts: axial; lateral; and medial. The medial mesoderm (cervical region) gives rise to ten paired tubular structures arranged segmentally. These nephric ducts grow laterally and open into the celome on one side while on the opposite end they form a longitudinal duct on either side of the midline. The resulting structure (or pronephros) degenerates at approximately the fourth week to be replaced by another system of ducts (mesonephros) that arises from the medial mesoderm and extends from the inferior cervical segments to the posterior lumbar segments. These ducts

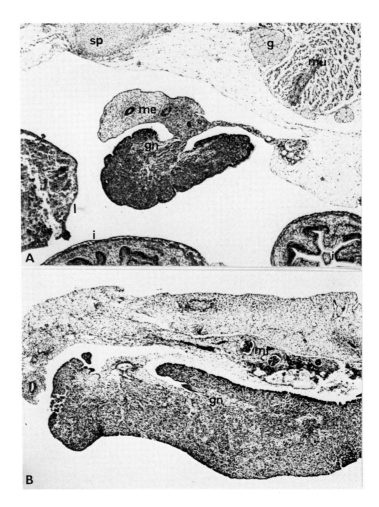

FIGURE 1–2. *Male gonad at sixth week of development. A, Localization in a transversal section. B, Longitudinal section showing groups of epithelial-looking cells growing into the gonad (dark areas). Occasional mesonephric glomeruli (mf) are also seen (x25). (sp): spinal cord; g: cord ganglia; mu: skeletal muscle; l: liver; i: intestine; me: mesonephros; gn: gonad.*

connect with the mesonephric glomeruli. On the opposite side, the mesonephric ducts form a single excretory duct called the Wolffian duct. At the end of the second month of gestation the mesonephros also disappears to be replaced by the metanephros or definitive kidney (Fig. 1–1C). In the male, the Wolffian ducts (Fig. 1–1D) persist to form the excretory ducts (epididymis, vas deferens, and seminal vesicles) while in the female they normally degenerate (Orgebin-Crist, 1981).

The paired Müllerian ducts arise as a groove in the lateral aspect of the mesonephric ridge near its cranial extremity. These Müllerian ducts remain lateral to the Wolffian duct and eventually form a tube that remains open. Further on, each Müllerian duct crosses the Wolffian duct on each side until they both form the female genital duct. The latter extends further to reach the urogenital sinus posteriorly where it forms the Müllerian tubercle, between the openings of both Wolffian ducts (Figs. 1–4 and 1–5A).

DEVELOPMENT OF THE UNDIFFERENTIATED EXTERNAL GENITALIA

The external genitalia arise from the primitive urogenital sinus that derives in turn from the cloaca. The latter becomes

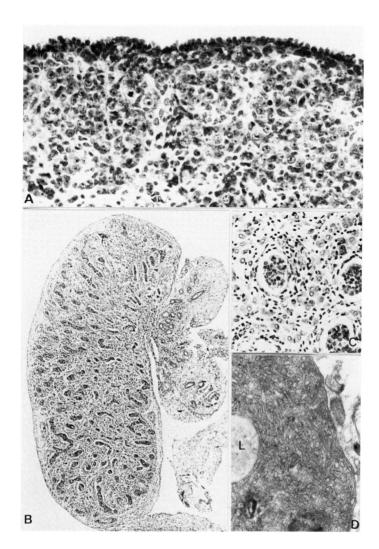

FIGURE 1-3. *A*, Detail of gonadal epithelium and testicular cords during the sixth week of development (x250). *B*, During the third month the male gonad already shows the outline of the testis including the presence of early defined seminiferous tubules (x25). *C*, Seminiferous tubules still devoid of lumina. There are Leydig cells in the interstitial space (x125). *D*, Detail of the cytoplasm of a Leydig cell during the third month showing abundant smooth endoplasmic reticulum and (L) lipid inclusions (x30,000).

established toward the end of the 17th day of embryonic development as a dilatation of the caudal end of the hindgut. The allantois also develops at this time anteriorly in the form of a saccular dilatation. During the third week of embryonal development the cloacal fold develops from the outer aspect of the cloacal membrane and a medial eminence or "cloacal eminence" is formed.

From the fifth week onward the cloaca is divided into two separate cavities, the primitive urogenital sinus with the urogenital membrane anteriorly and the anorectal canal with the anal membrane posteriorly (Figs. 1-5A and 1-6A).

During the sixth week the cloacal folds develop further into the genital or urethral folds that surround the urogenital membrane, and the anal folds which surround the anal membrane. The cloacal eminence will form the genital tubercle while, out of the genital folds, the genital swellings develop from two mesenchymal folds (Figs. 1-5A and 1-6A).

The primitive urogenital sinus also

FIGURE 1–4. *At about the sixth week each gonad has a pair of genital ducts: the mesonephric or Wolffian duct (W) and the paramesonephric or Müllerian duct (M). Both fuse before they reach the urogenital sinus (US) to form the utero-vaginal duct (UV). As they reach the urogenital sinus they form the tubercle of Müller (TM). The Wolffian ducts end in the urogenital sinus next to the uterovaginal duct. During the 7th and 8th weeks the Müllerian duct undergoes complete involution. This schematic drawing shows the mesonephric ducts connecting the sex cords to the Wolffian ducts as well as other mesonephric ducts in the process of involution.*

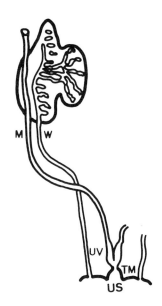

FIGURE 1–5. *Schematic drawing of the distal end of the genital tract and of the external genitalia at six weeks (A) and at ten weeks (B). Sagittal view;* **ub**: *urinary bladder;* **U**: *ureter;* **W**: *Wolffian duct;* **M**: *Müllerian ducts ending in the tubercle of Müller;* **um**: *urogenital membrane;* **D**: *vas deferens;* **SV**: *seminal vesicle;* **P**: *phallus;* **GF**: *genital folds.*

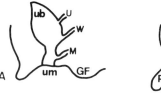 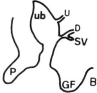

FIGURE 1–6. *Schematic drawing of external genitalia. A, At six weeks. B, At ten weeks. C, At birth.* **t**: *genital tubercle;* **g**: *genital folds and genital swellings;* **a**: *anal folds;* **m**: *urogenital membrane;* **p**: *penis;* **u**: *urethral groove;* **sf**: *scrotal folds;* **g**: *glans;* **r**: *scrotal raphe;* **s**: *scrotum.*

 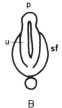 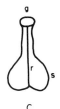

develops into two sections: a superior one (or vesicourethral duct) that eventually becomes the bladder and urethra while the allantois atrophies and remains as the uracus and an inferior one, the portion of the urogenital sinus that eventually differentiates according to the gonadal sex.

DEVELOPMENT OF THE TESTIS

Although genetic sex is determined by the XY chromosomal constitution at the time of conception, it still has to become expressed into gonadal sex (Jost, 1981). Thus, the indifferent gonad develops into the future testis in embryos with the XY chromosomal constitution while the development of phenotypic male differentiation depends on the secretion and metabolism of testosterone. The lack of testerone or the lack of response to it, results in female development, even in the presence of a Y chromosome and actual testis (see Chapter 17) (Opitz, 1980; Wachtel, 1979). Figure 1–7 illustrates the sequence of events in sex determination.

The initial changes leading to the development of the testis from the indifferent gonad are seen in embryos of 44 to 48 days (crown–rump 15 to 19 mm) (Fig. 1–1B, C, and D). At this stage there is rapid proliferation of sex cords developing inside the genital folds. Each cord becomes a seminiferous tubule when surrounded by a well-defined basement membrane (seventh week). At this point there is a loss of continuity between the epithelium that covers the gonad and the underlying seminiferous tubules. In fact, the epithelium

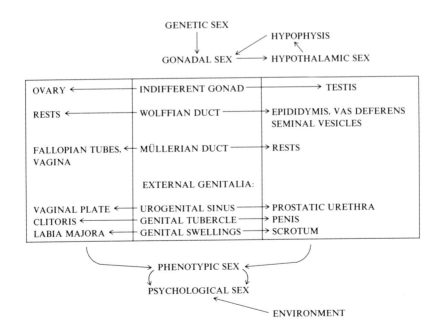

FIGURE 1–7. *Sequence of Sex Determination.*

gradually flattens and converts to a mesothelial lining.

The transformation of the primitive gonadal blastema into sex cords is induced by germinal cells with the XY chromosomal constitution. Evidence has recently been developed to suggest that testicular differentiation is invariably associated with the presence of an antigen (H–Y antigen), which is specified on the Y chromosome. In fact, it has been suggested that the presence of H–Y antigen is sufficient to induce testicular differentiation even in the absence or partial loss of the Y chromosome (Wachtel, 1979).

Although germ cells do not enter meiosis until puberty, the testicular differentiation progresses more rapidly than that of the ovary where, by comparison, cellular organization is considerably delayed. An interesting theory has been developed in the last decade (Jost and co-workers, 1974; Byskov and Saxen, 1976; Wartenberg, 1981). The gonadal blastema consists of light (epithelial) cells and dark (mesonephric) cells. Both cell-types would represent a dualistic system, exercising either a stimulating (dark cells) or a inhibitory (light cells) effect on the germ cell mitosis and meiosis. Unlike conditions in the female gonad, the light mitosis–and meiosis–preventing cells regains dominance in the sex cords, and meiosis is arrested before it starts.

In the initial stages of development the testis show four types of cells: germ cells; epithelial cells of the testicular cords; and two types of mesenchymal cells—one type among the testicular cords, and the other type between the testicular cords and the mesonephros corresponding to the early framework of the rete testis.

In the embryo of 48 to 60 days (crown–rump 18 to 32 mm) the mesenchymal cells located between the testicular cords evolve into the connective tissue elements that will surround the testicular cords and the rete testis. This connective tissue shows active proliferation to become arranged between the celomic epithelium and the testicular cords and form the tunica albuginea. The latter remains as the testicular capsule and illustrates the final stage of the transformation of the indifferent gonad into the actual testis.

The tunica albuginea is composed of three layers: (1) the visceral layer, which is strictly mesothelial; (2) the tunica albuginea proper, which includes almost the entire thickness of the capsule; and (3) the vascular layer, which supports the blood vessels, lymphatics, and nerves (Figs. 1–3B and 2–8). The albuginea is somewhat thicker along the posterior aspect of the testis. It is here that it forms the mediastinum testis, containing the rete and the initial segments of the efferent ducts.

During fetal life the seminiferous tubules are solid and disclose two types of cells—germinal cells and Sertoli or sustentacular cells (Figs. 1–3B and C; and 1–8). The germinal cells consist of three types: gonocytes, intermediate, and fetal spermatogonia (Fukuda, 1976; Gondos and Golbus, 1976; Gondos and Hobel, 1971; Holstein and co-authors, 1971; Wartenberg and others, 1971) (Fig. 1–8).

The gonocytes are those with the highest nucleo-cytoplasmic ratio. The nucleus is round and exhibits a single central and prominent nucleolus. The cytoplasm has a well developed Golgi apparatus, lipid droplets, and a rough endoplasmic reticulum with short cisternae and numerous microfilaments, the latter particularly abundant in the proximity of the cytoplasmic membrane. The intermediate cells are somewhat similar but they display a lower nucleo-cytoplasmic ratio, more cytoplasmic processes, and wider cisternae in the rough endoplasmic reticulum. These cells are connected by intercellular bridges. Fetal spermatogonia also have intercellular bridges, but they have the lowest nucleo-cytoplasmic ratio and a more condensed nuclear chromatin.

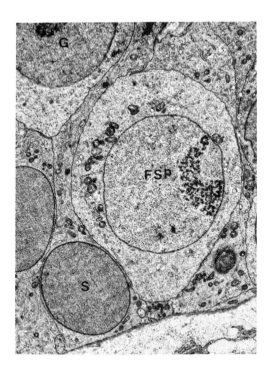

FIGURE 1–8. *Gonocyte (G) and fetal spermatogonia (FSP) among immature Sertoli cells (S) (x10,000).*

The nuclear membrane is smooth while that of the primordial cells is usually indented. The mitochondria usually surround the nucleus and they are bound together by a homogenous electron dense substance. Finally these cells display scant endoplasmic reticulum and lipid droplets (Fig. 1–8). Common to the three types of germinal cells is the presence of abundant cytoplasmic glycogen, polysomes, and chromatoid bodies, the latter composed of finely granular material surrounded or mixed with larger granules approximately the size of ribosomes. Until the 10th week of pregnancy, most of the germ cells are gonocytes. Around the 15th week the intermediate cells become predominant, while gonocytes are still present. At this age a few fetal spermatogonia are also seen. After the 22nd week, most of the germ cells are fetal spermatogonia and typical gonocytes are absent (Fukuda, 1976).

Fetal Sertoli cells also show significant changes during the process of testicular maturation. About the 13th week they reveal scalloped edges with long cytoplasmic processes. They rest on the basal lamina where they are interconnected by desmosomes. Their nucleus is ovoid and indented and the chromatin is finely granular. The nucleolus is rather inconspicuous at this time. The cytoplasm is dense and shows abundant ribosomes and microfilaments and the rough endoplasmic reticulum shows numerous cisternae arranged in parallel fashion. There are also microtubules, elongated mitochondria and a well defined Golgi apparatus. With time, Sertoli cells become gradually elongated, the nucleolus gains prominence and the cytoplasm develops a lighter texture. The rough endoplasmic reticulum becomes more dense and so does the amount of lipids and lysosomes. The microfilaments still remain, but they tend to become oriented toward the basal side of the cell (see Fig. 1–8) (Fukuda and others, 1975).

The interstitial or Leydig cells appear

rather late (Fig. 1–3**C** and **D**). They originate from the fibroblastic-looking mesenchymal cells and towards the 42 to 45 days (crown–rump 15 to 17 mm) they are already differentiating in appreciable numbers.

Characteristic fetal Leydig cells are already seen with the electron microscope in embryos measuring 29 mm and in those measuring 30 to 32 mm at 56 to 60 days they can be distinguished already by their polyhedric shape and by their tendency to cluster. During fetal life these cells are eosinophilic and they have abundant cytoplasmic granules rich in glycoproteins and lipids. Their ultrastructure shows a well-developed smooth endoplasmic reticulum and a number of mitochondria with tubular cristae and a variable amount of lysosomes and lipid droplets (Fig. 1–3**D**) (Gondos and Golbus, 1976). At this stage they already have a significant content of acid phosphatase, glucose-6-phosphatase, and 3-beta-hydroxysteroid dehydrogenase.

Fetal Leydig cells under the influence of placental human chorionic gonadotrophin (HCG) undergo complete differentiation from elongated precursor mesenchymal cells to cells with polygonal shape and round nucleus (see Fig. 2–5**B**) (Gondos and Golbus, 1976). Their cytoplasm is rich in lipids and oxidative and hydrolytic enzymes. Later on they develop cytoplasmic vacuolization especially at the periphery of the cell, and there is 3-beta-hydroxysteroid dehydrogenase activity. Full differentiation of Leydig cells is finally accomplished at the 12th week.

At a later stage there is further increase of cytoplasmic vacuolization and the cells retain their content in lipids but histochemical detection of 3-beta-hydroxysteroid dehydrogenase becomes invariably negative, a finding which has been interpreted as indicative of cellular involution. Electron microscopy during this sequence of events in the developments of Leydig cells has also demonstrated a gradual increase of cytoplasmic structures, especially the ones involved in steroid synthesis, namely the smooth endoplasmic reticulum, the mitochondrial cristae and the lipid droplets (see Figs. 1–3**D** and 2–9**C**). At this time Leydig cells together with Sertoli cells assume the control for the development of the male genital tract. This is accomplished by the formation of two different substances, one produced by Sertoli cells, which is responsible for the involution of the Müllerian ducts, and a second one the result of androgen secretion by Leydig cells (Holstein and co-workers, 1971).

Development of Excretory Ducts

The mesonephric tubules located at the level of the testis lose their glomerules and shorten their length and connect with the rete testis to form the efferent ducts (embryos of 48 to 60 days) (Fig. 1–4). The mesonepheric tubules caudal to the testis persist until the end of the third month when they split from the Wolffian duct and remain as blind ending tubules of the paradidymis.

The Wolffian duct remains in its entire length to form the excretory system except in its cephalic end where its vestiges remain as the appendix of the epididymis.

At the caudal region, where efferent ducts are not formed, the excretory duct increases in length and becomes convoluted to form the duct of the epididymis. A further evagination close to the caudal end forms the seminal vesicles (Fig. 1–6**B**).

The Müllerian ducts under the influence of the Müllerian Inhibitory Substance secreted by Sertoli cells begins its involution in embryos of 56 to 63 days (crown–rump 30 to 35 mm). This involution usually starts at the caudal end of the testis, progresses rapidly and the only remaining vestiges are the appendix testis in the cranial end and the prostatic utricle in the opposite end (Josso, 1972; Picard and others, 1978; Vigier and others, 1983).

The involution of the Müllerian ducts occurs simultaneously to the development of the tunica albuginea but each testis is responsible for the inhibition of the Müllerian duct on its own side and not for the contralateral one (Jirasek, 1970; Josso and co-workers, 1977).

DEVELOPMENT OF MALE EXTERNAL GENITALIA

Masculinization of external genitalia begins in fetuses of 65 to 70 days (crown–rump 35 to 40 mm). The primitive urogenital sinus is divided into an upper and a lower portion. The upper portion will form the prostatic urethra while the lower portion will result in the formation of the penile urethra and external genitalia. The prostate gland originates from a series of epithelial buds that appear on the urethral surface. Rapid development and elongation of the genital tubercle forms the penis (Figs. 1–5B and 1–6B and C). This also results in elongation of the urethral folds and the formation of the urethral groove, which eventually becomes the penile urethra. Closure of the urethral or genital folds over the groove is accomplished approximately 80 to 90 days after fertilization. Finally, the urethral epithelium derives from the endodermal lining of the inner surface of the urethral groove.

Neither the urethral groove nor the penile urethra that results from its closure reach the distal end of the penis (glans). Within the 4th month the terminal end of the urethra is formed from ectodermal cells of the glans, which invaginate and form a special duct in continuity with the penile urethra. At this time the genital swellings have migrated anteriorly and develop to form the scrotum on both sides of the midline or scrotal raphe (Fig. 1–6).

During the first three months of fetal development control of the process of masculinization of the external genitalia is exercised by androgen secretion of Leydig

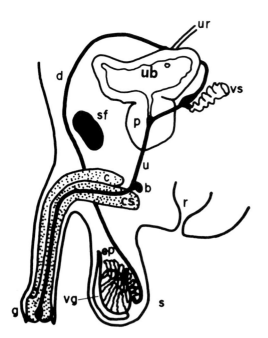

FIGURE 1–9. *Male genital system at birth. ur: ureter; ub: urinary bladder; p: prostate; vs: seminal vesicle; u: urethra; b: bulbourethral glands; c: corpora cavernosum; cs: corpora spongiosum; r: rectum; vg: vaginalis testis; t: testicle; ep: epididymis; sf: symphysis pubica; g: glans; s: scrotum.*

cells in response to HCG stimulation. During the second half of pregnancy the hypothalamo-pituitary axis plays an important role in the control of testosterone secretion by Leydig cells (Jost, 1970). In fact, in the absence of the pituitary gland, masculinization of the external genitalia may take place, but they fail to attain full-size. Hypothalamic male development proceeds during the third trimester and its absence will be followed by a female pattern of gonadotropin secretion. In the case of anencephaly, absence of hypothalamus results in changes similar to those brought about by hypophysectomy; namely, immature testes, decreased Leydig cell population, and frequent hypoplasia of penis and scrotum (Orgebin-Crist, 1981).

DESCENT OF THE TESTIS

In embryos of 70 to 80 days of gestation (crown–rump 50 mm) the testes leave their abdominal wall location and begin to descend into the retroperitoneal space. About the early part of the sixth month they are already close to the inguinal canal, where they remain until the seventh month. At this time they descend through the canal to reach the scrotum (Figs. 1–9 and 1–10).

The testicular descent is directed by the gubernaculum testis. This appears as an accumulation of mesenchymal cells extending from the genital ridges to the presumptive inguinal region, at the sixth week. From the second to the seventh month, the gubernaculum becomes surrounded by a skeletal muscle coat, originated from the internal oblique abdominal muscle. The gubernaculum is attached to the epididymis by one end, and to the scrotum by the opposite end. During the seventh month, its volume increases greatly, exceeding that of the testis. This enlargement is due to the increase in hyaluronic acid, which permits the testis to slip through the inguinal canal. At birth, the sole rest of the gubernaculum testis is the scrotal ligament; this ligament is fibrous and extends from the epididymis to the scrotal basis. The muscular layer surrounding the scrotal ligament is the origin of the cremaster muscle.

The mechanisms involved in testicular descent are not yet well known, and several mechanical and hormonal agents have been suggested (Hadziselimovic,

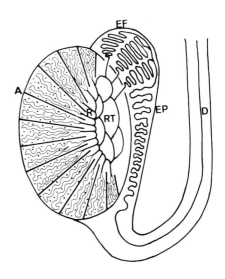

FIGURE 1–10. *Diagram of testis and epididymis at birth. D: vas deferens; EP: epididymal duct; EF: ductuli efferentes RT: rete testis; R: tubuli recti; A: albuginea (Seminiferous tubules and Leydig cells are represented within testicular lobules).*

1982). The main mechanical factors might be: (1) the high intraabdominal pressure, which would push the testis through the myxoid component of the gubernaculum testis; (2) the muscular component of the gubernaculum testis, which would pull the testis along the inguinal canal; and (3) the balloon swelling of the gubernaculum that should be the main downward force for testicular descent. Other authors have considered that the gubernaculum is only a guiding factor and not a motor of testicular descent. The formation of the processus vaginalis and the sinking of the testis in the gubernacular ground substance were the moving forces. Hadziselimovic (1982) and Mininberg and Schlossberg (1983) have shown that a fusion with the epididymis is essential to a normal descent of the testis.

The successful hormone treatments with HCG or LH-RH of undescended testes suggest that the testicular descent is an androgen dependent process. Hadziselimovic (1982) studies postulate that impaired intrauterine gonadatropin secretion leads to insufficient testosterone and dihydrotestosterone production thus resulting in epididymal malformations and cryptorchidism.

REFERENCES

1. Ando Y, Fujimoto T: Ultrastructural evidence that chick primordial germ cells leave the blood-vascular system prior to migrating to the gonadal ridge. Develop Growth Differ. 25:345, 1983
2. Byskov AG, Saxén L: Induction of meiosis in fetal mouse testis in vitro. Dev Biol 52:193, 1976
3. Forest MG: Development of the male reproductive tract. In White R, (ed) Aspects of Male Infertility. Williams & Wilkins. Baltimore 1982, pp. 1-60
4. Fujimoto T, Miyayama Y, Fuyuta M: The origin, migration and fine morphology of human primordial germ cells. Anat Rec 188:315, 1977
5. Fukuda T, Hedinger C, Groscurth P: Ultrastructure of developing germs cells in the fetal human testis. Cell Tissue Res 161:155, 1975
6. Fukuda T: Ultrastructure of primordial germ cells in human embryo. Virchows Arch B Cell Path 20:85,1976
7. Gondos B, Golbus MS: Ultrastructural changes in human fetal Leydig cells at midgestation. Andrologia 8 [Suppl] 1:116,1976
8. Gondos B, Hobel CJ: Ultrastructure of germ cell development in the human fetal testis. Z. Zellforsch 119:1, 1971
9. Gropp A, Ohno S: The presence of a common embryonic blastema for ovarian and testicular parenchymal (follicular, interstitial and tubular) cells in cattle, Bos taurus, Z Zellforsch 74:505, 1966
10. Grünwald P: The development of sex cords in the gonads of man and mammals. Am J Anat 70:359, 1942
11. Holstein AF, Wartenberg H, Vosameyer J: Zur Cytologie der pränatalen Gonadenentwicklung beim Menschen.III. Die Entwicklung der Leydigzellen in Hoden von Embryonen und Feten. Z. Anat Entwickl Gesch 135:43, 1971
12. Jirasek JE: The relationship between differentiation of the testicle, genital ducts and external genitalia in fetal and postnatal life. In Rosenberg E, Paulsen CA, (eds) The Human Testis. New York: Plenum Press 1970, p. 19
13. Josso N: Evolution of the Müllerian-inhibiting activity of the human testis. Effect of fetal, peri-natal and post-natal human testicular tissue in the Müllerian duct of the fetal rat in organ culture. Biol Neonate 20:368, 1972
14. Josso N, Picard JY, Trah D: the antimüllerian hormone. Recent Prog Horm Res 33:117, 1977
15. Jost A: Fetal sexual differentiation. In Biochemical and Social Bases of Pediatrics. Masson Inc. New York 1981, pp 39-48
16. Jost A: Hormonal factors in ther sex differentiation of the mammalian fetus. Philos Trans R Soc London Ser B 259:119, 1970
17. Jost A, Magre S, Crescent M, Perlman S: Sertoli cells and early testicular differentiation. In Mancini RE, Martini L, (eds) Male Fertility and Sterility. Proceedings of the Serono Symposia, Vol. 5. Academic Press. New York, 1974
18. Hadziselimović F: Pathogenesis and treatment of undescended testes. Eur J Pediatr 139:255, 1982

19. Mininberg DT, Schlossberg S: The role of the epididymis in testicular descent. J Urol 129:1207, 1983
20. Opitz JM: Comments on some genetic abnormalities of sex determination and sex differentiation in *Homo sapiens*. Eur J Pediatr 133:79, 1980
21. O'Rahilly R: The timing and sequence of events in the development of the human reproductive system during the embryonic period proper. Anat Embryol (Berl) 166:247, 1983
22. Orgebin-Crist MC: The influence of testicular function on related reproductive organs. In: Burger H, de Kretser D, (eds) The Testis. Raven Press. New York 1981, pp. 239–253.
23. Picard JY, Tran D, Josso N: Biosynthesis of labelled anti-Müllerian hormone by fetal testis: evidence for the glycoprotein nature of the hormone and for its disulfide-bounded structure. Mol and Cell Endocrinol 12:17, 1978
24. Vigier B, Tran D, du Mesniul du Buisson F, Heyman Y, Josso N: Use of monoclonal antibody techniques to study the ontogeny of bovine anti-Müllerian hormone. J Reprod Fertil 69:207, 1983
25. Wachtel SS: Primary sex determination. Arthritis and Rheumatism 22:1200, 1979
26. Wartenberg H: Differentiation and development of the testes. In Burger H, de Kretser D, (eds) The Testis. Raven Press, New York 1981, pp. 39–80
27. Wartenberg H: Human testicular development and the role of the mesonephros in the origin of a dual Sertoli cell system. Andrologia 10:1, 1978
28. Wartenberg H, Holstein AF, Vossmeyer J: Zur Cytologie der pränatalen Gonadenentwicklung beim Menschen. II Elektronenmikroskopische Untersuchungen über die Cytogenese von Gonocyten und fetalen Spermatogonien im Hoden. Z Anat Entwicklungsgesch 134:165, 1971
29. Witschi E: Migration of the germ cells of human embryos from the yolk sac to the primitive gonadal folds. Carnegie Contyr Embryol 32:67, 1948

2

DEVELOPMENT OF THE TESTIS FROM BIRTH TO PUBERTY

The extent of testicular development that takes place during gestation is not sufficient to accomplish full testicular maturity. This is not finally attained until puberty when the testis can participate fully in the process of reproduction, which requires the formation of spermatozoa and the secretion of male hormones. During the 14 years between birth and puberty further changes will take place gradually, and these will involve both the seminiferous tubules and the interstitial space. An account of these changes should include the structure of the testis at birth followed by each one of the stages of its evolution to adult age. These stages include: (1) a resting phase, from birth till approximately four years of age; (2) the phase of active growth, from four years till the age of nine; and (3) the maturation phase, from nine years to adulthood (Mancini, 1968; Nistal and others, 1984).

The Testis in the Newborn

Histological study of the testis during the first few months following birth (Fig. 2–1A) demonstrates the following features: The seminiferous tubules are only slightly tortuous when compared to those of the adult testis. They average 80 microns in diameter (Fig. 2–2) and they are still arranged in solid cords devoid of lumina (Fig. 2–1B). They are surrounded by a thin basement membrane composed of electron dense basal lamina displaying a homogeneous structure with fine granules and filaments and further surrounded by a delicate network of reticulin fibers. The basement membrane is also surrounded by scattered myofibroblasts (myoid cells) with numerous bundles of characteristic cytoplasmic microfilaments and a relatively well-developed rough endoplasmic reticulum (Fig. 2–3) (DeKretser and others, 1975; Hadziselimovic, 1977).

Within the seminiferous tubules at this stage there are two types of cells: immature Sertoli cells and germ cells. Immature Sertoli cells predominate and they are arranged in the form of a pseudostratified cylindrical epithelium (Figs. 2–1B and 2–3). Two variants of Sertoli cells have been distinguished by electron microscopy (Hadziselimovic and Seguchi, 1974; Nistal and Paniagua, 1983). The first variant is oval or round and reveals a single nucleus located in the center of the cell. The nuclear chromatin is finely granular surrounding an eccentric nucleolus. The cytoplasm has the usual organelles with no specific characteristics. The second variant of Sertoli cell is elongated. The nucleus is also elongated and frequently indented. The nucleolus displays a well-defined electron-dense spherical body surrounded by the usual nucleolar trabecular texture. The cytoplasm has elongated mitochondria and there is a generous amount of free ribosomes and glycogen. Toward the basal portion of the cell there are microfilaments and pinocytotic vesicles, whereas in the apical portion there are cisternae of rough endoplasmic reticulum, a well-developed Golgi apparatus, and high-density vesicles probably corresponding to secretory granules (Fig. 2–3B). Some authors have suggested that immature Sertoli cells may produce hormones of a non-steroid nature (Gondos, 1980). In addition, there is a moderate amount of smooth endoplasmic reticulum with no specific features. The

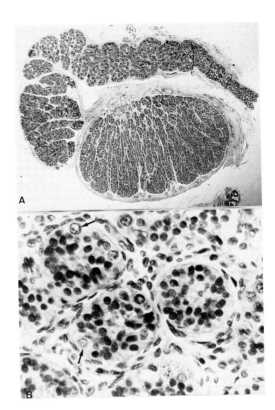

FIGURE 2–1. *A, Testis and epididymis at birth (x10). B, Close-up of seminiferous tubules at birth. They are composed of spermatogonia and Sertoli cells. Spermatogonia (arrows) show light nuclear texture (x250).*

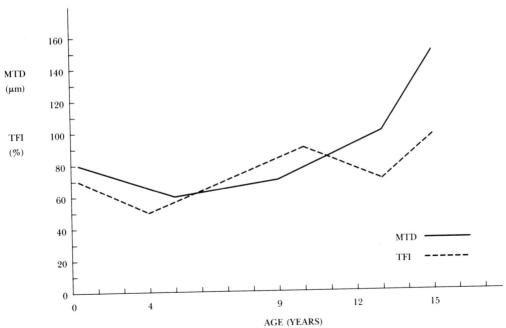

FIGURE 2–2. *Relationship of testicular mean tubular diameter (MTD) and tubular fertility index (TFI) to age.*

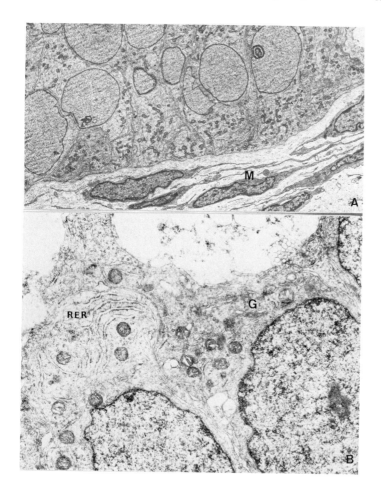

FIGURE 2–3. *A, Basal portion of the seminiferous tubule from a newborn showing immature Sertoli cells and the basement membrane surrounded by myofibroblasts (M) (x3,000). B, Apical portion of immature Sertoli cells showing a developed Golgi complex(G) and supranuclear cisternae of rough endoplasmic reticulum (RER) (x20,000).*

cytoplasm of this second type of Sertoli cell can be clear or dark, which rather than indicating two different types, seems to correspond to different functional stages. Both types of Sertoli cells show small points of occlusions resembling desmosome junctions between the cytoplasms of adjacent cells. Both Sertoli cell variants seem to correspond to a single Sertoli cell type which when distributed forms a pseudostratified epithelium. The morphological differences between basal and columnar Sertoli cells may be attributed to such a distribution (Nistal and Paniagua, 1983). Although some authors have described the presence of occasional mitoses in Sertoli cells in the testis of the newborn (Steinberger and Steinberger, 1977). A recent study (Nistal and others, 1982) suggests that the Sertoli cell number per testis does not change from birth to adulthood, and mitoses in these cells were not observed.

The second type of cell encountered in the seminiferous tubules corresponds to the germ cells. These include fetal spermatogonia and A spermatogonia (Seguchi and Hadziselimovic, 1974). The former are usually located in the central portion of the tubules and can be distinguished from others by their large size and their clear cytoplasmic features, and the developed, centrally located nucleolus. Their ultrastructural features have been reported in the first chapter (Figs. 2–4A and B).

The second variant of germ cells is the A spermatogonia which derive from

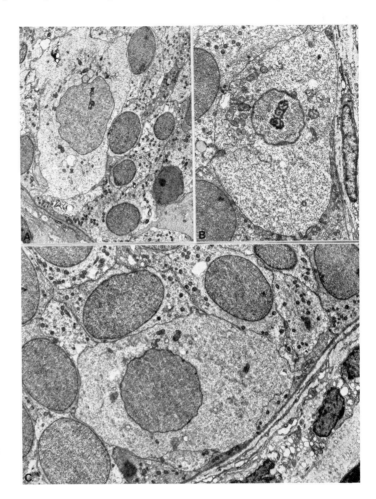

FIGURE 2–4. *Germ cells in infantile testes. A, Fetal spermatogonium surrounded by immature Seretoli-cells (x5,000). B, Fetal spermatogonia showing a developed central nucleolus (x8,000). C, Ad Spermatogonium similar to that of the adult testis (x10,000).*

the fetal spermatogonia but displays a smaller size and characteristic location in contact with the basal lamina of the seminiferous tubule (Figs. 2–1B and 2–4C and 5A), although some spermatogonia can occupy a higher position. Both Ap and Ad spermatogonia, similar to those that will be described in the next chapter, are seen since birth (Hadziselomovic, 1977) (Figs 2–4C and 5A). A gradual growth and proliferation of the population of A spermatogonia is followed by a corresponding withdrawal of fetal spermatogonia. Mitotic activity has been demonstrated in both (Fig. 2–6A) (Vilar, 1970).

The interstitial space of the testis is made up of loose connective tissue with abundant immature fibroblasts, reticulin fibers, blood vessels, lymphatics, and interstitial cells (Figs. 2–1B and 2–5B). The number of mature Leydig cells is considerably lower than in the fetal testis since they regress after the third month of gestation following the decreasing levels of HCG (Fig. 2–7). Regressing Leydig cells are fairly abundant together with other fibroblastic-looking elements that contain abundant microfilaments, smooth endoplasmic reticulum, and lipid inclusions (Fig. 2–5B). These fibroblast-like cells are probably precursors of the adult Leydig cells. The fetal Leydig cells are common through the first two years after birth. They are generally arranged in clusters of two or three cells. Compared to adult Ley-

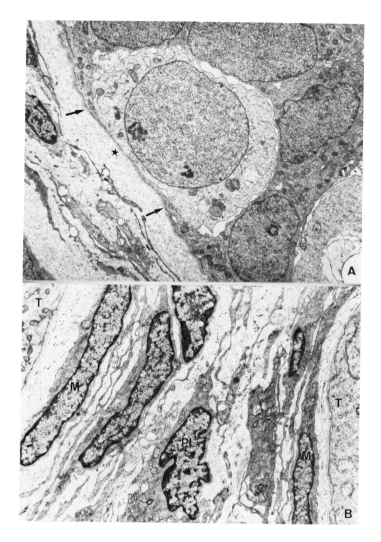

FIGURE 2–5. *A*, Ap spermatogonium of a newborn surrounded by Sertoli cells. The latter show cytoplasmic projections separating the spermatogonium from the basal lamina (arrows). In some areas, however, the spermatogonium establish direct contact with the lamina (asterisk) (x10,000). *B*, Detail of the interstitial space of the testis of a newborn demonstrating myofibroblasts (*M*) and fibroblast-looking cells. Some of them show a shorter configuration and early differentiation into Leydig cells with less abundant cytoplasmic projections. They are the precursors of the adult Leydig cells (*PL*). Seminiferous tubule (*T*) (x6,000).

dig cells they have a more abundant rough endoplasmic reticulum. Small concentrations of testosterone have been measured in the testicular and epididymal tissues during the first two years of life; the maximal levels were found between 1 to 3 months of age with peak values similar to those found in pubertal tests. (Bidlingmaier and others, 1983; Vilar, 1970)

The tunica albuginea at this stage shows only a partial development of the collagen fibers (Mancini, 1968, Vilar, 1970). It measures 300 microns in thickness and contains three layers in increasing proportion of fibers, ground substance, and cells (Figs. 2–1A, and 2–8). In continuity with the albuginea a number of connective tissue septae divides the testicular parenchyma at this stage in approximately 250 lobules. Scattered foci of extramedullary hematopoiesis are found in the albuginea and in the interstitial space (Fig. 2–8B).

RESTING PHASE

During the first four years after birth the seminiferous tubules demonstrate a basement membrane similar, but slightly

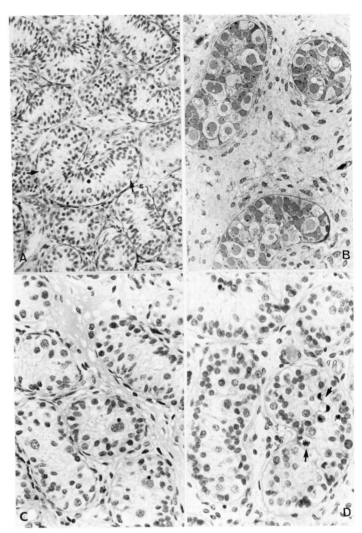

FIGURE 2–6. *A*, Microscopic appearance of testis at one year of age. The seminiferous tubules are populated by immature Sertoli cells, basal spermatogonia (arrows) and scattered germ cells (asterisk) in the central portion of the tubule. No luminal development is seen at this time (x125). *B*, Testis at three years of age. Seminiferous tubules still devoid of lumen show proliferating germ cells. There are no Leydig cells in the interstitial space (Toluidine blue, x250). *C*, Testis at seven years. The seminiferous tubules have developed a central lumen and they are lined by enlarged and binucleated (asterisks) spermatogonia (x250). *D*, Testis at eight years. Germ cells show mitoses (arrows) (x250).

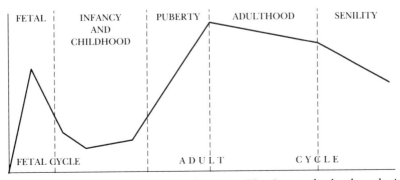

FIGURE 2–7. *Two cycles of Leydig cells in the testis. The first cycle develops during fetal life, reaches its peak about the third month, and gives rise to fetal Leydig cells which eventually disappear. The second cycle begins at puberty and gives rise to the permanent adult Leydig cells.*

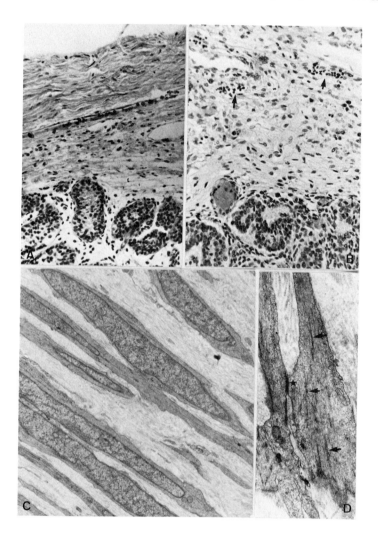

FIGURE 2–8. *Albuginea of the newborn. A, The albuginea is composed of three layers demonstrating a gradual decrease of their collagen content. The innermost layer is markedly vascularized (x125). B, Albuginea showing foci of hematopoiesis (arrows) (x125). C, Detail of smooth muscle cells alternating with collagen fibers (x7,000). D, Detail of the cytoplasm of two myofibroblasts demonstrating zones of electron density (arrows) and gap junctions (asterisk) (x20,000).*

thicker than the one in the newborn. The average diameter of the tubules decreases from 80 to 60 microns (Fig. 2–2). Sertoli cells are identical to those in the newborn.

With increasing age there is a decrease of the number of fetal spermatogonia and a gradual increase of A spermatogonia. Many of them, however, seem to undergo involution as indicated by the presence of abundant spermatogonia with pyknotic nuclei and acidophilic cytoplasm along with swollen and binucleated forms. This could be interpreted as an initial failure of germinal cell differentiation followed by an attempt of spermatogonium proliferation about three to four years of age (Mancini, 1968) (Fig. 2–5B). The spermatogonium proliferation might be controlled by chalones that produce the germ cells (Thumann and Bustos-Obregon, 1982). At this time an increase in the number of mast cells are observed in the testis (Nistal and others, 1984).

The interstitial tissue does not show any significant changes in the newborn except for a gradual increase of collagen deposition. Fetal Leydig cells have almost disappeared by this time and only degenerating cells and the precursors of adult Leydig cells remain (Hadziselimovic, 1977).

The tunica albuginea becomes slightly thinner despite some increased collagenization of the connective tissue, especially in the outer and middle layers. The inner layer retains its character of loose connective tissue. The fibroblasts in the two outer layers become more scarce and they lose their functional activity. Finally, there is also a decrease of ground substance, which is almost totally covered by a generous amount of collagen fibers arranged in an orderly fashion (Mancini, 1968, Vilar, 1970).

PHASE OF ACTIVE GROWTH

Between four and nine years of age, the seminiferous tubules and the interstitial tissue of the testis show a period of active growth and development (Fig. 2–6C and D). The seminiferous tubules increase their length considerably and their diameter also increases progressively to reach an average of 75 microns by the age of eight (Fig. 2–2). Furthermore, the tubules develop a central lumen (Fig. 2–6C).

The tubular epithelium becomes more cylindrical and less pseudostratified (Nistal and Paniagua, 1983). The Sertoli cells retain their previous appearances, but with age they gradually increase their smooth and rough endoplasmic reticulum and their lipid inclusions while their nuclei also become more frequently indented. The number of Sertoli cells, which average 26 in the newborn, is no more than 10 in cross sections of adult seminiferous tubules. Yet it is quite likely that the absolute number of Sertoli cells remains constant and the alleged decrease is probably the result of their separation as the tubular structures expand their caliber and increase their length (Nistal and others, 1982).

Next to the A spermatogonia, a second type develops gradually. It corresponds to the B spermatogonia similar to those found in the adult testis (see Chapter 3). Occasional spermatocytes can also be observed. All the spermatogonial types demonstrate the presence of intercellular bridges. Later on, the large spermatogonia reappear, many of them with two nuclei and with degenerative features similar to those previously described in the infant. After the age of seven to eight years, there is usually a second attempt at germinal cell maturation (Fig. 2–6, C and D). In the interstitial tissue there is a gradual increase of collagen fibers and a decrease of young fibroblasts. Fetal Leydig cells have disappeared by now and they have not yet been replaced by their adult counterpart, although precursor Leydig cells and occasional differentiating Leydig cells can be seen (Hadziselimovic, 1977).

The collagen content of the albuginea also increases and although the latter becomes progressively thinner during the first part of this phase of testicular growth up until the age of six to eight years, at this time it begins a process of gradual thickening that will continue through puberty (DeKretser, 1968; Franchi and Mandl, 1964; Mancini, 1968).

PHASE OF MATURATION

The most striking testicular changes since birth occur during puberty, a period that is variable in each individual case but tends to take place between the years of 9 to 15 and includes the transformation of a nonfunctional infantile testis into an adult, fertile organ. This transformation represents the response of the testicular tissues to the pituitary secretion of gonadotrophins under hypothalamic control (Faiman and Winter, 1974; Kulin and Santner, 1977; Swerdloff and Heber, 1981).

The seminiferous tubules undergo significant changes leading to active spermatogenesis (Figs. 2–9 and 2–10). Their caliber increases to a maximum of about 150 microns (Fig. 2–2) and the basement

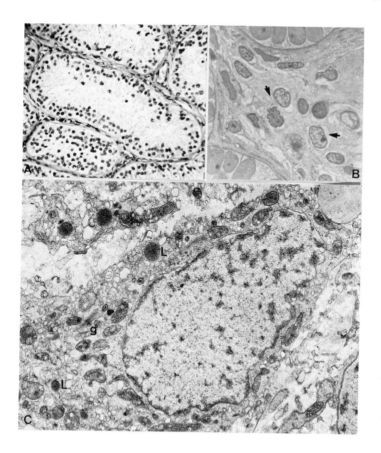

FIGURE 2–9. Testis of 13-year-old male during pubertal development. A, Seminiferous tubules disclose numerous primary spermatocytes in various stages of the first meiotic division (x125). B, Interstitial space demonstrating fibroblast-looking cells intermingled with others with lighter nuclei (arrows) and more plump in shape, suggestive of Leydig cells during early stages of differentiating (x450). C, Electron micrograph of differentiating Leydig cell. The smooth endoplasmic reticulum is fairly well developed and there are mitochondria with parallel cristae and lysosomes (L); g: Golgi complex (x13,000).

membrane also increases in thickness as it gains further complexity (Mancini, 1968). On the one hand there is an increase of collagen fibers along with the number of myofibroblasts that surround the basal lamina and some elastic fibers make their initial appearance.

In the seminiferous tubules the immature Sertoli cells still present at this time begin their gradual transformation into adult cells (Fig. 2–10A) (Hadziselimovic, 1977; Nistal and Paniagua, 1983) under hypophysary stimulation (Chemes and associates, 1979). The nucleus becomes indented and irregular, the chromatin is finely granular, and the nucleolus displays a moderately electrodense spherical body (fibrilar center), a compact granular portion, and a trabecular part containing both granular and fibrilar portions (see Fig. 3–3B). The cytoplasm is clear and contains numerous enlarging mitochondria with straight or tortuous shapes and longitudinally arranged cristae, distributed predominantly in the basal portion of the cell (Fig. 2–10A). Concentric laminar formations (see Fig. 3–3A) begin to appear from rough endoplasmic reticulum (Paniagua and co-authors, 1984). At this time there are also cisternae of smooth endoplasmic reticulum attached to the cytoplasmic membrane oriented in such a way that they face the ones in the adjacent cell. This reveals the formation of the Sertoli-Sertoli specialized tight junctions that may be demonstrated by means of freeze fracture and lanthanum tracer studies (Camatini and others, 1979 and 1981). In addition there are lysosomes, lipid inclusions, and crystalloid structures referred to as "Charcot-Böttcher crystals." These are made up of fine microtubules of 150 Å thickness arranged in parallel bundles of 10 × 25 microns (see Fig. 3–2). Mi-

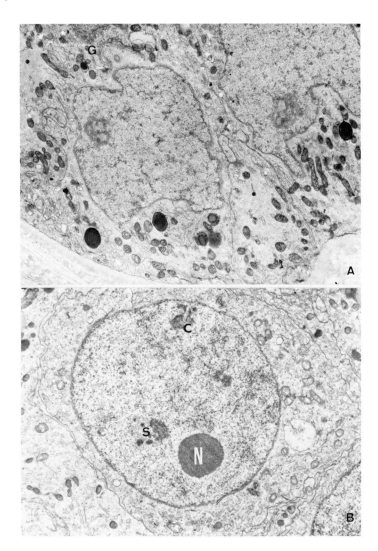

FIGURE 2–10. Thirteen-year-old testis during puberty. A, Sertoli cells show gradual maturation with increasing nuclear irregularity and elongation of mitochondria, which concentrate predominantly in the basal portion of the cell. There are lysosomes and lipid inclusions. The rough endoplasmic reticulum appears more scarce while the smooth reticulum has expanded. The Golgi complex (G) is prominent and there are abundant microfilaments (asterisks), characteristic of residual immaturity (x13,000). B, Primary spermatocyte during pachytene stage of the first meiotic division. N: nucleolus; C: synaptinemal complex; S: sex vesicle (x13,000).

crofilaments already abundant in early puberty become gradually scarce as the cell matures. With puberty, Sertoli cells develop cytoplasmic projections that surround neighboring germinal cells.

Regarding histochemical features, there is a gradual increase of acid phosphatase and aminopeptidase together with phosphorylase and glucose-6-phosphatase. The amount of glycogen and lipid also increases while a proportionate decrease of cytoplasmic RNA has been documented (Mancini, 1968; Vilar, 1970).

With approaching puberty there is a decrease of spermatogonia that show increasing degenerative features. From the beginning of puberty the spermatogonia make a third and this time successful attempt to develop the rest of the germinal cell line to be dealt with in the study of the adult testis. Spermatogenesis with production of spermatozoa is not fully accomplished until the end of puberty.

At the beginning of puberty, coinciding with the development of the seminiferous tubules, there is a simultaneous reactivation of growth activity in the interstitial tissue and in the albuginea. The interstitial tissue in response to pituitary secretion of Luteinizing hormone (LH) which considerably increase at this time (Swerdloff and Heber, 1981), discloses gradual transformation of precursor Leydig cells into adult forms (Fig. 2–9**B** and **C**). This development can be followed both histochemically and ultrastructurally (Fawcett and Burgos, 1960; Nistal and Paniagua, 1979).

Histochemical techniques demonstrate increasing enzymatic activity characteristic of cells engaged in steroid synthesis such as lipase, esterases, dehydrogenases, and oxidative enzymes. Furthermore, the number of microfilaments decreases as the cells increase their content of lipids, lipofuscins and smooth endoplasmic reticulium.

The end point of their differentiation is heralded by the appearance of Reinke crystalloids (see Figs. 3–17**A** and **B**) (Nistal and Paniagua, 1979). In a small percentage of these cells there are microcrystalline structures instead of the Reinke crystalloid. These structures measure from 200 to 250 microns in thickness, and resemble parallel laminas, which result from several foldings of a single lamina. These microcrystals are usually found in groups and they are related to the components of the Reinke crystalloids, the structure of which will be detailed later (see Figs. 3–18**C** and **D**) (Yamada, 1962).

Toward the beginning of puberty there is increased fibroblastic growth and activity resulting in an increase of the intercellular substance along with some edema. At the end of this period, cellular activity also comes to an end and the edema subsides. Similar changes also take place in the connective tissue of the albuginea. Increased fibroblastic activity is followed by an expanded ground substance and by the deposition of new collagen. At the same time there is edema and escape of proteins. In early puberty the albuginea shows a rapid increase in thickness until it reaches 380 microns at which time there is a more gradual thickening to reach a final measurement of approximately 450 microns. At this point there is a decrease of the amount of edema fluid and a slow down of fibroblastic activity.

Accompanying these histological changes at puberty there is development of secondary male characteristics closely related to the synthesis of steroid hormones by the Leydig cells, which by now have nearly or fully completed their maturation process (Santen and Kulin, 1981).

REFERENCES

1. Bidlingmaier F, Dörr HG, Eisenmenger W, Kuhnle U, Knorr D: Testosterone and androstenodione concentrations in human testis and epididymis during the first two years of life. J Clin Endocrinol Metabol 57:311, 1983
2. Camatini M, Franchi E, Decurtis I: Sertoli junctions in human testes: a freeze fracture and lanthanum tracer study, J Submicr Cytol 11:511, 1979
3. Camatini M, Franchi E, Decurtis I: Differentiation of inter-Sertoli junctions in human testis. Cell Biol Int Rep 5:109, 1981
4. Chemes HE, Dym M, Raj HG: Hormonal regulation of Sertoli cell differentiation. Biol Reprod 21:251, 1979
5. DeKretser DM: The fine structure of the immature human testis in hypogonadotropic hypogonadism. Virchows Arch B Cell Path 1:283, 1968
6. DeKretser DM, Kerr JB, Paulsen CA: The peritubular tissue in the normal and pathological human testis. An ultrastructural study. Biol Reprod 12:317, 1975
7. Faiman C, Winter JSD: Gonadotropins and sex hormone patterns in puberty. In Grumbach MM, Grave GD, Mayer FE, (eds) The Control of the Onset of Puberty. John Wiley and Sons. New York 1974, pp. 32–55
8. Fawcett DW, Burgos MH: Studies on the fine structure of the mammalian testis. II. The human interstitial tissue. Am J Anat 107:245, 1960

9. Franchi LL, Mandl AM: The ultrastructure of germ cells in foetal and neonatal male rats. J Embryol Exp Morph 12:289, 1964
10. Gondos B: Testicular Development: Structure and Function. In Steinberger A, Steinberger E, (eds). Raven Press New York 1980, pp. 3–20
11. Hadziselimovic F, Seguchi H: Ultramikroskopische Untersuchungen an Tubulus Seminiferous bei Kindern von der Geburt bis zur Pubertät. II. Entwicklung und Morphologie der Sertolizellen. Verh Anat Ges 68:149, 1974
12. Hadziselimovic F: Crypotorchidism: ultrastructure of normal and cryptorchid testes. In: Advances in Anatomy, Embryology and Cell Biology, Vol. 53. Springer-Verlag. New York 1977, pp. 1–72
13. Kulin HE, Santner SJ: Timed urinary gonadotropin measurements in normal infants, children and adults, and in patients with disorders of sexual maturation. J Pediatr 90:760, 1977
14. Mancini RE: Bases histofisiológicas de la función testicular. In Fundación para el fomento de estudios endocrinológicos y metabólicos de Rosario (ed): Testículo humano. Buenos Aires: Panamericana Médica, 1968, p. 11
15. Nistal M, Abaurrea MA, Paniagua R: Morphological and histometric study on the human Sertoli cell from birth to the onset of puberty. J Anat 134:351, 1982
16. Nistal M, Paniagua R: Leydig cell differentiation induced by stimulation with HCG and HMG in two patients affected with hypogonadotropic hypogonadism. Andrologia 11:211, 1979
17. Nistal M, Paniagua R: The postnatal development of the human Sertoli cells. Z Mikrosk Anat Forsch 97:732, 1983
18. Nistal M, Santamaria L, Paniagua R: Mast cells in the human testis and epididymis from birth to puberty. Acta Anat (Basel) (In press) 1984
19. Paniagua R, Nistal M, Bravo MP: The formation of annulate lamellae in the human Sertoli cell. Arch Androl (In press) 1984
20. Santen RJ, Kulin HE: Hypogonadotropic hypogonadism and delayed puberty. In Burger H, de Kretser D, (eds). The Testis. Raven Press, New York 1981, pp. 329–356
21. Seguchi H, Hadziselimovic F: Ultramikroskopische Untersuchungen am Tubulus seminiferus bei Kinder von der Geburt bis zur Pubertät. I Spermatogonien-entwicklung. Verh Anat Ges 68:133, 1974
22. Steinberger A, Steinberger E: The Sertoli cells. In Johnson AD, Gomes R, (eds) The Testis, Vol 4. Academic Press. New York 1977, pp. 371–399
23. Swerdloff RS, Heber D: Endocrine control of testicular function from birth to puberty. In Burger H, de Kretser D, (eds). The Testis. Raven Press, New York 1981, pp. 107–140
24. Thumann A, Bustos-Obregon E: "In vitro" assay of rat spermatogonial chalone in prepubertal seminiferous tubules. Andrologia (Berlin) 14:35, 1982
25. Vilar O: Histology of the human testis from neonatal period to adolescence. In Rosemberg E, Paulsen CA (eds): Advances in experimental medicine and biology vol. 10 The human testis. New York: Plenum Press, 1970, p. 95
26. Yamada E: Some observations on the fine structure of the interstitial cell in the human testis. In Breese SS (ed): 5th International conference on electron microscopy. New York: Academic Press, 1962, Vol. 2

3

ADULT TESTIS

The end of puberty marks the final stage of the process of testicular maturation. From here on the testis will function as a secretory gland capable of secreting spermatozoa and as an endocrine organ responsible for testosterone secretion related to the development of the secondary male characteristics.

The following is a brief account of the structure of the adult testis.

Supporting Structures

The testes are ovoid in shape and measure approximately $4 \times 3.5 \times 3$ cm each (Fig. 3–1A). They are suspended in the scrotal sac at the end of the spermatic cord. The scrotal wall is composed of skin, a thin layer of muscle (dartos), and a layer of connective tissue that includes some striated muscle (cremaster). The testes are freely movable in their location between the visceral and the parietal layers of the tunica vaginalis. The scrotal wall has a significant surface and includes abundant sweat glands. This wall provides an environment with a temperature lower than that of the adjacent body. Cold temperatures result in contraction of the dartos muscle, which wrinkles the skin and decreases the total size of the scrotal sac.

The visceral layer of the tunica vaginalis is made up of mesothelial cells lining the albuginea or thick capsule that completely surrounds the testis except at the upper part of the posterior testicular edge where the large blood vessels are allowed to enter (Fig. 3–1A). It has been established that the albuginea has a more active role than the support and protection of testicular structures. It is capable of protein synthesis and it can actively contract under the stimulation of acetylcholine and noradrenaline. On the other hand it has been suggested that it can serve as a permeable membrane controlling the flow of spermatozoa to the epididymis and regulating changes of testicular size.

In the adult testis the three layers of the albuginea described in the infant have attained an organized arrangement. The outer layer, composed of dense connective tissue, is lined by mesothelium. The middle layer is less structured and contains abundant fibroblasts, whereas the inner one is composed of richly vascularized loose connective tissue. Contractile cells in the category of smooth muscle and myofibroblastic cells have been described, especially in the outer layer and in the peripheral portion of the middle one. Further elements of significance include encapsulated nerve endings similar to corpuscles of Meissner and Pacini.

Arising from the albuginea there are numerous trabeculae or septae dividing the testis in approximately 250 lobules. These septae provide the supporting framework for the blood vessels and nerve supply of the testis.

The inner or vascular layer of the albuginea covers the septae in continuity with the connective tissue of the interstitial space of the testis. The albuginea is particularly thick in the posterior aspect of the testis where it forms the mediastinum testis which also includes the rete testis (Fig. 3–1A) (Davis and others, 1970).

Seminiferous Tubules

Spermatogenesis is the main role of the seminiferous tubules. Each testicular lobule is composed of two to four tortuous

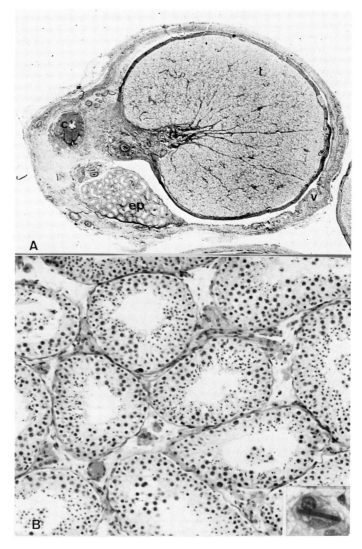

FIGURE 3-1. *A, Adult testis and epididymis. ep: epididymis t: seminiferous tubules; rt: rete testis; C vas deferens; v: tunica vaginalis testis (x2.5). B, Parenchyma of adult testis showing seminiferous tubules with active spermatogenesis and abundant capillaries and Leydig cells in the interstitial space (x100). Inset shows a close-up of a Leydig cell with Reinke crystalloid (x450).*

seminiferous tubules beginning on a blind end next to the albuginea and ending in the tubuli recti close to the mediastinum after a winding and convoluting course. The extension of each convoluted seminiferous tubule is not more than 1 cm^3 but its total length, when it is unfolded reaches about 1 m with an approximate diameter of 150 to 300 microns. The basement membrane maintains the structure described in the pubertal testis. Beyond this membrane there are several layers of myofibroblasts bound together by close (less than 150 Å) contact (Bustos-Obregón, 1974) and they serve as a barrier for the passage of substances between the tubules and the interstitial space. It has also been claimed that the contractility of myofibroblasts is related to the contractile movements described in the seminiferous tubules (Hamasaki and Murakami, 1979). Sertoli cells-myofibroblast contacts have been reported (Nistal and Paniagua, 1983). This is in accordance with the metabolic cooperation between Sertoli cells and myofibroblasts in culture (Huston, 1983). The maturation of myofibroblasts is dependant on normal pituitary function (Waites and Gladwell, 1982). The Sertoli cells and the spermatogonia are in direct contact with the basal lamina (Fig. 3–1**B**).

The observation of hypercurved seminiferous tubules in some cases of infertility (Averback, 1980) probably represents an extreme variation of the arrangement just mentioned, although the exact cause of this syndrome remains unknown.

Sertoli Cells

Cross sections of a seminiferous tubule usually demonstrate an average of ten Sertoli cells in each (Hadziselimovic and Seguchi, 1974). At puberty they have completed their maturation and show the following characteristics in the adult testis (Figs. 3–2, 3–3, and 3–4). The nucleus is generally located in the basal portion of the cell and it displays deep indentations (Fig. 3–2**A**). The nuclear chromatin is evenly distributed and the nucleolus is highly characteristic because along with the usual granular and fibrillar components of electron dense material it shows the presence of a spherical body (fibrilar center) composed of delicate fibrils of lesser density than the remainder of the nucleolus (Fig. 3–3**B**). The cytoplasm extends from the basal lamina to the lumen of the seminiferous tubule and it has an irregular contour in order to fill in the

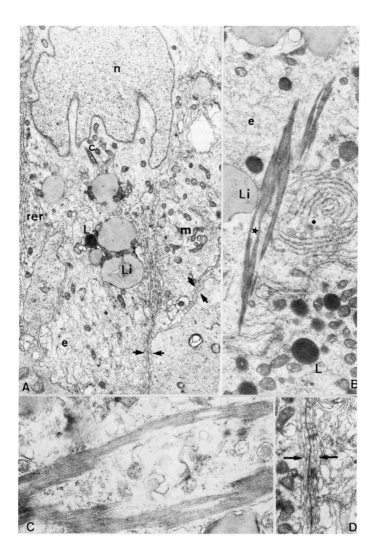

FIGURE 3–2. *A, Adult Sertoli cells. Basal portion of cell shows abundant smooth endoplasmic reticulum, some cisternae of rough endoplasmic reticulum, lipid inclusions and lysosomes. Junctions between Sertoli cells (arrows) include cisternae of smooth endoplasmic reticulum (x10,000). B, Detail of Charcot-Böttcher crystals (star), primary lysosomes, and concentric cisternae of smooth endoplasmic reticulum (asterisk) (x16,000). C, Higher magnification of Charcot-Böttcher crystals arranged in parallel bundles (x40,000). D, A pair of cisternae of smooth endoplasmic reticulum (one in each cell) is seen at the junction of two Sertoli cells. These cisternae are forming a triad (arrows) located close to and parallel to the edge of the cytoplasmic membrane. In between, there are microfilaments and electron dense material (x22,000). n: nucleus; c: centriole; Li: lipid; rer: rough endoplasmic reticulum; L: lysosomes; e: smooth endoplasmic reticulum; m: mitochondria.*

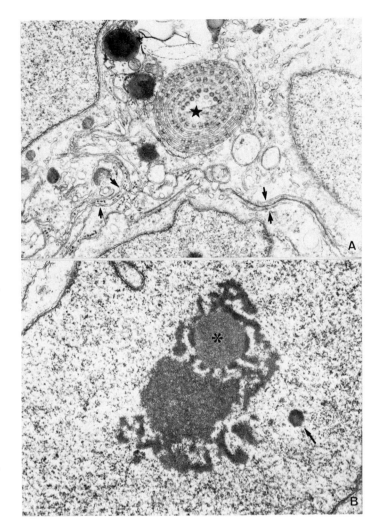

FIGURE 3–3. *Adult Sertoli cells. A, Concentric arrangement of annulate lamellae of smooth endoplasmic reticulum are seen in the center (star). Functions between Sertoli cells demonstrate the presence of microfilaments in cross sections (arrows) (x22,000). B, The nucleolus of mature Sertoli cells shows a special configuration. The center is occupied by an area of light density (asterisk) compared to the trabecular material around it. A spherical perichromatin body lies nearby (arrow) (x55,000).*

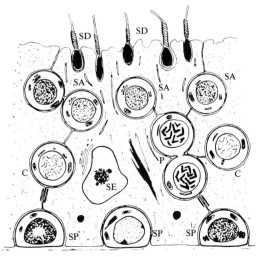

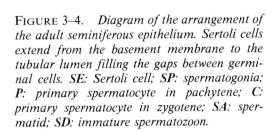

FIGURE 3–4. *Diagram of the arrangement of the adult seminiferous epithelium. Sertoli cells extend from the basement membrane to the tubular lumen filling the gaps between germinal cells. SE: Sertoli cell; SP: spermatogonia; P: primary spermatocyte in pachytene; C: primary spermatocyte in zygotene; SA: spermatid; SD: immature spermatozoon.*

gaps between the germinal cells (Fig. 3-4). This feature is probably related not only to the maintenance of the blood-testicular barrier for the protection of the germinal cells but also to the supply of their nutritional essentials and for the coordination of their development to spermatozoa. It has been established that the germinal cell line fails to progress in the absence of mature, adult Sertoli cells.

Sertoli cells are attached together by interdigitating and minimal intercellular spaces frequently enclosed by narrow junctions, which include the presence of two opposing cisternae of smooth endoplasmic reticulum arranged alongside each of the cytoplasmic membranes (Figs. 3-2A, D, and 3-3A) (Nagano and Suzuki, 1976). Between the cisternae and the cytoplasmic membranes there are a number of dense microfilaments (Fig. 3-3A). The narrow junctions include tight junctions, gap junctions and small desmosomes. These specialized junctions between Sertoli cells form the blood-testis barrier (Landon and Pryor, 1981; Waites and Gladwell, 1982). Gap junctions and desmosome like structures (Russell, 1980) without adjacent smooth endoplasmic reticulum cisternae have been observed between Sertoli cells and spermatogonia while those between Sertoli cells and mature spermatids that show an intercellular space measuring about 100 Å only demonstrate the presence of cisternae and microfilaments in the Sertoli cell (Burgos and others, 1970; Russell and Malone, 1980; Russell, 1980).

Other components include the presence of elongated mitochondria with parallel cristae and a relatively abundant smooth endoplasmic reticulum in the form of vesicles or tubules, and short cisternae. The rough endoplasmic reticulum is rather scarce and it is made up of a limited number of basally located cisternae arranged in continuity with the smooth endoplasmic reticulum (Fig. 3-2A). Scattered throughout the cytoplasm there are groups of free ribosomes. The number of microfilaments characteristically abundant in the immature Sertoli cell (Fig. 2-10A) is significantly reduced in the mature stage. Charcot-Böttcher crystals are found only in man (Fig. 3-2B and C) and consist of microtubules measuring approximately 150 Å in thickness arranged in bundles of 10 and are 25 microns in length. Further characteristic components of these cells include concentrically arranged annulate lamellae (Fig. 3-3A), lipid inclusions, lysosomes, and lipofuscin granules (Fig. 3-2A) (Bawa, 1963; Schulze, 1974).

Compared to germinal cells, Sertoli cells exhibit significant resistance to heat, radiation, and toxic agents and they have an abundant supply of enzymes, including phosphatases, DPN and TPN oxydases, dehydrogenase, nucleotidases, esterase, and lipase, all of them probably related to their interaction with germinal cells. An additional feature includes their phagocytic role in the incorporation and breakdown of residual material left over from the maturation of spermatids and the degeneration of a significant number of germinal cells. Finally, the role of Sertoli cells as primary target-cells of follicle stimulating hormone (FSH), and in the synthesis of both androgen-binding-protein (ABP) and steroids has been well established (Dorrington and Fritz, 1975; Lacy, 1973). Their ability to participate in the control of their own function and maturation by secreting FSH-inhibiting factor (inhibin) has also been well documented (Chemes and co-workers, 1979).

Germinal Cells

In the adult testis the germinal cell line is fully developed. Three types of spermatogonia develop from the prepubertal germ cells, spermatogonia type A pale, type A dark, and type B. The latter is responsible for maintaining the continuity with primary and secondary spermatocytes, spermatids and spermatozoa (Fig. 3-5).

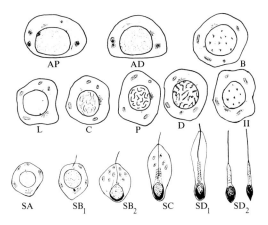

FIGURE 3–5. *Schematic drawing of different types and cellular stages of development encountered in the germinal cell line of the seminiferous epithelium. AP: spermatogonium type A, pale; AD: spermatogonium type A, dark; B: spermatogonium B; PL, L, C, P, D: primary spermatocyte during first meiotic division, preleptotene, leptotene, zygotene, pachytene, and diakinesis; II: secondary spermatocyte; SA, SB_1, SB_2, SC, SD_1 and SD_2: spermatids in successive stages of differentiation into spermatozoa.*

Spermatogonia

Type A spermatogonia are less numerous than type B and display an oval or round shape, a mean diameter of 12 microns and a characteristic location resting upon the basal lamina. The remainder of their surface is covered by the adjoining Sertoli cells (Fig. 3–6A). Most of them have a round nucleus with pale texture due to an evenly distributed and finely granular chromatin. A single nucleolus is usually attached to the nuclear membrane. Several types of nucleoli of the pale type have been described, probably representing different functional stages of the cell. The cytoplasm is somewhat clear and contains sparse organelles including round mitochondria with occasional cristae in a perinuclear arrangement. There are also vesicles of smooth endoplasmic reticulum, a small Golgi apparatus, and scattered ribosomes (Fig. 3–6).

There are, however, a number of features highly characteristic of the type A spermatogonia. Mitochondria are closely packed and hardly separated by homogeneous, electron dense material (Fig. 3–7C). Another feature in man is the presence of elongated cytoplasmic inclusions located close to the nucleus also known as Lubarsch crystals (Fig. 3–7A). These inclusions are made up of a group of parallel microfilaments alternating with a second group of granules or microfilaments that they cross at right angles. Other features characteristic of these spermatogonia are the presence of intercellular bridges from cell to cell and of membranous grooves in the nuclear chromatin (Burgos and others, 1970; Schulze, 1977).

All of these features correspond to the pale type (Ap) of spermatogonia A (Fig. 3–6B). A second type A or dark (Ad) has been distinguished also (Fig. 3–6A) and some authors have further described an elongated variant (Al)(Rowley and others, 1971) (Fig. 3–7A). Dark spermatogonia are separated from the others by the course character of their chromatin resulting in a higher nuclear density. Some of them also show a nuclear vacuole with no limiting membrane corresponding to a circumscribed focus of scarce chromatin. Dark and pale cells cannot be distinguished otherwise by their cytoplasmic features (Holstein, 1975).

Type B spermatogonia are the most numerous. They also rest upon the basal lamina but they are only partially attached to it since most of the cytoplasm is surrounded by the fine cytoplasmic projections of adjacent Sertoli cells. Otherwise, they have a round shape and a spherical nucleus located in the center of the cell. The latter contains one or two nucleoli generally detached from the nuclear membrane and in close relation to the surrounding chromatin. The cytoplasm is

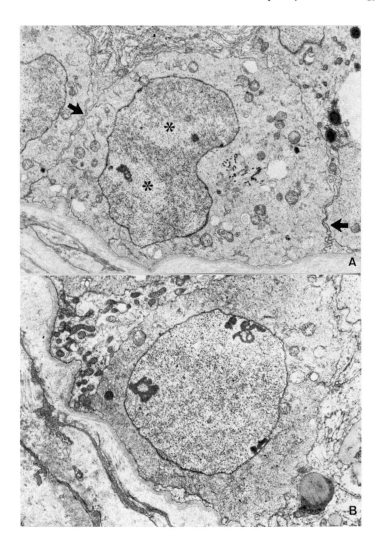

FIGURE 3-6. Adult spermatogonia. A, Spermatogonium type A, dark showing nuclear areas of light electron density (asterisks). Arrows indicate cytoplasmic extensions of Sertoli cells between spermatogonia (x15,000). B, Spermatogonia type A, pale with finely distributed chromatin and prominent nucleoli (x15,000).

very similar to that of type A spermatogonia although there are more abundant ribosomes (Fig. 3-7B).

According to the model proposed by Clermont (1963), and revised by Schulze (1979; 1977), pale type A spermatogonia represent the stem cells that by division produce both a new type A pale stem cell and a type A dark cell. The latter in turn would give rise to type B spermatogonia, which divides to form spermatocytes. Because of their long prophase, the latter show increasing condensation of their chromatin. Spermatocytes are still attached to each other by intercellular bridges, a feature that will remain at the level of spermatids providing a physical continuity of the entire germ cell line up to the formation of spermatozoa (Clermont, 1966; Holstein, 1975; Rowley and co-authors, 1971; Schulze, 1982).

Spermatogenesis

Type B spermatogonia give rise to primary spermatocytes through the process of conventional mitotic division. Primary spermatocytes will be the first to undergo meiotic division (Figs. 3-8 and 3-9). Up until this time they are very similar to spermatogonia, but they show a gradual increase in size to reach a diameter

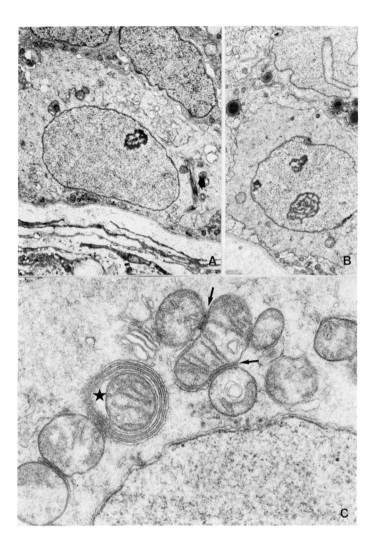

FIGURE 3-7. *Spermatogonium in the adult testis.* A, Spermatogonium, type A pale, elongated variant (Al). A crystal of Lubarsch is seen close to the nucleus (arrow) (x12,000). B, Spermatogonium, type B, separated from the basal lamina by the cytoplasm of a Sertoli cell. The nucleoli are centrally located (x12,000). C, Spermatogonium. Detail of mitochondria bound by electron dense material (arrows). Some of the mitochondria are surrounded by concentric lamellae of smooth endoplasmic reticulum (star) (x40,000).

of 18 microns. The cytoplasm shows few characteristic organelles distinct from those described in the cytoplasm of spermatogonia.

At the beginning of the first meiotic division, or *leptotene* stage, the chromatin is arranged in fine threads. The nucleolus remains prominent. Electron microscopy has shown at this time an increase of endoplasmic reticulum and Golgi complex (Nistal and others, 1980).

Pairing of homologous chromosomes takes place in the next stage, *zygotene*, when they are visualized as fine chromatin threads arranged in long loops against a pale cytoplasmic background. The nucleolus is still visible. Occasional segments of unpaired chromosomes appear as clumps of dense chromatin material. Ultrastructurally, the most significant features of this stage are the appearance of "synaptonemal complexes" the presence of a pair of sex chromosomes. With electron microscopy the latter are identified as the "sex vesicle." Synaptonemal complexes (Figs. 3-8A and 3-9A) are ribbon-like structures associated with the chromatin and apparently involved in chromosomal pairing and crossing-over. They appear as two-high density lines (lateral elements) connected by fine threads arranged alongside and running

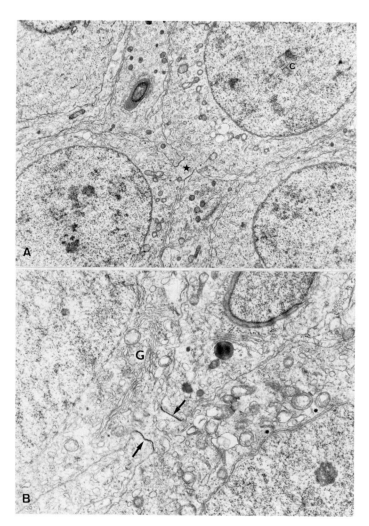

FIGURE 3–8. *Primary spermatocytes. A, Spermatocytes in pachytene attached to each other by cytoplasmic bridges (star). C: synaptonemal complex (x9,000). B, Detail of a cytoplasmic bridge between two spermatocytes. At this level the inner layer of cytoplasmic membrane is reinforced by electron dense material (arrows). The Golgi complex is well developed (G). The nucleus is surrounded by cisternae of endoplasmic reticulum attached to the nuclear membrane (asterisks) (x22,000).*

perpendicular to the lines. The sex vesicle (Fig. 3–9A) is a well-defined chromatin mass approximately the size of a nucleolus corresponding to the X and Y chromosomes. It also includes a number of fine fibers and dense filaments that correspond to the synaptinemal complexes already alluded to (Knibiehler and others, 1981). One or several rough endoplasmic reticulum cisternae surrounding the nuclear envelope are frequently seen in humans (Chemes and co-authors, 1978; Nistal and others, 1980).

The next stage, *pachytene*, is the longest. At this time all chromosomes have completed their pairing and become distributed throughout the nucleus. The synaptonemal complexes and the pair of sex chromosomes are still present. The nucleolus at this point may develop a characteristic configuration showing a dense and granular portion attached to a looser and partially fibrillar mass of chromatin (Fig. 3–9A) (Holm and Rasmussen, 1983).

The *diplotene* stage follows in which homologous chromosomes begin to split and remain connected only by chiasmata, which represent crossing-over sites. By now the nucleus has reached its maximum size and at the end of this stage the nucleolus has a limited size and begins to show a trabecular texture.

In the last stage of the prophase or *diakinesis* the chromosomes are short and

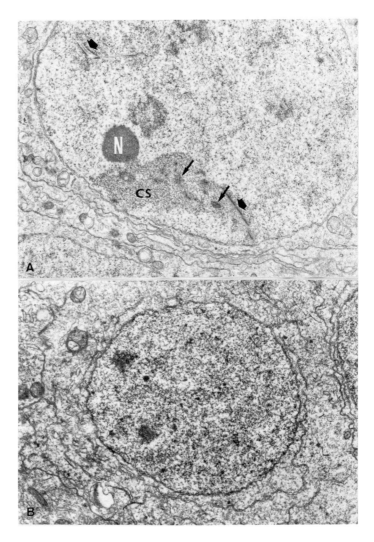

FIGURE 3-9. *Spermatocytes. A,* During the stage of pachytene in the first meiotic division the nucleus shows numerous synaptonemal complexes (thick arrows) and the so-called sex vesicle with several components: fibrillar chromatin of the sex chromosomes *(CS)* and irregular masses of heavy electron density that correspond to portions of the synaptinemal complex between both chromosomes (thin arrows). *N:* nucleolus (x22,000). *B,* Secondary spermatocyte with abundant endoplasmic reticulum and thick clumps of chromatin material (x16000).

thick and they become arranged around the nucleus following detachment of their chiasmatic connections. The nucleolus and nuclear membrane now disappear. Cytoplasmic synthesis of membrane material shows a steady progress throughout the prophase (Solari and Tres, 1967; Sotelo, 1969).

At the end of the prophase the chromosomes occupy the equatorial region of the cell (metaphase). Eventually each homologous chromosome along with two chromatids migrates to one pole of the cell. During the telophase the nuclear membrane is fully established surrounding the two newly formed nuclei. Chromosomal spindles are no longer visible and the chromosomes themselves gradually fade away.

The two resulting cells are secondary spermatocytes and they are also attached to each other by cytoplasmic bridges. These cells are also round and measure approximately 12 microns in diameter (Fig. 3-9B). Their nucleus shows dense chromatin clumping with interconnecting chromatin threads. They are difficult to observe because their interphase has a short duration. Within a few hours they undergo a second meiotic division resulting in the formation of spermatids. The latter are haploid cells no longer capable of division evolving gradually into spermatozoa. This process represents the final step of spermatogenesis and is also referred to as spermiogenesis. Histometric studies have shown that from 36 to 45 percent of primary spermatocyte loss occurs during the meiotic process (Johnson and co-authors, 1983).

Spermiogenesis

In their early stage, spermatids are round and relatively small (8 microns diameter). Their nucleus shows either delicate chromatin threads or dense clumps of homogeneous material approximately the size of nucleoli. Very soon, the nucleus decreases gradually in size and shows features of involution. The cytoplasm shows abundant vesicles of smooth endoplasmic reticulum, small mitochondria at the periphery of the cell and a well-developed Golgi complex. The rough endoplasmic reticulum is rather sparse and there is a characteristic chromatin body located in the neighborhood of the nucleus and probably related to it. This chromatoid body (Fig. 3–10**B**) exhibits two distinctly separate and irregular zones; one is densely fibrous, the other granular (Courot and Loir, 1968). Histochemically it shows the tinctorial characteristics of ribonucleoproteins.

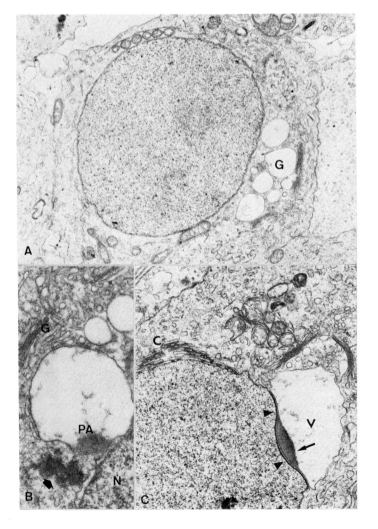

FIGURE 3–10. *Immature spermatids. A, The differentiation of spermatids into spermatozoa is heralded by the presence of a developed Golgi complex (G) next to abundant endoplasmic reticulum (x16,000). B, Large vesicles containing electron dense material detach themselves from the Golgi complex and form the acrosomal granule (PA) next to the nucleus. The chromatoid body (arrow) is found also close to it. G: Golgi apparatus; N: nucleus (x33,000). C, Formation of the acrosomal vesicle (V) is the next step in the maturation of the spermatids. The acrosomal granule is seen inside the vesicle (arrows). The inner layer of the nuclear membrane is thickened at this level (arrowheads). Above the nucleus and partially attached to the nuclear membrane there are groups of annulate lamellae of endoplasmic reticulum (C) (x22,000).*

The beginning of spermiogenesis is heralded by the formation of dense vesicles in the region of the Golgi complex that surrounds the nucleus (proacrosomal granules) (Fig. 3–10A and B). Blending of these vesicles results in the formation of a single large one (acrosomal vesicle), which becomes attached to a nuclear groove. Correspondingly, an area of increased density begins to appear in the inner side of the nucleus and against the nuclear membrane facing the acrosomal vesicle. A certain number of flattened cisternae of smooth endoplasmic reticulum separated by electron dense material begin to appear above the nucleus in close proximity to the acrosomal vesicle (Fig. 3–10C) (Nistal and co-workers, 1980). As the new proacrosomal granules incorporate to the acrosomal granule the acrosomal vesicle becomes attached to the nuclear surface in the form of a cap (Fig. 3–11A). This structure gradually flattens out to increase the length of its nuclear attachment (Fig. 3–11B). The electron dense material of the acrosomal granule extends throughout the acrosomal vesicle to form the acrosome (Fig. 3–11C and D). The latter becomes oriented towards the nuclei of the adjacent Sertoli cells. The acrosome has abundant glycoproteins and glycolipids as well as carbohydrates (galactose, manose, fructose) and enzymes (hyaluronidase, acid phosphatase, nucleotidase) (Sinowatz and co-workers, 1982). The cytoplasmic membrane over the acrosome

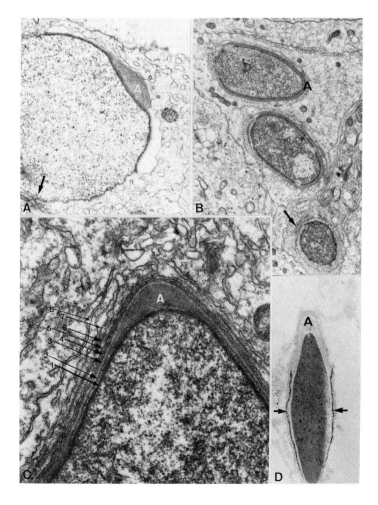

FIGURE 3–11. *Differentiation of mature spermatids into spermatozoa. A, B, C, and D show successive stages of spermiogenesis including development of the acrosome (A), condensation of chromatin and elongation of the nucleus. The latter develops numerous dense granules before it becomes hyperchromatic. Some of them correspond to DNA, others to RNA. A and B show groups of annulate lamellae (arrows) attached to the nucleus. C shows each of the different membranes of the spermatid: 1: nuclear membrane; 2: inner layer of the acrosomal sheath; 3: outer layer of the acrosomal sheath; 4: plasmalemma of the spermatid; 5: cytoplasmic membrane of adjacent Sertoli cell; 6: filaments of Sertoli cell; 7 and 8: cisternae of endoplasmic reticulum of Sertoli cell. D: silver stain of the postacromosomal sheath (arrows)(courtesy of D B Krimer) (A ×18,000; B ×6,000; C ×42,000; D ×6000).*

develops a number of tubular projections which become attached to the Sertoli cell (tubulo-bulbar complexes) (Russell and Malone, 1980).

During the formation of the acrosome two significant changes take place in the nucleus: on the one hand the chromatin becomes condensed and increasingly granular (Figs. 3–11 and 3–12) until it becomes a homogeneous mass devoid of structure, while the nucleolus disappears. This process progresses from the periphery to the center and from the subacrosomal region to the opposite. On the other hand, the centrioles migrate to the nuclear side opposing the acrosome. One of them becomes perpendicular to the nuclear axis, and the nuclear membrane becomes thickened at this level (Figs. 3–12D and 3–13B). The other centriole occupies a more external position and later becomes the basal corpuscle of the flagellum. Initially, the chromatoid body remains close to it but soon disappears (Fig. 3–12E). In the early stages the flagellum has a structure similar to cilia. It is called axonema or filamentous axial complex (Fig. 3–13C, D, and E).

Toward the distal end of the acrosome the cytoplasmic membrane develops

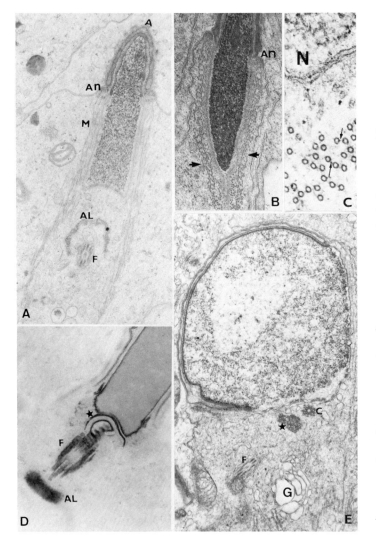

FIGURE 3–12. *Differentiation of spermatozoon. A, Spermatid with elongated nucleus and fully formed acrosome. A: acrosome; An: Nuclear ring; M: manchette; AL: annulus; F: flagellum (x18,000). B, Manchette microtubules (arrows), oblique and cross section. An: nuclear ring. C, Closeup of microtubules in cross section. Some of them show interconnecting filaments (arrows). N: Nucleus (x60,000). D, Silver stain demonstrating the connecting piece (star), the proximal end of the flagellum (F), and the annulus (AL) (x35,000). E, Residual cytoplasmic structures surrounding the early part of the flagellum. Membranous structures suggest remnants of Golgi complex. C: centriole; asterisk: chromatoid body; F: flagellum (x27,000) (courtesy of D B Krimer).*

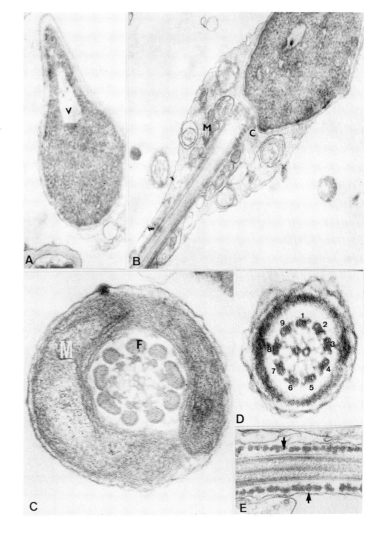

FIGURE 3–13. *Differentiated spermatozoon. A, Elongated head with acrosome and condensed nucleus. The nuclear vacuole (V) is frequently seen and probably corresponds to an artifact (x30,000). B, Neck of spermatozoon and beginning of the middle piece. The initial part of the flagellum is outlined by the connecting piece (C). The connecting piece shows a mitochondrial sheath (M) surrounding the axonema and the dense longitudinal fibers (x30,000). C, Cross section of the middle piece demonstrating the mitochondrial sheath (M) and the dense fibers (F) surrounding the nine peripheral doublets and the pair of central microtubules (x120,000). D, Cross section of the distal principal piece. The dense outer fibers have disappeared. The peripheral double microtubules of the axoneme have been numbered (x120,000). E, Longitudinal view of the main section of the flagellum. The fibrous sheath has a discontinuous character (arrows) (x33,000).*

an invagination that extends close to the nuclear membrane. This invagination surrounds the nucleus like a ring and it is called nuclear ring (Fig. 3–12A and B) (Elder and Hsu, 1982). At this time, bundles of microtubules develop from the cytoplasmic membrane to surround the nucleus and even reach the level of the centrioles. They correspond to the caudal sheath, or manchette, which will disappear later coinciding with the total condensation of the chromatin (Fig. 3–12A, B, and C).

At the origin of the flagellum the cytoplasmic membrane develops another invagination to form a membranous ring that surrounds the base of the flagellum. The inner lamina of the invagination shows deposition of a dense material the nature of which has been related to the chromatoid body. This structure has been called the annulus or centriolar ring, not to be confused with the nuclear ring (Fig. 3–12A and D).

A new structure called the connective piece surrounds the pair of centrioles toward the nuclear groove. It is composed of nine striated columns with a common attachment at their proximal end. At the level of the axonema each striated column continues in the form of a dense outer longitudinal fiber extending almost to the caudal end of the flagellum (Fig. 3–13B, C, and D) (Irons and Clermont, 1982). It consists of several proteins with a high cysteine content (Olson and Sammons, 1980).

Longitudinal sections of dense fibers show a helical striation at an angle of 60° to the long axis, which results in a 400 Å periodic structure (Paddock and Woolley, 1980). According to some authors the latter results from helicoidal arrangement of each fiber.

Another structure called the external fibrous sheath extends from the annulus to the distal end of the flagellum surrounding the latter in the form of two segmented columns. Cross sections show two triangular shaped processes, or ribs, stemming from each column. They are the longitudinal columns (Fig. 3–13D and E). Later on the annulus is displaced toward the distal end of the flagellum and with it it draws the invagination of the cytoplasmic membrane. The space between the origin of the flagellum and the annulus is filled by mitochondria (Fig. 3–13B and C). When the rest of the cytoplasm is discarded leaving a residual body that contains lipid droplets and RNA, the spermatozoa is fully developed. The residual body is now phagocytized by Sertoli cells (Burgos and co-authors, 1970; Fawcett, 1965).

Structure of the Spermatozoon

When fully developed in the seminiferous tubule, the spermatozoon has the following structure:
1. The head, which includes a pear-shaped nucleus with a tapered acrosomal end surrounded by a narrow strip of cytoplasm devoid of organelles. The head measures approximately 5 microns. The acrosome located in the anterior region forms a widened cap that covers about two-thirds of the nuclear surface. The acrosome shows some subacrosomal material beneath it and ends in the postacrosomal sheath (Pedersen, 1972) (Fig. 3–11D), a protein rich structure that can be stained with PAS and silver.
2. The neck is a narrow segment in continuity with the head and it includes the base of the flagellum. This encroaches upon a nuclear groove (articular fossa) and includes the connecting piece with the proximal and distal centrioles. The latter is the basal body of the flagellum (Fig. 3–12D and 3–13B).
3. The middle piece extends for a distance of approximately 10 microns and includes the proximal end of the flagellum (Fig. 3–13B). At this level it is composed of the axonema, which has the structure of a regular cilium consisting in nine peripheral microtubule doublets surrounding a pair of central microtubules (Fig. 3–13C). The microtubules are numbered by tracing a line that crosses the two central tubules. A second perpendicular line will split one of the peripheral double microtubules. This pair of microtubules is identified as number 1 and the others are numbered clockwise if they are to the left of the dinein arms or counterclockwise if their situation is the opposite. The peripheral double microtubules are surrounded by the dense fibers. Each pair of microtubules has a corresponding fiber and the latter are numbered following the same system (Fig. 3–13C and D). Rather than symmetrical in relation to a certain axis, the fibers are placed in relation to an imaginary line, which splits fiber number 1 and reaches the opposite side between fibers numbered 5 and 6. Fibers numbered 1, 5, and 6 are the largest. The dense fibers are surrounded by the mitochondrial sheath composed of elongated mitochondria displaying parallel cristae, a moderately dense matrix, and a double helicoidal arrangement (Fig. 3–13C). Usually there is a small amount of cytoplasm between the mitochondrial sheath and the surrounding external membrane (Fig. 3–13B).
4. The middle piece is followed by the principal piece, which is the longest seg-

ment of the flagellum. At this level of the principal piece, the mitochondrial sheath has been replaced by the fibrous sheath already described (Fig. 3–13D and E). The dense fibers become smaller as they approach the distal end of the flagellum and those numbered 8 and 3 totally disappear.
5. The terminal end of the flagellum measures two microns and shows no trace of fibrous sheath or dense fibers. Except for the absence of some microtubules the structure of this flagellum is very similar to that of a regular cilium (Fawcett, 1965).

Associations of the Seminiferous Epithelium

It has been noted for some time that each of the cell types represented in the germinal line can be identified in random sections of any seminiferous tubule. However, the arrangement of the germinal cells, far from capricious, is characteristically organized in six cellular associations as detailed in Table 3–1 and Figures 3–14 and 3–15.

Each association is indicated in Roman numerals and includes the successive arrangement of the different cell types in a column. Their order reflects the arrangement in which they are encountered in the seminiferous epithelium from basement membrane to the lumen of the tubule. Following the terminology of Clermont (1963) the initials correspond to: Ap: Spermatogonia A pale; Ad: Spermatogonia A dark; B: Spermatogonia type B; I: Primary spermatocytes in interphase; L: Primary spermatocytes in leptotene; Z: Primary spermatocytes in zygotene; P: Primary spermatocytes in pachytene; II: Secondary spermatocytes in interphase; Sa, Sb_1, Sb_2, Sc, Sd_1 and Sd_2, spermatids in progressive steps of maturation (from undifferentiated spermatid Sa, to fully differentiated spermatozoon, Sd_2) (Fig. 3–5).

These six associations occur in such a way that in a single cross section of several seminiferous tubules each may display a combination of up to four of these associations. Furthermore, atypical associations do also occur, due to accelerated or delayed maturation of some of the cells. The patterns of associations in human seminiferous tubules is apparently irregular, in contrast to that in other mammals (Figs. 3–14 and 3–15). However, Schulze (1982) has recently reported that the distribution of associations in two-dimensional maps of the human seminiferous tubules reveal the presence of helically arranged sequences. These findings suggest the existence of a spermatogenetic wave in humans similar to the occurance in other mammals.

Cycle of the Seminiferous Epithelium

The numbering of these associations is not arbitrary. The portion of a seminiferous tubule showing an association I has to follow each of the other five associations before I is repeated. This series of changes is called the cycle of the seminiferous epithelium. Since the appearance of a spermatogonium Ap until its final maturation into a spermatozoon, a number of successive associations will take place to complete 4.6 cycles as illustrated in Figure 3–16.

Autoradiography studies with the use of tritiated thymidine and nuclear incorporation of DNA have elucidated the duration of each of these associations and cycles. Duration of the associations I through VI is 4.8; 3.1; 1; 1.2; 5, and 0.8

TABLE 3–1. *Associations of the Seminiferous Epithelium*

I	II	III	IV	V	VI
A_p	A_p	A_p	A_p	A_p	A_p
A_d	A_d	A_d	A_d	A_d	A_d
B	B	I	L	A_d	B
P	P	P	P	L–Z	Z–P
Sa	Sa	Sb_1	Sb_2	P	II
Sd_1	Sd_2			Sc	So

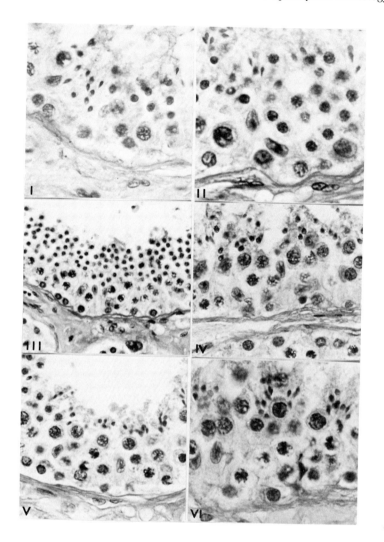

FIGURE 3–14. *I through VI show successive examples of the six associations of the seminiferous epithelium. I: x700; II: x900; III: x300; IV: x600; V: x700; VI: x900.*

days respectively. The length of a complete cycle is the sum of the duration of the six associations which represents a total of 15.9 days. Since spermatogenesis consists of 4.6 cycles, its total duration should be $15.9 \times 4.6 = 74$ days (Fig. 3–16).

TESTICULAR INTERSTITIUM

Leydig Cells

Between the seminiferous tubules there is a loose connective tissue which includes reticulin fibers and to a lesser extent, collagen fibers. Characteristic cells of this connective tissue are fibroblasts (not especially active in this case), macrophages, polymorphonuclear leucocytes, mast cells, and lymphocytes. There are also abundant blood vessels, lymphatics, and nerves. The most significant component of this connective tissue, however, is the interstitial or Leydig cell, which is responsible for the secretion of male steroid hormone (testosterone) under LH stimulation (Van der Molen and others, 1983; Ewing and Zirkin, 1983).

Leydig cells are found singly or in groups, almost invariably around capillaries for a more effective blood interac-

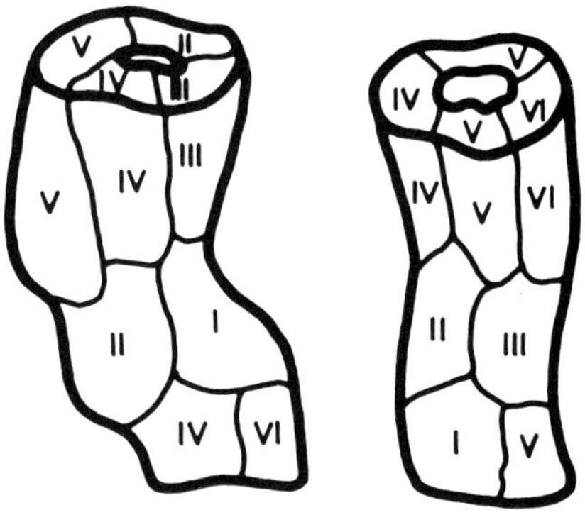

FIGURE 3–15. *The six associations of the human seminiferous epithelium have an irregular arrangement in mosaic form. The maturation of the seminiferous tubules is apparently not synchronous. Cross sections of the tubules demonstrate at least four different associations.*

tion (Figs. 3–1 and 3–17**A** and **B**). Their cytoplasm is generally polygonal and the nucleus is oval, eccentric and slightly irregular. The nuclear chromatin is arranged in the form of a dense peripheral band attached to the nuclear membrane. The nucleolus, usually well developed, is close to the nuclear membrane. Cells with two nucleoli are not unusual. The cytoplasm is vacuolated and acidophilic and it is almost totally occupied by smooth endoplasmic reticulum, mitochondria, lipid inclusions, lysosomes, and crystals of Reinke (Fig. 3–17C).

The smooth endoplasmic reticulum consists of a tight network of anastomosing tubules. If the tissue has not been fixed properly, the endoplasmic reticulum may look vesicular (Fig. 3–17C). Other organelles are also embedded in between the tubules of the smooth reticulum. Normal Leydig cells do not show any specific characteristics of their smooth endoplasmic reticulum, such as concentric cisternae frequently seen in mammals and abnormal human testes (see Fig. 11–5B).

The rough endoplasmic reticulum is rather sparse in adult Leydig cells, where it is generally found in close proximity to the nucleus. There are also free ribosomes, some of them grouped as polyribosomes. The Golgi apparatus is not particularly developed. Mitochondria are often large and pleomorphic with predominance of elongated or curved forms. Their cristae are tubular and have a clear matrix. Normal Leydig cells may show occasional electron dense inclusions (DeKretser, 1967).

Lysosomes are quite abundant throughout the cytoplasm, some of them forming lipofuscin granules (Fig. 3–17C). Lipid inclusions, often large, are also frequent (Fig. 3–18F). Microfilaments, abundant in immature Leydig cells (Fig. 3–18C), tend to decrease as the cells mature.

FIGURE 3–16. *Diagram of the different cellular stages accounting for each of the associations of the seminiferous epithelium and of the sequence of spermiogenesis. Completion of spermiogenesis includes more than four cycles lasting for approximately 74 days. Each of the associations is indicated in Roman numerals followed by its corresponding duration. Cell types are represented with the same initials used in Fig. 3–5.*

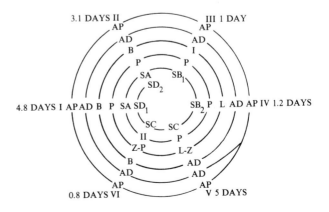

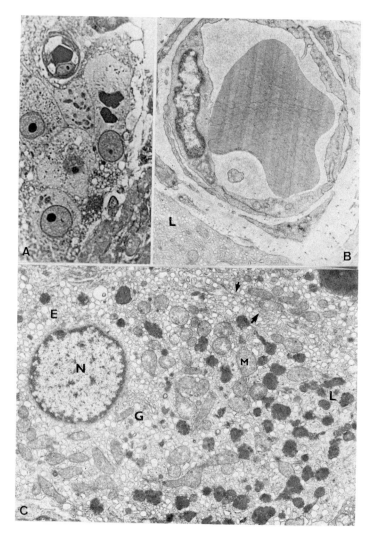

FIGURE 3–17. Adult Leydig cells. A, Semithin section (one micron) showing groups of Leydig cells in the interstitial space between tubules (x1,500). B, One of abundant blood capillaries in the interstitial space where Leydig cells empty their hormonal secretion (x12,000). C, Leydig cells demonstrating a round nucleus (N). Their condensed chromatin (heterochromatin) is predominantly attached to the nuclear membrane. The cytoplasm is predominantly filled with smooth endoplasmic reticulum (E); mitochondria with tubular cristae (M); and lipofuscin (L). The Golgi complex is not particularly developed (G). Attachments between Leydig cells are indicated by arrows (x15,000).

Reinke crystals are peculiar to man (Figs. 3–1B and 3–18A and B). These are composed of hexagonal or rectangular prisms, each measuring 10 to 20 microns in length and 2 to 3 microns in width. High magnification shows each prism composed of microtubules measuring approximately 150 Å in diameter, arranged in two series of parallel tubules, each crisscrossing the other. The distance between two microtubules is approximately 190 Å (Fig. 3–18A) (Fawcett and Burgos, 1960). Another kind of Reinke crystal shows a hexagonal or honey-comb lattice (Fig. 3–18B).

Some of the adult Leydig cells exhibit paracrystalline structures, which have been described in the differentiating Leydig cell (see Chapter 2) instead of the Reinke crystalloids (Rubin and others, 1971). Leydig cells occurring in clusters are bound together by interdigitations of the cytoplasmic membrane as well as by gap junctions (Fig. 3–18D and E). Cytoplasmic projections are particularly abundant in the cytoplasmic side facing the connective tissue. Next to the cytoplasmic membrane there are scattered vesicles lined by a filamentous material (Nagano and Suzuki, 1976). The presence of abundant smooth endoplasmic reticulum, mitochondria with tubular cristae, lipid

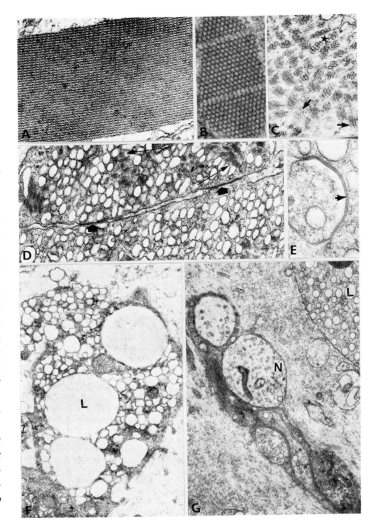

FIGURE 3—18. *Adult Leydig cells. A, Reinke crystal composed of two series of parallel microtubules crossing each other in the form of a tridimensional network (x100,000). B, Closeup of Reinke crystal illustrating a hexagonal lattice (x200,000). C, Groups of paracrystalline inclusions. Each is made up of six microfilaments arranged longitudinally along the section (arrows). The upper part of the photograph shows their profile in cross section (star) revealing that each microcrystal is a single laminae that undergoes five foldings (x100,000). D, Junctions between Leydig cells (thick arrows) (x250,000). E, Detail of gap junctions between Leydig cells (x80,000). F, Cytoplasm of a Leydig cell showing lipid inclusions (L) (x25,000). G, Nonmyelinated nerve with synaptic vesicles (N) in close proximity to a Leydig cell (L) (x10,000).*

inclusions, and lipofuscin in the Leydig cells is generally regarded as evidence of active steroid hormone synthesis (Ewing and Zirkin, 1983). Different Leydig cell populations are present in the testes. They can be characterized by quantitatively and qualitatively different responses to hormones (Rommerts and Brinkman, 1981).

The dark and fusiform cells described in the adult testis as related to Leydig cells, most likely correspond to examples of immature Leydig cells in different stages of development as they have been previously characterized in the infantile and in the pubertal testes (see Chapter 2).

Leydig cells identical to those in the interstitial space can also be encountered in ectopic locations including the albuginea, testicular septa, epididymis, and spermatic cord. Although infrequently, they can also be located within nerves (see Fig. 6–14C). This has been explained on the basis of cellular migration along the nerves, but they could have derived also from local precursor mesenchymal cells already present within nerves that develop simultaneously with those in the interstitial location (Halley, 1960; Nistal and Paniagua, 1979b).

The association of macrophages to Leydig cells, and the endocyte and immunological activity of the former, suggests that macrophages could have a role in testicular functions (Miller and co-authors, 1983).

Blood Supply of the Testis

The testes receive their arterial supply from the testicular artery, which derives from the abdominal aorta. The testicular arteries bifurcate after reaching the spermatic cord (Juskiewnski and Vaysse, 1978) and they divide further into main branches to reach beyond the albuginea into the interlobular septa. Furthermore, each of these vessels give several smaller branches to reach the rete testis (centripetal arteries). Other branches leave the centripetal arteries in the form of a loop to run in the opposite direction (centrifugal arteries) (Fig. 3–19). Both centripetal and centrifugal arteries display considerable spiral arrangement (Fig. 3–20). Also, both groups of arteries continue branching out into smaller vessels that maintain their spiral profile until their caliber decreases to 50 microns. At this point they end up in the interstitial space in the form of arterioles. The group of capillaries originating from these arterioles will form an anastomotic network in the interstitial space (intertubular capillaries) (Figs. 3–1B, 3–17B) or around the tunica propria of the seminiferous tubules (peritubular capillaries). In relation to those capillaries, groups of veins run through the septa toward the testicular capsule. Those located deeply travel to the rete testis (centripetal veins) while those draining the more superficial zone go toward the albuginea (centrifugal veins). Both groups of veins eventually merge and leave the testis to form the pampiniform plexus of the spermatic cord, which is identified as a group of vein's surrounding the testicular artery. At this level there are no arteriovenous shunts (Kormano and Suoranta, 1971). The albuginea is supplied from branches of the testicular artery including those for the albuginea alone and those derived from the epididymal arteries. The latter predominate in the portion of the testis next to the epididymis.

The development of the lymphatic drainage of the testis begins during fetal life. During infancy there are already lymphatic capillaries within the lobules and within the interlobular septa. The development of lymphatics is actually completed at the beginning of puberty (Hundeiker, 1969). In other mammals the lymphatic capillaries form a peritubular network that courses through the septa and drains into collecting lymphatics, which reach the albuginea or the rete testis along with the vessels. There are two types of peritubular lymphatics in these mammals. One is made up of actual capillaries lined by endothelial cells and a second type is composed of paralymphatic spaces surrounded by fibroblasts and located next to the basement membrane of seminiferous tubules. These fibroblasts fulfill the role of a discontinuous endothelial lining (Fawcett and others, 1969; Wrobel and others, 1981). In the human testis the lymphatic capillaries are only seen within the interlobular septa, but not around the seminiferous tubules. The lymphatic capillaries show a discontinuous endothelium

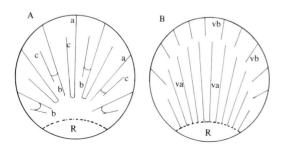

FIGURE 3–19. Vascularization of the testis. A, Arterial distribution in the testicular parenchyma. a: main branches of testicular arteries; b: centripetal branches; c: centrifugal branches. B, Distribution of veins: va: centripetal veins; vb: centrifugal veins. (Modified from M Kormano and H Suoranta.)

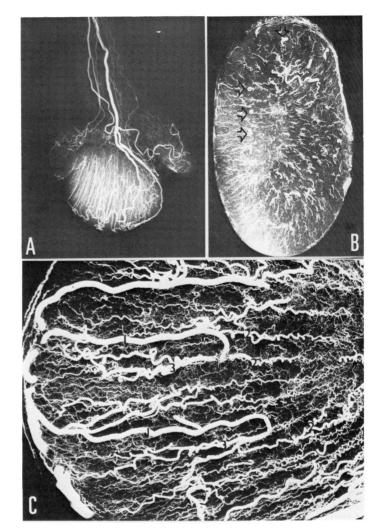

FIGURE 3-20. Vascularization of adult testis demonstrated by angiography of testicular artery. A, The testicular artery divides at the level of the albuginea and the branches are directed to the testicular parenchyma forming the main branches as well as the centripetal and centrifugal branches (x1.2). B, Cross section of the testis shows the arrangement of the main branches of the testicular artery (arrows). They keep the same distance from the albuginea and from each other. C, Close view demonstrates the main branches (1), the centrifugal (2), and centripetal (3) branches (x5).

supported by a discontinuous basal lamina (Holstein and co-workers, 1979).

Nerve Supply of the Testis

While the innervation of the scrotum and cremasteric muscle is strictly somatic, the innervation of the testis derives from sympathetic postganglionic and visceral afferent fibers. Although some nerves reach the testis directly, most of them do so indirectly from the lumbar and thoracic splanchnic nerves and send fibers to the prevertebral plexuses and ganglia. These in turn send fibers to form the internal spermatic plexus that accompanies the spermatic artery. One or two small ganglia are usually located next to the origin of the testicular artery (Hodson, 1970).

Nerves of the internal spermatic plexus follow the testicular artery to the testis and they surround this organ after branching out at the level of the albuginea. From here they innervate the interlobular septa to reach the interstitium along with the blood vessels. Most of these nerves are nonmyelinated and have a small caliber (Fig. 3-18G). Some of the axons are partially lined by Schwann cells and they display varicosities containing abundant vesicles characteristic of synaptic junctions. These vesicles correspond to three types: some have a diameter of 400 to 600 Å and have an electrodense content. Others,

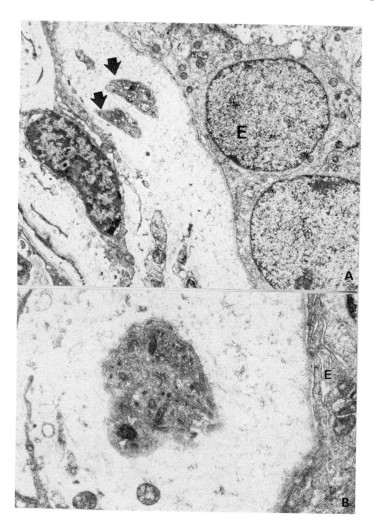

FIGURE 3–21. *A, Nonmyelinated nerve fibers with partial loss of Schwann cells (arrows) have gone through the basement membrane approaching the seminiferous epithelium (E) (x6,000). B, Next to the seminiferous epithelium (E) nerve axons contain several vesicles. Some are clear, measuring 400 to 600 Å; others (measuring 300 Å and 1,000 Å) contain dense granules (x35,000).*

having the same dimensions, display a more clear content and a third type measures 1,000 to 1,200 Å and contain small, dense granules (Fig. 3–21). Occasionally, some of these described swellings extend through the lamina propria to touch the basement membrane of the seminiferous epithelium. Although no true synaptic junctions with the germinal epithelium have been described, these nerves may still exercise some form of control over the seminiferous tubules, possibly by the discharge of neurohumoral transmitter substance in the basement membrane. The same applies to Leydig cells in which proximity there are similar nerve varicosities also displaying characteristic vesicles (Fig. 3–18G). In this location, however, some authors have described the presence of occasional connections between nerve fibers and Leydig cells (Baumgarten and Holstein, 1967; Nistal and Paniagua, 1979a; Nistal and others, 1982). On the other hand, there is still no convincing evidence to indicate nerve control over spermatogenesis or over the maintenance or the function of Leydig cells. There are sensory nerve endings not only in the scrotum but also in the albuginea in the form of encapsulated endings similar to the corpuscles of Meissner and Pacini and displaying the presence of a cellular body in the dorsal ganglia of the spinal cord (Kreutz, 1964).

REFERENCES

1. Averback P: Histopathological diagnosis of hypercurved seminiferous tubules. Histopathology 4:75, 1980
2. Baumgarten HG, Holstein AF: Catecholaminhaltige Nervenfasern in Hoden des Menschen. Z Zellforsch 79:398, 1967
3. Bawa SR: Fine structure of the Sertoli cell of the human testis. J Ultrastruct Res 9:459, 1963
4. Burgos MH, Vitale-Calpe R, Aoki A: Fine structure of the testis and its functional significance. In Johnson AD, Gomes WR, Vandemark NL, (eds): The testis I. New York: Academic Press, 1970, p. 551
5. Bustos-Obregón E: Description of the boundary tissue of human seminiferous tubules under normal and pathological conditions. Verh Anat Ges 68:197, 1974
6. Chemes HE, Dym M, Raj HGM: Hormonal regulation of Sertoli cell differentiation. Biol Reprod 21:251, 1979
7. Chemes HE, Fawcett DW, Dym M: Unusual features of the nuclear envelope in human spermatogenic cells. Anat Rec 192:493, 1978
8. Clermont Y: The cycle of the seminiferous epithelium in man. Am J Anat 112:35, 1963
9. Clermont Y: Renewal of spermatogonia in man. Am J Anat 118:509, 1966
10. Courot M, Loir M: Ultrastructure du corps chromatoide pendent la phase d'allongement de la spermatide chez le belier. 6th International Congress on Animal Reproduction. Paris, 1968
11. Davies AG: Role of FSH in the control of testicular function. Arch Androl 7:97, 1981
12. Davis JR, Langford GA, Kerby PJ: The testicular capsule. In Johnson AD, Gomes WR, Vandemark NL (eds): The testis I. New York, Academic Press, 1970, p. 282
13. De Kretzer MD: Changes in the fine structure of the human testicular interstitial cells after treatment with human gonadotropins. Z Zellforsch 80:344, 1967
14. De Kretser DM, Au CL, Le Gac F, Robertson DM: recent studies on inhibin. In D'Agata R, Lipsett MB, Polosa P, van der Molen HJ, (eds) Recent Advances in Male Reproduction: Molecular Basis and Clinical Implications. Raven Press. New York 1983, pp 101-112
15. Dorrington JH, Fritz IB: Cellular localization of 5-alfa-reductase and 3-alfa-hydroxysteroid dehydrogenase in the seminiferous tubule of the rat testis. Endocrinology 96:879, 1975
16. Elder FFB, Hsue TC: Observations on the argentophilic properties of mammalian spermatids. Cytogenet Cell Genet 34:48, 1982
17. Ewing LL, Zirkin B: Leydig cell structure and steroidogenic function. Recent Prog Horm Res 39:599, 1983
18. Fawcett DW, Burgos MH: Studies on the fine structure of the mammalian testis. II The human interstitial tissue. Am J Anat 107:245, 1960
19. Fawcett DW: The anatomy of the mammalian spermatozoon with particular reference to the guinea pig. Z Zellforsch 67:279, 1965
20. Fawcett DW, Heideger PM, Leak LV: Lymph vascular system of the interstitial tissue of the testis as revealed by electron microscopy. J Reprod Fertil 19:109, 1969
21. Gulizia S, Sanborn BM, D'Agata R, Steinberger E: Androgen-binding species in human testes. In D'Agata R, Lipsett MB, Polosa P, van der Molen HJ, (eds) Recent Advances in Male Reproduction: Molecular Basis and Clinical Implications. Raven Press: New York 1983, pp. 47-52
22. Hadziselimovic F, Seguchi H: Ultramikroskopische Untersuchungen an Tubulus Seminiferous bei Kindern von der Geburt bis zur Pubertät. II Entwicklung und Morphologie der Sertolizellen. Verh Anat Ges 68:149, 1974
23. Halley JBW: Relation of Leydig cells in the human testicle to the tubular and testicular function. Nature 195:865, 1960
24. Hamasaki M, Murakami M: SEM observation of the contractile cells of japanese monkey seminiferous tubules treated with HCL-collagenase. J Electron Microsc. (Tokyo) 28:154, 1979
25. Hansson V, Jegou B, Attramadal H, Jahnsen T, Le Gac F, Tvermyr M, Froysa A, Horn R: Regulation of Sertoli cell function and response. In D'Agata R, Lipsett MB, Polosa P, van der Molen HJ. (eds) Recent Advances in Male Reproduction: Molecular Basis and Clinical Implications. Raven Press. New York 1983, pp. 53-68
26. Hodson N: The nerves of the testis, epididymis and scrotum. In Johnson AD, Gomes WR, Vandemark NL (eds): The Testis I. New York, Academic Press, 1970, p. 47
27. Holm PB, Rasmussen SW: Human meiosis. Carlsberg Res Commun 48:351, 1983
28. Holstein AF: Fakten und Probleme der Spermatogenese (eine Orientirunshilfe für den Unterricht). Verh Anat Ges 69:857, 1975
29. Holstein AF, Orlandini GE, Möller R: Distribution and fine structure of the lymphatic system in the human testis. Cell Tissue Res 200:15, 1979
30. Hundeiker M: Lymphatic vessels in the par-

enchyma of human testis. Arch Klin Exp Derm 235:271, 1969
31. Hutson JC: Metabolic cooperation between Sertoli cells and peritubular cells in culture. Endocrinology 112:1375, 1983
32. Irons MJ, Clermont I: Formation of the outer dense fibers during spermiogenesis in the rat. Anat Rec 202:463, 1982
33. Johnson L, Petty CS, Neaves WB: Further quantification of human spermatogenesis: germ cell loss during postprophase of meiosis and its relationship to daily sperm production. Biol Reprod 29:207, 1983
34. Juskiewnski S, Vaysse P: Arterial vascularization of the testes and surgery for undescended testicles (testicular ectopia). Anat Clin 1:127, 1978
35. Knibiehler B, Mirre C, Hartung M, Jean P, Stahl A: Sex vesicle-associated nuclear organizers in mouse spermatocytes: localization, structure, and function. Cytogenet Cell Genet 31:47, 1981
36. Kormano M, Suoranta H: Microvascular organization of the adult human testis. Anat Rec 170:31, 1971
37. Kreutz WV: Ueber das Vorkommen korpuskulärer Nervenendigungen in der Tunica Albuginea Testis des Menschen. Anat Anz 115:27, 1964
38. Lacy D: Androgen dependency of spermatogenesis and the physiological significance of steroid metabolism in vitro by the seminiferous tubules. In Jones UHT, Serio M, Martini L (eds): The Endocrine Function of the Human Testis. New York: Academic Press, 1973, vol. 1, p. 493
39. Landon GV, Pryor JP: The blood-testis barrier in men of diverse fertility status: an ultrastructural study. Virchows Arch (Pathol Anat) 392:355, 1981
40. Miller SC, Bowman BM, Rowland HG: Structure, cytochemistry, endocytic activity, and immunoglobulin (Fc) receptors of rat testicular interstitial-tissue macrophages. Am J Anat 168:1, 1983
41. Nagano T, Suzuki F: Freeze-fracture observations on the intercellular junctions of Sertoli cells and of Leydig cells in the human testis. Cell Tissue Res 166:37, 1976
42. Negro-Vilar A, Lumpkin MD: Inhibin: central and peripheral effects to regulate folicle-stimulating hormone secretion. In Negro-Vilar A, (ed) Male Reproduction and Fertility. Raven Press. New York 1983, pp. 159–170
43. Nistal M, Paniagua R: Leydig cell differentiation induced by stimulation with HCG and HMG in two patients affected with hypogonadotropic hypogonadism. Andrologia 11:211, 1979
44. Nistal M, Paniagua R: Histogenesis of human extraparenchymal Leydig cell. Acta Anat 105:188, 1979b
45. Nistal M, Paniagua R: The postnatal development of the human Sertoli cells. Z Microsk Anat Forsch 97:732, 1983.
45b. Nistal M, Paniagua R, Abaurrea MA: Varicose axons bearing "synaptic" vesicles on the basal lamina of the human seminiferous tubules. Cell Tissue Res 226:75, 1982
46. Nistal M, Paniagua R, Esponda P: Development of the endoplasmic reticulum during human spermatogenesis, Acta Anat 108:238, 1980
47. Olson GE, Sammons DW: Structural chemistry of outer dense fibres of rat sperm. Biol Reprod 22:319, 1980
48. Paddock SW, Woolley DM: Helical conformation of dense fibres from mammalian spermatozoa. Exp Cell Res 126:199, 1980
49. Pedersen H: The postacrosomal region of the spermatozoa of man and *Macaca arctoides*. J Ultrastruct Res 40:366, 1972
50. Rommerts FFG, Brinkman AO: Modulation of steroidogenic activities in testis Leydig cells. Mol Cell Endocrino 21:15, 1981
51. Rowley MJ, Berlin JD, Heller CG: The ultrastructure of four types of human spermatogonia. Z Zellforsch. 112:139, 1971
52. Rubin P, Cesarini JP, Mattei, A, Laffargue P, Vague J:Etude en microscopie electronique de la cellule de Leydig chez l'homme normal. Ann Endocr 32:661, 1971
53. Russell LD, Malone JP: A study of Sertoli-spermatid tubulobulbar complexes in selected mammals. Tissue & Cell 12:263, 1980
54. Russell LD: Sertoli-germ cell interrelations: a review. Gamete Research 3:179, 1980
55. Sanborn BM, Wagle JR, Steinberger A, Lamb DJ: Sertoli cell as an androgen target. In D'Agata R, Lipsett MB, Polosa P, van der Mole HJ, (eds) Recent Advances in Male Reproduction: Molecular Basis and Clinical Implications. Raven Press. New York 1983, pp. 69–78
56. Schulze C: On the morphology of the human Sertoli cell. Cell Tissue Res 153:339, 1974
57. Schulze C: Morphological characteristics of the spermatogonial stem cells in man. Cell Tiss Res 198:191, 1979
58. Schulze W: Evidence of a wave of spermatogenesis in human testis. Andrologia 14:200, 1982
59. Schulze W: Licht- und elektronenmikroskopische Studien an der A-Spermatogonien von Männern mit intakter Spermatogenese und bei Patienten nach Behandlung mit Antiandrogenen. Andrologia 10:307, 1977
60. Sinowatz F von, Friess AE, Wrobel KH: His-

tochemische, Zytochemische und ultrastrukturelle Untersuchungen zur Spermiogenese. Acta Histochem. [Suppl] (Jena) 25:137, 1982
61. Solari AJ, Tres LL: The ultrastructure of the sex vesicle in the mouse. Chromosoma 22:16, 1967
62. Sotelo JR: In Lima deFaria A (ed): Handbook of Molecular Cytology. Amsterdam-London: North Holland Publ Co, 1969
63. Steinberger A, Steinberger E: Secretion of FSH inhibiting factor by cultured Sertoli cells. Endocrinology 99:918, 1976
64. Van der Molen HJ, Bakker GH, Rommerts FFG: Biochemical actions of luteinizing hormone in the regulation of testicular steroid-production. In D'Agata R, Lipsett MB, Polosa P, van der Molen HJ, (eds) Recent Advances in Male Reproduction: Molecular Basis and Clinical Implications. Raven Press. New York 1983, pp. 91-100
65. Waites GMH, Gladwell RT: Physiological significance of fluid secretion in the testis and blood-testis barrier. Physiol Rev 62:624, 1982
66. Wrobel KH, Sinowatz F, Mademann R: Intertubular topography in the bovine testis. Cell Tissue Res 217:289, 1981

4

EPIDIDYMIS AND SPERMATIC DUCTS

The spermatic ducts include all the structures that contribute to the passage of the spermatozoa and testicular fluid to the surface. The role of the spermatic ducts is not only passive since they actively contribute to the motility of spermatozoa, to the composition of the seminal fluid, and to the final step of maturation of spermatozoa.

The spermatic ducts can be divided in intratesticular and extratesticular segments. The former include the straight ducts (ductuli recti) in continuity with the seminiferous tubules and the rete testis in continuity with the straight ducts. From the rete testis the testicular fluid reaches the epididymis, which is the beginning of the extratesticular spermatic ducts (see Fig. 1–10). The epididymis is a paired organ, semilunar in shape, and it is surrounded by a capsule. It originates on the superior pole of each testis and extends partially along one side. It is essentially composed of a loose fibrous connective tissue stroma embedding the efferent ducts that converge to form the epididymal duct. The efferent ducts are located predominantly in the head of the epididymis, which is immediately adjacent to the upper pole of the testis. From this area the epididymal duct continues through the body of the epididymis to become the vas deferens almost at the level of the lower pole of the testis (see Figs. 1–10, 3–1). The vas deferens leaves the testis and for some distance runs parallel to the blood vessels and nerves of the testis. Together they cross the anterior abdominal wall through the inguinal canal and continue within the spermatic cord, which consists of the vas deferens, together with blood vessels, lymphatic vessels and nerves, embedded in a loose connective tissue. In the pelvis the vas leaves the spermatic cord and continues to the posterior aspect of the bladder where it dilates to become the ampulla of the vas. From this point it joins with the terminal portion of the seminal vesicle where it continues as the ejaculatory duct, which then descends through the prostate gland, reaches the prostatic urethra, and converges with the opposite ejaculatory duct from the other testis at the verumontanum. From here the prostatic urethra is continuous with the penile urethra to the urethral meatus. (see Fig. 1–9) (Ladman, 1973).

Straight Ducts (Ductuli Recti)

The seminiferous tubules follow a highly tortuous course, converging in each lobule as a straight duct located next to the mediastinum testis (Fig. 4–1A). In their initial segment, the straight ducts form an ampulla which is lined by Sertoli cells. Toward their distal portion, however, the epithelium becomes cuboidal, consisting of modified Sertoli cells that have extensive, vacuolated, cytoplasmic processes that almost occlude the lumen. Although it has been postulated that the ampullary segment probably acts as a valve to limit the back flow of spermatozoa to the seminiferous tubules (Cavicchia and Burgos, 1976), a possible reabsorptive or secretory function has also been suggested for these cells (Waites and Gladwell, 1982). In some animals, the straight ducts and rete testis are capable of phagocytic activity (Osman and Plöen, 1978; Sinowatz and others, 1979).

Rete Testis

The straight ducts open into a system of anastomosing channels coursing through the mediastinum to form the rete

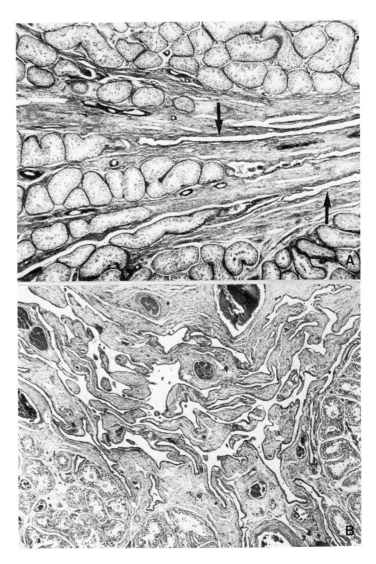

FIGURE 4-1. *A,* Straight ducts (ductuli recti) (arrows) distal to seminiferous tubules (x60). *B,* Rete testis located in the mediastinum testis and composed of a network of anastomosing channels at the end of the straight ducts (ductuli recti) (x60).

testis (Fig. 4-1B). These channels are transversed by fine strands (chordae) containing myoid cells and capillaries (Roosen-Runge and Holstein, 1978) (Fig. 4-2). The epithelial lining is largely made up of cuboidal cells with occasional groups of columnar cells each possessing a single cilium. Furthermore, those cells lining the deeper ducts also may show phagocytic activity. The seminiferous fluid and spermatozoa reach the epididymis through the rete testis, but the mechanism of this flow remains obscure since no musculature is found in the wall of the rete. On the other hand, this may be explained on the basis of pressure differences between the rete testis and the seminiferous tubules. Reference has also been made to a possible participation of the connective tissue of the mediastinum testis and the albuginea, both of which contain specialized contractile cells (Burgos and Cavicchia, 1975; Bustos-Obregon and Holstein, 1976; Dym, 1976; Kormano, 1977). The fluid of the rete testis differs from that of the seminiferous tubules in iron, protein, and steroid composition and in sperm concentration. Although, whether this contribution to testicular fluid is by a secretory process or by a

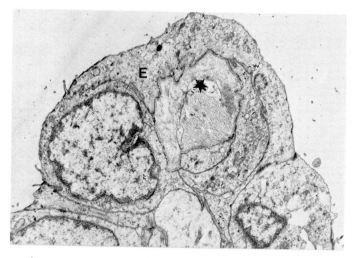

FIGURE 4–2. *Chordae testis in the rete testis consisting of connective tissue strands (star) covered by a flattened or cuboidal epithelial lining (E) (x10,000).*

passive transportation is unclear. Physiological studies suggest that the fluid entering the rete testis is the result of active solute transport (mainly sodium) which sets up an osmotic gradient (Waites and Gladwell, 1982). Although the rete testis epithelial cells can phagocytose and digest spermatozoa, experimental studies indicate that these cells lack absorptive activity (Goyal, 1982).

EFFERENT DUCTS

The channels of the rete testis converge to form 10 to 15 efferent ducts, which leave the testis to reach the head of the epididymis (Fig. 4–3A). The efferent ducts are also referred to as "efferent cones" because of their cone shape when they become coiled around themselves (Fig. 1–10). The space between the cones is filled by the connective tissue stroma of the epididymis. At this level, the epithelial lining of the ducts is somewhat scalloped due to the uneven size of the cytoplasm of alternating groups of the cuboidal and cylindrical epithelial cells (Fig. 4–3B). There is a mixture of ciliated and nonciliated (principal) cells. Ciliated cells show a large, spherical apically located nucleus and dense apical aggregations of mitochondria. The principal cells present a basally located nucleus, supranuclear aggregates of large granules, and microvilli. Beneath the basement membrane there is a thin layer of circularly arranged muscle cells. The contribution of these structures to the flow of testicular fluid is indicated by the presence of smooth muscle and cells provided with large cilia which are oriented toward the epididymal duct. A gradual change in function of the principal cells from secretion in the proximal regions to absorption in the distal regions of the efferent ducts are reflected in the ultrastructural features of cells from each region. Granules of principal cells lining the proximal efferent ducts show a clear floccular content, while granules of principal cells lining the distal efferent ducts are heteromorphic and contained an heterogenous content, resembling secondary lysosomes. It has been calculated that more than 90 percent of the fluid secreted by the testis is absorbed into and across the epithelial cells in these regions (Waites and Gladwell, 1982) (Fig. 4–4). Unlike other mammals, no secretory function has yet been demonstrated in the principal cells (De Kretser and others, 1982). Like in the rete testis, epithelial phagocytosis of the sperm has been observed in some mammals (Goyal, 1982).

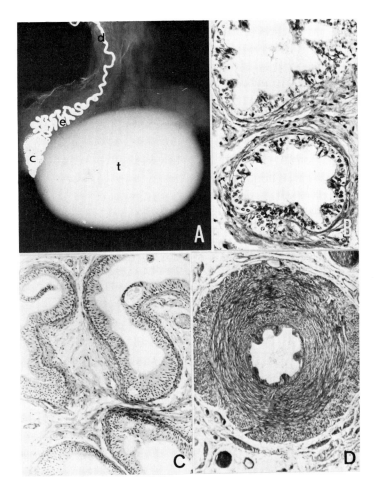

FIGURE 4-3. *A*, The efferent ducts (*c*), the epididymal duct (*e*), and the vas deferens (*d*) are clearly outlined with contrast medium (*t:* testis) (×1.3). *B*, Efferent ducts. The epithelium is somewhat scalloped because of the combination of cuboidal and columnar cells (×125). *C*, The epididymal duct appears composed of several ducts on sectioning due to its special tortuosity. The lining epithelium is pseudostratified and cylindrical and displays numerous stereocilia. It is encircled by muscle. The connective tissue in the stroma of the epididymis demonstrates abundant blood vessels (×60). *D*, Vas deferens with an epithelial lining similar to the epididymis, surrounded by three muscle layers (×60).

Epididymal Duct

The efferent ducts of the testis converge into a single duct, the epididymal duct. This duct is extremely long, approximately 5 meters, but occupies only a limited space because of pronounced tortuosity and spiralling (Fig. 4–3A). Its trajectory determines the presence of a number of lobules separated by connective septa, which are continuous with the capsule and have a thick texture when compared to the surrounding stroma (see Fig. 2–1A).

The epididymal duct is lined by a columnar epithelium displaying slender microvilli also called stereocilia and abundant lysosomes in their apical portion (Figs. 4–3C, 4–5A). Smaller, basal cells are also present resting on the basement membrane. There is a thin lamina propria with abundant fenestrated capillaries (Fig. 4–5B and C) surrounded by circularly arranged smooth muscle fibers thicker than those in the efferent ducts (Fig. 4–3C). Approaching the vas deferens the muscle layer becomes increasingly thick, developing an additional layer of longitudinal smooth muscle fibers (Bedford and others, 1975; Holstein, 1976).

The epididymal duct, provided with long stereocilia, contributes to the reabsorption of testicular fluid and to electrolyte transport. Microperfusion techniques have demonstrated absorption at this level of salt and water as well as secretion of

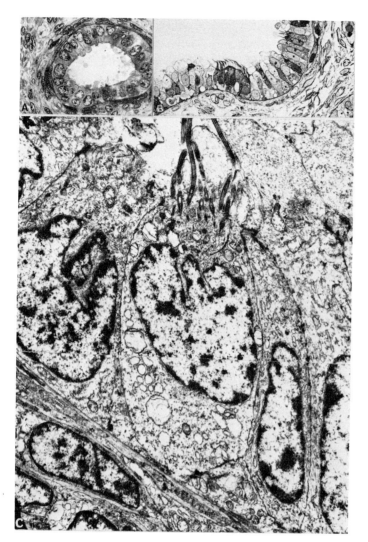

FIGURE 4–4. *Efferent duct. 1 μm thick section of an efferent duct in a child (A) and in an adult (B). The latter shows a taller epithelial lining than that of the infant. The pseudostratified distribution and the presence of ciliated cells are more prominent in the adult A and B (x850). C, Fine structure of an adult efferent duct showing a ciliated cell between two principal cells (x10,000).*

potassium, especially in the head of the epididymis (Wong, and co-authors, 1978). The synthesis of some, but not all, protein that secretes the epididymis is androgen-dependent (Brooks, 1983).

The spermatozoa develop numerous changes along the epididymal duct that result in the acquisition of their partial fertilizing ability (Turner, 1979). At this time they also initiate their motility (Hoskins and others, 1978), and there are changes of their metabolism, their acrosomal membrane and their nuclear structure (Dacheux and Paquignon, 1980; Laufer and co-workers, 1979). During this maturation process they also demonstrate an increase of cyclic AMP (Dacheux and Paquignon, 1980; Hoskins and co-authors, 1978) followed by a gradual disarray of the particles that surround the acrosome of the epididymal cells in the form of a glycocalyx (Suzuki and Nagano, 1980; Jones and co-workers, 1983; Brown and associates, 1983). All of these changes are controlled by the epididymal epithelium under androgenic influence and take place progressively as the spermatozoa pass through the epididymis. Spermatozoa isolated form the caput epididymis are unable to fertilize ova; as the spermatozoa descend to the corpus epididymis, they begin to acquire their fertilization capacity

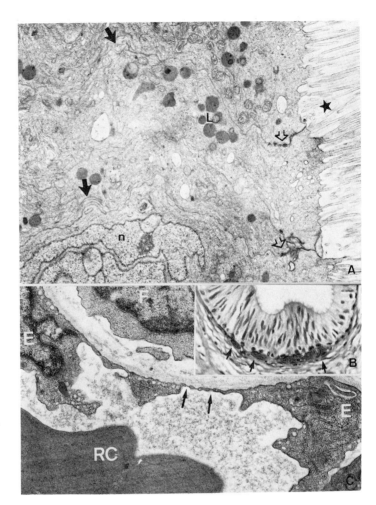

FIGURE 4–5. **A**, Epididymal epithelium showing irregular nuclei (**n**), extensive interdigitations (arrows), junctional complexes (open arrows) between adjacent cells, numerous lysosomes (**L**) and stereocilia (star) (x6,000). **B**, Section of the epididymal duct showing numerous capillaries immediately beneath the epithelium (x125). **C**, Detail of one of the capillaries demonstrating the presence of pores partially occluded by a thin diaphragm (arrows). **E**: endothelium, **F**: fibroblast, **RC**: red blood cell (x30,000).

(Setty, 1979). However, the spermatozoa leaving the male genital tract are not yet completely capable of fertilizing the ova, and "capacitation" in the female reproductive tract is required before full fertilizing potential is accomplished. Some authors have also called attention to the presence of spermiophage cells in the epithelial lining of the epididymal duct (Phaedke, 1975). Intraepithelial lymphocytes have also been reported (Wang and Holstein, 1983).

VAS DEFERENS

The vas deferens is in continuity with the epididymal duct (Fig. 4–3**A**), and it is also composed of a cylindrical epithelium displaying stereocilia and a layer of basal cells. It shows three types of cylindrical cells: (**a**) chief cells with abundant lysosomes; (**b**) dark cells with dense nucleus; and (**c**) cells with abundant mitochondria (Hoffer, 1976). All three types of cells have highly irregular nuclei (Fig. 4–6**A**, **B**, and **C**). During infancy the vas only shows columnar undifferentiated cells with short stereocilia and small basal cells (Fig. 4–6**D**) (Paniagua and co-authors, 1981 and 1983).

The lumen of the vas is more irregular than in the epididymal duct. The epithelium moving away from the testis develops increasing epithelial folds and the muscle coat becomes thicker (1 to 4.5 mm thickness) and is composed of three layers: in-

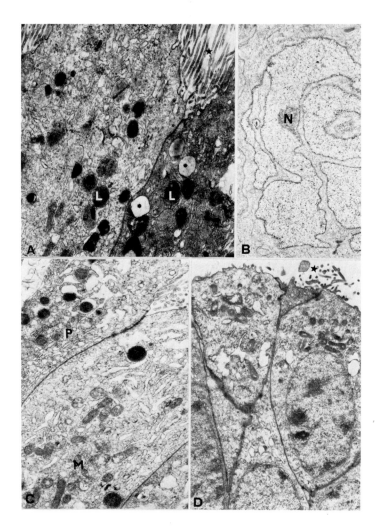

FIGURE 4–6. Ultrastructure of vas deferens. A, Principal cell (left side of picture) with abundant lysosomes (L) and endoplasmic reticulum. Dark cell (right side of picture) with lipid vacuoles (asterisk) and electron dense cytoplasm. Both show numerous stereocilia (star) (x15,000). B, Nucleus of a principal cell showing lobulated nuclear contour. N: nucleolus (x15,000). C, Mitochondria-rich cell (M) next to a principal cell (P) (x15,000). D, Vas deferens in the newborn showing undifferentiated cells, regular nuclei, and poorly developed stereocilia (star) (x5,500).

ner, outer, and middle. The thickness of the muscle coat decreases gradually along the duct. Beyond the muscle there is the adventitia composed of loose connective tissue in continuity with neighboring structures (Fig. 4–3D).

The vas forms an ampulla next to the junction of the prostate and seminal vesicle. The ampulla is histologically similar to the remainder of the vas except for the presence of more abundant elastic fibers. The role of the ampulla is that of storing spermatozoa between ejaculations (Aumüler and Bruhl, 1977; Cossu and others, 1983).

It has been pointed out that the vas is not only a passive duct for the passage of spermatozoa but it also plays an active role in the maturation of spermatozoa and in the final composition of the seminal fluid. This can also be concluded by the presence of significant regional morphological changes along the vas. From the epididymis to the ampulla the chief cells decrease in number while there is a corresponding increase of both dark cells and mitochondrion-rich cells. The chief cells appear to be specialized for the recovery of protein from the testicular fluid, whereas the dark cells appear to be predominantly involved in the maintenance of osmosis. Furthermore, there is evidence to indicate that the dark cells probably represent degenerate chief cells (Paniagua and co-authors, 1981).

VASCULARIZATION OF SPERMATIC DUCTS

The rete testis is poorly vascularized although it receives some arterial branches from the hilum of the testis or even from the centripetal arteries. At any rate, the capillaries are less abundant than in the testis.

The superior and inferior epididymal branches of the testicular artery are responsible for the blood supply of the head and part of the body of the epididymis. The remainder of the epididymis is supplied from branches of the artery of the vas deferens, and some of them are connected to the arteries of the head of the epididymis. In addition, there are also arterial branches of testicular origin that connect with those of the epididymis (see Fig. 3-20A).

All of these arteries run along the surface of the epididymis, but they also give off special branches that reach the interlobular septa of the epididymis. These minor arteries show significant spiralling in the adult, and the complexity of their spiralling seems to increase with age. The spiral arteries do not show excessive branching but they give out a number of arterioles of lesser caliber and no spiralling which, after a short distance, became arranged in a network of fenestrated capillaries located in the connective tissue between the efferent ducts or around the epididymal duct (Fig. 4-3C) (Kormano and Reijonen, 1976).

The efferent ducts are surrounded by a dense capillary network at the head of the epididymis, and this is even more striking among the ducts located closer to the testis where they tend to display greater caliber and less conspicuous musculature. The epididymal duct is provided with a lighter capillary network, and this is even further organized in the form of fenestrated capillaries arranged around the duct in a circular fashion. The epididymal capillaries enter a venous plexus that follows a similar course than the arteries except for the absence of a spiralling arrangement.

The vas deferens has a double capillary network: one surrounding the outer aspect of the muscle layer and a second one that reaches the lamina propria where it forms a capillary network that surrounds the epithelium (Kormano and Reijonen, 1976).

The testicular and epididymal venous flow drains into the spermatic plexus, forming three principal drainage systems: a) internal spermatic vein (anterior group), which accompanies the internal spermatic testicular artery, and opens into either the cava (right side) or the renal vein (left side); b) deferential vein (central group), which runs along the vas deferens beside the deferential artery; and c) cremasteric or internal spermatic vein (posterior group), which drains into the inferior epigastric and pudendal veins. There are numerous anastomoses between the three groups of veins.

In the spermatic cord near the testis there are a number of lymphatic capillaries in relation to the vas deferens. These capillaries are arranged in the form of an alveolar framework drained by collecting lymphatics. These are located predominantly toward the periphery of the pampiniform plexus and decrease considerably as they approach the inguinal canal. In their wall there are scattered smooth muscle cells (Möller, 1980).

NERVE SUPPLY OF SPERMATIC DUCTS

The nerve supply of the epididymis derives indirectly from the intermesenteric and the lower mesenteric plexuses, eventually forming the middle spermatic plexus, which reaches the testis along with the testicular artery. In fact, its course is similar to the superior spermatic plexus except for the distal end where it reaches the epididymis. In addition, there are fibers of the pelvic pelvus that contribute to the inferior spermatic plexus. The latter surrounds and supplies the spermatic cord, following it down to the tail of the epididymis. It includes a combination of sympathetic and parasympathetic fibers. There are communicating fibers between the pelvic and the hypogastric plexuses.

Reaching the epididymis, the nerve fibers traverse the capsular tissue and branch out within the epididymal septa. Here they divide further into finer branches to surround the blood vessels, the efferent ducts, the epididymal duct, and finally penetrate the interstitial space. Adrenergic fibers are more abundant than cholinergic fibers although both have a very similar distribution (Baumgarten and others, 1968; Hodson, 1970). Groups of axons partially lined by Schwann cells become embedded in special "gaps" provided by the smooth muscle cells (Fig. 4–7A and B). These axons form numerous varicosities which contain a number of

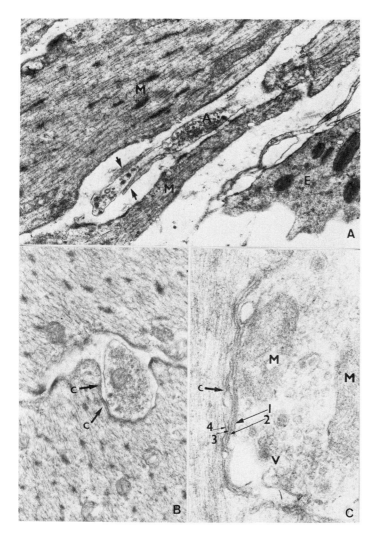

FIGURE 4–7. *Fine structure of the innervation of the vas deferens. A, Non-myelinated axon (A) embedded among smooth muscle cells (M). The axon is partially surrounded by Schwann cells (arrows). E: eosinophilic leukocyte (x28,000). B and C, Detail of the junction of an axon with a smooth muscle cell. Within the latter there is a cisterna of smooth endoplasmic reticulum (C) arranged along the sarcolemma at a distance of less than 100 Å. The synaptic vesicles of the axon (V) are light or dark measuring 400–600 Å in diameter. In addition, there are larger vesicles (approximately 1,000 Å), containing a small dense granule (200 Å). M: mitochondria, 1: Axon membrane; 2: sarcolemma; 3: outer surface of the sarcolemmal cisterna; 4: inner surface of same (B x35,000; C x62,000).*

vesicles that can be categorized as either clear or as a combination of clear and dark. Some of these varicosities almost come in contact with the sarcolemma of the muscle cell (less than 100 Å). Sometimes a cisterna of smooth endoplasmic reticulum lies beneath the sarcolemma running along the entire length of the synapsis and separated from it by less than 100 Å (Fig. 4-7B and C) (Nistal and Paniagua, 1977).

REFERENCES

1. Aumüller G, Bruhl B: Ueber den Bau der Ampulla ductus deferens des Menschen. Verh Anat Ges 71:561, 1977
2. Baumgarten HG, Falck B, Holstein AF, Owman C, Owman T: Adrenergic innervation of the human testis, epididymis, ductus deferens and prostate: A fluorescence microscopic and fluorimetric study. Z Zellforsch 91:402, 1968
3. Bedford JM: In Astwood EB and Greep RO (eds): Handbook of Physiology Section on Endocrinology. Bethesda: American Physiol Soc, 1975
4. Brooks DE: Epididymal function and their hormonal regulation. Aust J Biol Sci 36:205, 1983
5. Brown CR, von Glos KI, Jones R: Changes in plasma membrane glycoproteins of rat spermatozoa during maturation in the epididymis. J Cell Biol 96:256, 1983
6. Burgos MH, Cavicchia JC: Phagocytic activity in the epithelium of the rete testis. Proc tenth int cong of anat Science council of Japan p. 444, 1975
7. Bustos-Obregon JE, Holstein AF: The rete testis in man: ultrastructural aspects. Cell Tissue Res 175:1, 1976
8. Cavicchia JC, Burgos MH: Tridimensional reconstruction and histology of the intratesticular seminal pathway in the hamster. Anat Rec 186:493, 1976.
9. Cossu M, Marcello MF, Usai E, Testa-Riva F, Riva A: Fine structure of the epithelium of the human ejaculatory duct. Acta Anat (Basel) 116:225, 1983
10. Dacheux JL, Paquignon M: Relations between the fertilizing ability, motility and metabolism of epididymal spermatozoa. Reprod Nutr Develop 20:1085, 1980
11. De Kretser DM, Temple-Smith PD, Kerr JB: Anatomical and function aspects of the male reproductive organs. In Bandhauer K, Frick J, (eds) Disturbances in Male Fertility, Springer-Verlag: Berlin-Heidelberg-New York 1982, pp. 1-131
12. Dym M: The mammalian rete testis. A morphological examination. Anat Rec 186:493, 1976
13. Goyal HO: Light microscopic and ultrastructural evidence of epithelial phagocytosis of sperm in the rete testis and ductuli efferentes in the bull. Am J Vet Res 43:785, 1982
14. Hodson N: The nerves of the testis, epididymis and scrotum. In Johnson AD, Gomes WR, and Vandemark NL (eds): The testis I. New York: Academic Press, 1970, p. 47
15. Hoffer AP: The ultrastructure of the ductus deferens in man. Biol Reprod 14:425, 1976
16. Holstein AF: Structure of the human epididymis. In Hafez ESE, (ed) Human Semen and Fertility Regulation in Men. C. V. Mosby and Sons. St Louis 1976, pp. 23-30
17. Hoskins DD, Brandt H, Acott TS: Initiation of sperm motility in the mammalian epididymis. Federation Proc 37:2534, 1978
18. Jones R, von Glos KI, Brown CR: Changes in the protein composition of rat spermatozoa during maturation in the epididymis. J Reprod Fertil 67:299, 1983
19. Kormano M, Reijonen K: Microvascular structure of the human epididymis. Amer J Anat 145:23, 1976
20. Kormano M: The rete testis. In Johnson AD and Gomes WR (eds): The testis IV. New York: Academic Press, 1977, p. 461
21. Ladman AJ: Male reproductive system. In Greep RO and Weiss L (eds): Histology 3rd ed. London: McGraw-Hill, 1973
22. Laufer N, May JY, Segal S, Grover NB: Size of rat spermatozoa during maturation along the epididymis. Arch Androl 3:293, 1979
23. Möller R: Arrangement and fine structure of lymphatic vessels in the human spermatic cord. Andrologia 12:564, 1980
24. Nistal M, Paniagua R: Ultraestructura de las sinapsis neuromusculares en el conducto deferente de rata. Anal Anat 26:483, 1977
25. Osman DI, Plöen L: The mammalian tubuli recti: ultrastructural study. Anat Rec 192:1, 1978
26. Paniagua R, Regadera J, Nistal M, Abaurrea MA: Histological, histochemical and ultrastructural study along the length of the human vas deferens before and after puberty. Acta Anat (Basel) 111:190, 1981
27. Paniagua R, Regadera, J, Nistal M, Santamaría L: Elastic fibres of the human ductus deferens. J Anat 137:467, 1983

28. Phaedke AM: Spermiophage cells in man. Fertil Steril 26:760, 1975
29. Roosen-Rungen EC, Holstein AF: The human rete testis. Cell Tissue Res 189:409, 1978
30. Setty BS: Regulation of epididymal function and sperm maturation. Endocrine approach to fertility control in males. Endokrinologie 74:100, 1979
31. Sinowatz F, Wrobel KH, Sinowatz S, Kugler P: Ultrastructural evidence for phagocytosis of spermatozoa in the bovine rete testis and testicular straight tubules. J Reprod Fert 57:1, 1979
32. Suzuki F, Nagano T: Epididymal maturation of rat spermatozoa studied by thin sectioning and freeze-fracture. Biol Reprod 22:1219, 1980
33. Turner TT: On the epididymis and its function. Invest Urol 16:311, 1979
34. Waites GMH. Gladwell RT: Physiological significance of fluid secretion in the testis and blood-testis barrier. Physiol Rev 62:624,1982
35. Wang YF, Holstein AF: Intraepithelial lymphocytes and macrophages in the human epididymis. Cell Tissue Res 233:517, 1983
36. Wong PYD, Au CL, Ngai HK: Electrolyte and water transport in rat epididymis; its possible role in sperm maturation. Int J Androl 2:608, 1978

5

HORMONAL CONTROL OF TESTICULAR FUNCTION

J.J. Vazquez

The testis goes through a period of rest from birth until puberty. The first three years are followed by a period of slow growth and development characterized by increasing caliber and length of seminiferous tubules and by a gradual rise of the tubular fertility index (see Chapter 2).

At puberty, the testis speeds up the maturation process to assume two clearly different functions—one reproductive, the other hormonal. The reproductive function or spermatogenesis takes place in the germinal epithelium of the seminiferous tubules, which account for about 90 percent of the testicular volume. Male gametogenesis is an active and organized process, basically consisting of the transformation of spermatogonia or immature cells into mature male gametes (Clermont, 1972). This process involves a series of sequential steps from spermatogonia evolving into primary and secondary spermatocytes, spermatids and spermatozoa. The interstitial or Leydig cells, because of their ability to synthesize male hormone (testosterone), are fully responsible for the testicular hormonal function or steroidogenesis.

Although spermatogenesis and steroidogenesis are actually two separate processes, they are somewhat related to each other even though the exact mechanisms of this interaction are not fully known. Testosterone, basically secreted by Leydig cells, can be mentioned as an example because it is also related to Sertoli cells. The latter are provided with the appropriate enzymatic makeup to convert testosterone into estrogens. This newly formed estradiol may in turn regulate the production of testosterone since it is established that Leydig cells have estrogen receptors.

Our present knowledge about hormonal control of testicular function is shaped by the following three factors (Van der Molen and others, 1979):

1. The development of highly sensitive radioimmunoassay techniques for detecting levels of gonadotropins and steroids;
2. The ability to isolate seminiferous tubules from the surrounding interstitial tissue and to extract pure Leydig cells from any other testicular components; and
3. More sophisticated knowledge regarding the molecular mechanisms involved in the control of steroidogenesis.

Hypothalamo-pituitary Axis

The testis is subjected to the control and regulation of other secretory organs, namely the pituitary, the hypothalamus—leading organ regarding endocrine control—and possibly the central nervous system beyond the hypothalamus.

Adenohypophysis

Two hormones, Follicle Stimulating Hormone (FSH) and Luteinizing Hormone or Interstitial Cell Stimulating Hormone (LH) are secreted by the anterior pituitary and have a testicular effect. Both are gonadotropins of glycoproteic nature and in the male their secretion is not subjected to a cyclic rhythm (Fig. 5-1) (Lincoln, 1979). Other hormones such as prolactin (Gray and others, 1981; Drago and Scapagnini, 1983), growth hormone (Zipf and Wukie, 1983) and thyrotropin (Hutson and Stocco, 1981) also plays a significant although secondary role.

FSH has a stimulating effect upon the germinal epithelium of the testis while LH is strictly related to steroidogenesis by stimulation of Leydig cells. Both gonadotrophins are released into the blood circulation, but their effect is restricted to the testis. LH has an average life of one hour, while the average duration of FSH is approximately five times longer.

Hypothalamus

A certain number of active peptides are synthesized at the level of the hypothalamus for the control of the pituitary hormones. These peptide substances reach the adenohypophysis through the descending venous system of the Popa and Fielding (Jeffcoate, 1975).

Contrary to the anticipated finding of two releasing factors, one for FSH and a second one for LH, to this date only one releasing factor has been identified. This is a decapeptide so-called Gn-RH (gonadotropin releasing hormone) also known as LH-RH since it is capable of releasing LH to a greater extent than FSH.

In fact, highly specific receptors for LH-RH have been demonstrated at the level of the adenohypophysis, which, by stimulating adenylate cyclase of the cellular membrane, would result in an elevation of cyclic AMP. It is quite likely that the presence of calcium ions and prostaglandins is essential for this reaction (Marchetti and others, 1983).

STEROIDOGENESIS

Testosterone biosynthesis from acetate and cholesterol takes place through two different pathways: Δ (Hyppa and others, 1971), with pregnenolone, 17-dihydroxy pregnenolone, dehydroepiandrosterone and Δ (Hyppa and others, 1977), androstendiol acting as intermediate metabolites; and Δ (Hashimoto and co-workers, 1975) with successive steps to progesterone, 17-hydroxy progesterone and androstenedione. There is some evidence to indicate that some of these intermediate moieties, particularly dihydroepiandrosterone and androstenedione, are secreted directly into spermatic veins (Fig. 5-2).

Under the influence of LH testicular Leydig cells undergo protein synthesis and mitochondrial production of pregnenolone following breakage of the lateral

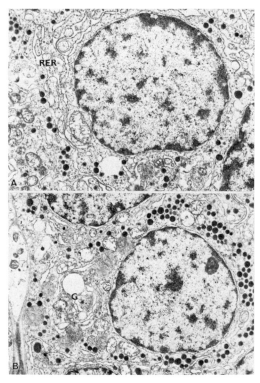

FIGURE 5-1. *Adenohypophysis. Gonadotropin secreting cells. Scattered throughout the cytoplasm there are numerous secretory granules, intensely osmophylic, measuring approximately 250 nm in diameter. Also shown are an abundant rough endoplasmic reticulum (**RER**) and a well-developed Golgi apparatus (**G**) (A and B x3000).*

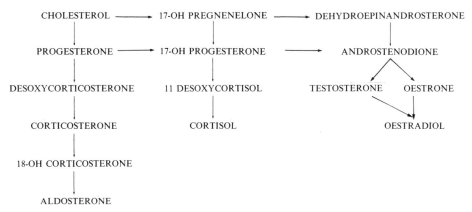

FIGURE 5–2. *All the necessary enzymes for the transformation of acetate into cholesterol are present in the smooth endoplasmic reticulum except those involved with breaking the lateral chains of cholesterol.*

chains of cholesterol (Ewing and co-authors, 1983). The function of Leydig cells is not necessarily synchronized among themselves, and they can show considerable variation in their response to LH (Bergh, 1983). The presence of FSH potentiates the release of testosterone by LH. Yet, in order to maintain normal steroidogenesis, the presence of prolactin is also essential, probably to increase the number of LH receptors of Leydig cells (Purvis and Hansson, 1978; Zipf and Wukie, 1983).

Plasma testosterone is bound to globulin and although not clearly defined yet, its synthesis seems to follow a circadian rhythm (Bellastella and associates, 1983). It is largely metabolized in the liver, most of it converted to 17-ketosteroids, and the remainder is metabolized in the form of estradiol (E_2). It should be pointed out that only 30 percent of urinary ketosteroids are from testosterone derivation. The remaining 70 percent are of adrenal origin (Paulsen, 1974).

In as much as testosterone is essential for the seminiferous tubules, it is very likely that Leydig cells select the lymphatic route for their hormonal supply. The effects of testosterone on tissues generally take place in one of the following molecular forms: as testosterone; as dihydrotestosterone in the presence of 5-alpha reductase; or as estradiol (E_2) particularly effective on the central nervous system.

The following are the most important effects of testosterone or its metabolites:

1. *External genitalia*: Development of penile and testicular size. Pigmentation and wrinkling of scrotal skin.
2. *Secondary sex organs*: Enlargement of prostate gland and seminal vesicles.
3. *Hair distribution*: Growth of beard and moustache in the male. Body hair (axillary, trunk, extremities, and pubic hair).
4. *Growth*: Pubertal growth to reach an average of 7.5 cm per year.
5. *Voice*: The voice changes to a lower pitch following hypertrophy of the larynx and vocal cords.
6. *Sexual attitude*: Increases in libido and sexual potency.

All of the above changes appear during puberty coinciding with the release of significant amounts of male hormone.

The development of spermatogenesis largely reflects the effect of testosterone and pituitary hormones, chiefly FSH. The

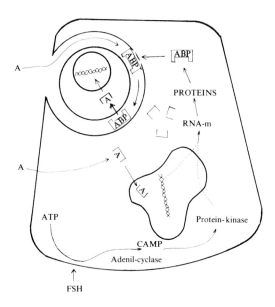

FIGURE 5–3. *Diagram of FSH effect on Sertoli and germinal cells.* ABP: *Androgen binding protein;* A: *Androgens.*

effects of this hormone on germinal cells seem to take place through Sertoli cells rather than directly (Fig. 5–3) (Means and others, 1978). A coadjuvent effect on spermatogenesis stimulation through Sertoli cells has also been attributed to thyrotropin (TSH) (Hutson and Stocco, 1981).

REGULATORY CYCLES

The testes are not only subjected to direct stimuli from the pituitary or the hypothalamus, but they soon establish a functional relationship with them upon the basis of a feedback mechanism similar to other endocrine glands (Fig. 5–4) (Means and others, 1978).

Steroidogenesis and Release of Testosterone

It is well established that testosterone and related metabolic products have a negative feedback effect upon the release of pituitary LH. Of the four hormones secreted by the testis only two of them, testosterone and estradiol, play an important role in the regulation of LH. Many of the inhibitory effects of testosterone are related to its peripheral conversion to estradiol (Purvis and Hansson, 1978; Kalra and Kalra, 1983).

Spermatogenesis and Release of FSH

The precise mechanisms responsible for the release of FSH from the pituitary gland are not yet completely understood. For many years, there has been some speculation about a feed-back mechanism controlling the FSH release by means of a FSH-inhibitory factor (inhibin), synthesized by the seminiferous tubules. Yet, the constant observation of elevated FSH levels and incomplete germinal cell line in some testicular disorders such as Klinefelter's and Del Castillo's syndromes suggests that complete spermatogenesis may be an essential requirement for the release of inhibin.

Recent studies have further characterized and clarified the role of inhibin. It is a water soluble, low molecular weight polypeptide, synthesized by the Sertoli cells (Backer and Hudson, 1976; Swerdloff and co-authors, 1973). Inhibin is secreted into the testicular fluid, and is reabsorbed through the epithelial cells of the ductus of the epididymis (Backer and Hudson, 1976). Inhibin levels are markedly dimin-

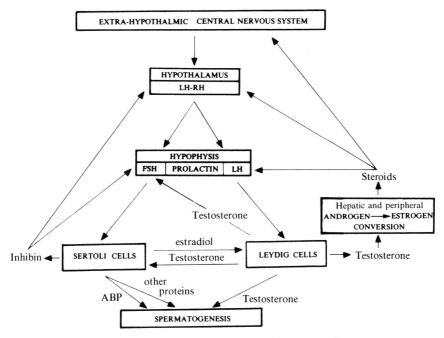

FIGURE 5-4. *Diagram of regulatory mechanisms of testicular function.*

ished in azoospermic or oligospermic patients (Steinberger, 1983). These peptides have been isolated from several avian and mammalian species and appeared to be biologically and chromatographically similar (Bandivdekar and others, 1982). Recent studies on factors that moderate inhibin secretion by cultured Sertoli cells suggest that androgens accutely stimulate the production of Sertoli cell inhibin (Verhoeven and Franchimont, 1983).

Nevertheless, inhibin is not the sole hormone controlling the hypophysary FSH release. After clinical treatments, such as testicular irradiation or intense chemotherapy, which damage the seminiferous epithelium, FSH levels are found to be only slightly increased. On the other hand, experimental studies on testosterone administration to castrated laboratory animals revealed that these animals were capable of controlling FSH levels. These observations suggest that testosterone is the principal hormone controlling FSH release.

Pituitary Control of the Hypothalamus

Control of the hypothalamus by the pituitary gland so-called "short circuit" has been so far demonstrated only in the rabbit and the rat.

Intrahypothalamic Control

There is evidence to indicate the presence of an "ultrashort circuit" in the rat whereby the LH-RH releasing factor controls its own secretion (Hyppa and others, 1971).

Several mechanisms have been proposed to explain this system of hypothalamic control, but the most favored one relates to the presence of *peptidases* located in the hypothalamus and capable of inhibiting LH-RH. It is also possible that the effect of both steroids and LH may be mediated by the peptidase system.

It should be emphasized that there still remains a great amount to learn about the control of testicular function which some have looked upon as the "Cinderella of the endocrine glands." Two areas in which further knowledge is required include the germinal epithelium control of FSH and the accepted concept that a single hypothalamic factor may control the release of two seemingly different gonadotropins.

Tests of Testicular Function

A detailed clinical history is essential for the detection of hypogonadism. Features of diagnostic relevance include the onset of puberty the study of hair distribution, osseous development, penile size and especially the evaluation of testicular size by the use of Prader's orchimeter (Takihara and others, 1983). In addition the study of the chromosomal constitution (karyotype) and the testicular biopsy (to be described in Chapter 7) are essential for proper classification of male gonadal dysfunction.

Testicular function tests are usually directed to provide information about gametogenesis or hormonal secretion. During a study of seminal fluid the patient should abstain from intercourse during three days before the test. The sample should be obtained by masturbation since the one obtained from interrupted coitus is usually unsatisfactory because it frequently misses the initial part of the ejaculate, which generally contains the largest number of spermatozoa. The use of a rubber contraceptive should also be discouraged because it tends to jeopardize spermatozoal motility. The masturbation sample should be kept at room temperature and transported to the laboratory as soon as possible.

A complete examination of the seminal fluid should include the following aspects:

1. *Volume.* Normal values range between 2 and 5 ml.
2. *Number of spermatozoa.* Normal density of sperm is usually above 50 million/ml. Figures below 20 million/ml usually reflect significant oligospermia.
3. *Sperm motility.* Normal seminal fluid shows spermatozoal motility in 70 percent of the cells two hours after ejaculation. Percentages below 40 are frequently associated with sterility.
4. *Morphology of spermatozoa.* Again, the presence of a significant number of abnormal forms, so-called teratospermia, is usually associated with infertility. Abnormal spermatozoa, however, can also be encountered in significant numbers in patients during febrile episodes.
5. *Chemistry of seminal fluid.* Determination of pH of the fluid and values of fructose, citric acid and acid phosphatase generally reflects the secretory status of the prostate and seminal vesicles.

Most useful is the evaluation of testosterone and gonadotropins. The determination of urinary 17 ketosteroids is not a sensitive index of Leydig cell function since approximately 70 percent of urinary ketosteroids is of adrenal origin and only the remainder is directly related to testosterone metabolism. Chromatographic techniques provide little additional information.

Gonadotropins. Modern techniques of radioimmunoassay have made possible the accurate determination of LH and FSH in plasma and urine. Far from uniform, their secretion occurs in "pulses" and their levels reveal considerable fluctuations during a given day. The level of gonadotropins seems to show a tendency to rise with age. Occasionally it may be difficult to differentiate low levels from normal. FSH and LH levels, however, are very useful to differentiate between hypergonadotropic and hypogonadotropic hypogonadism.

Testosterone. Gas chromatographic techniques have been surpassed by radioimmunoassay because of its accuracy and sensitivity. Normal testosterone values tend to be low in the child, increase after puberty and decrease steadily after the age of 40. Normal values between 18 and 40 years are 605 ± 180 ng/100 ml, (Smals and co-workers, 1978) although fluctuations from 350 to 1200 ng/100 ml have also been reported. (Backer, 1976). These values are obviously lower in patients with hypogonadism.

Estrogens. Values of plasma estradiol in the adult male are below 40 pg/ml.

Response Tests. Similar to other endocrine glands, there are a number of stimulation tests which enable a precise evaluation of the function of the hypothalamus-hypophysis-testicular axis providing valuable information in regard to the secretory potential of gonadotropin-secreting pituitary cells and of Leydig cells. On the basis of their practical value, the following tests should be described.

Test of Stimulation with Chorionic Gonadotropin (HCG). Because of LH activity, HCG can stimulate Leydig cells to secrete testosterone. In the classical test intramuscular administration of 3,000 IU of chorionic gonadotropin during four consecutive days brings about a progressive elevation of testosterone levels. The most useful purpose of this test is the demonstration of functional tissue in cryptorchid patients. Its value is more limited for the differential diagnosis of primary and hypogonadotropic hypogonadism (Traub, 1981). In an effort to simplify the test, Smals and co-authors (1979) suggest the administration of a single dose of 1,500 IU of HCG, which results in a significant elevation of plasma testosterone in controls as opposed to patients with hypogonadotropic hypogonadism.

Test of stimulation with Gn-RH, which consists of monitoring elevations of LH and FSH following the administration of 100 ng of Gn-RH decapeptide. In normal males there is a significant rise of LH levels reaching the highest peak in approximately 25 minutes. The rise of FSH is even more significant, but it is generally delayed. There is also an elevation of plasma testosterone, but this is even more delayed and irregular. Figure 5-5 shows the changes of plasma LH and FSH obtained in our laboratory with the test of stimulation with 100 µg Gn-RH.

Theoretically it should be a useful test for the differential diagnosis of pituitary versus hypothalamic hypogonadism. Characteristically there should be no response in the former while in case of hypothalamic disorders there should be a moderate decrease of values. Some paradoxical responses have been described, however, and in order to improve detection of cases with no actual hypophyseal damage, some have proposed the administration of repeated doses of Gn-RH

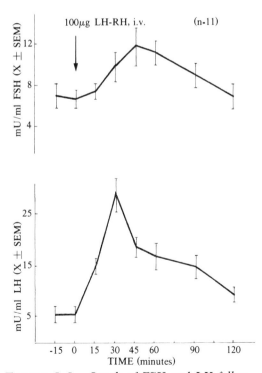

FIGURE 5-5. *Levels of FSH and LH following IV administration of 100 micrograms of LH-RH.*

(Snyder and co-workers, 1979). For this purpose the initial values of LH and FSH are recorded in response to an intravenous dose of 250 µg Gn-RH. This is followed by repetitive intravenous infusion of 500 µg Gn-RH for seven consecutive days and a second intravenous dose of 250 µg at the end. At this point the increased levels of LH are considerably more objective.

Others (Brenne and Paulsen, 1977) have proposed prolonged intravenous administration of Gn-RH to obtain a more accurate evaluation of gonadotropin values and even a steroid response from the testis (McNeil and others, 1979).

Chronic stimulation of pituitary cells by high doses of Gn-RH or its agonists may result in an inhibition of testicular androgen secretion (Belanger and coworkers, 1983). This has been attributed to "desensitization" of the pituitary cells with decreases in circulating gonadotropins (Hsueh, 1982).

Clomiphene Test. Clomiphene brings about release of pituitary gonadotropins apparently by interfering at a hypothalamic level with steroid feedback inhibition of gonadotropin secretion. The most widely accepted method of this test uses an oral dose of 50 µg twice a day for seven days. LH and FSH levels are determined on the 0, 7, and 10 days. Normally, a 50 percent elevation of LH takes place about the seventh day, while no changes are observed in boys before puberty or in patients with hypogonadotropic hypogonadism. Other studies have dealt with the LH and FSH rebound to the combined administration of Gn-RH and clomiphene citrate (Hashimoto and others, 1975). There are also some references regarding testicular tissue changes following administration of clomiphene (Rönnberg, 1980).

REFERENCES

1. Backer HW, Hudson B: Disfunción gonadal masculina. In Bayliss RI (ed): Clínica endocrinológica Barcelona: Salvat, 1976, p. 83
2. Bandivdekar AH, Vijayakshmi S, Moodbidri SB, Sheth AR: Low-molecular-weight inhibin from sheep, human, rat, and chicken testes. Int J Androl 3:140, 1982
3. Bélanger, A, Labrie F, Séguin C, Cusan L, Carmichael R, Caron S: Inhibition of testicular Δ^4-androgen secretion by treatment with luteinizing hormone-releasing hormone agonists in the rat. In Negro-Vilar A, (ed) Male Reproduction and Fertility. Raven Press. New York 1983, pp. 127–139
4. Bellastella A. Criscuolo T, Mango A, Perrone L, Sinisi AA, Faggiano M: Circannual rhythms of plasma luteinizing hormone, follicle-stimulating hormone, testosterone, prolactin and cortisol in prepuberty. Clin Endocrinol (Oxf) 19:453, 1983
5. Bergh A: Paracrine regulation of Leydig cells by the seminiferous tubules. Int. J Androl 6:57, 1983
6. Brenne WJ, Paulsen CA: Prolonged intravenous infusions of LH-releasing hormone into normal men. Horm Metab Res 9:13, 1977
7. Clermont Y: Kinetics of spermatogenesis in mammals: seminiferous epithelium cycle and spermatogonial renewal. Physiol Rev 52:198, 1972
8. Drago F, Scapagnini U: Prolactin and behavior: a neurochemical substrate. In D'Agata R, Lipsett MB, Polosa P, van der Molen HJ, (eds) Recent Advances in Male Reproduction: Molecular Basis and Clinical Implications. Raven Press. New York 1983, pp. 299–304
9. Ewing LL, Wing TY, Cochran RC, Kromann N, Zirkin BR: Effect of luteinizing hormone on Leydig cell structure and testosterone secretion. Endocrinology 112:1763, 1983
10. Gray P, Franken DR, Slabber CF, Potgieter GM: A possible relationship between prolactin and spermatogenesis in humans. Andrologia 13:127, 1981
11. Hashimoto T, Mikai K, Matsumoto K, Izumi K, Kumahara Y: LH and FSH response to synthetic LH-RH after consecutive administration of clomiphene citrate in normal males. J Clin Endocrinol 41:1110, 1975
12. Hsueh AJW: Direct effects of gonadotropin releasing hormone on testicular Leydig cell functions. Ann N Y Acad Sci 383:249, 1982

13. Hutson JC, Stocco DM: Regulation of Sertoli cell function by thyrotropin. Biol Reprod 25:303, 1981
14. Hyppa M, Motta M, Martini L: "Ultrashort" feed-back control of follicle-stimulating hormone-releasing factor secretion. Neuroendocrinology 7:227, 1971
15. Jeffcoate SL: The control of testicular function in the adult. Clinics in Endocrinology and Metabolism p. 521, 1975
16. Kalra SP, Kalra PS: Modulation of luteinizing hormone-releasing secretion by gonadal steroids in the male rat. In Negro-Vilar A, (ed) Male Reproduction and Fertility. Raven Press. New York 1983, pp. 35–44
17. Lincoln GA: Pituitary control of the testis. Brit Med Bull 35:167, 1979
18. Marchetti B, Labrie F, Pelletier G, Proulx-Ferland L, Reeves JJ: Hormonal control of pituitary luteinizing hormone-releasing hormone receptors. In D'Agata R, Lipsett MB, Polosa P, van der Molen HJ, (eds) Recent Advances in Male Reproduction: Molecular Basis and Clinical Implications. Raven Press. New York 1983, pp. 215–226
19. McNeil LW, McKenna TJ, Lacroix A, Benveniste R, Ravin D: Seventy two-hour infusions of LH-RH in normal men: Gonadotropin and testicular steroid responses. J Clin Endocrinol Metab 49:149, 1979
20. Means AR, Dedman JR, Tindall DJ, Welsh MJ: Hormonal regulation of Sertoli cells. Int J Androl (Suppl 2) 1:403, 1978
21. Paulsen CA: The testes. In Williams RH (ed): Textbook of Endocrinology 5th ed Philadelphia: Saunders Co, 1974, p. 323
22. Purvis K, Hansson V: Hormonal regulation of Leydig cell function. Mol Cell Endocrinol 12:123, 1978
23. Rönnberg L: The effect of clomiphene citrate on different sperm parameters and serum hormone levels in preselected infertile men: a controlled double-blind cross-over study. Int J Androl 3:479, 1980
24. Smals AGH, Kloppenborg PW, Pieters GF, Losekoot DC, Benraad T: Basal and human chorionic gonadotropin-stimulated 17 alpha-hydroxyprogesterone and testosterone levels in Klinefelter's syndrome. J Clin Endocrinol Metab 47:1144, 1978
25. Smals AGH, Pieters GF, Drayer JI, Benraad T, Kloppenborg PW: Leydig cell responsiveness to single and repeated human chorionic gonadotropin administration. J Clin Endocrinol Metab 49:12, 1979
26. Snyder PJ, Rudenstein RS, Gardner DF, Rothman JG: Repetitive infusion of gonadotropin-releasing hormone distinguishes hypothalamic from pituitary hypogonadism. J Clin Endocrinol Metab 48:865, 1979
27. Steinberg A: In vitro model for study of testicular inhibin. In Negro-Vilar A, (ed) Male Reproduction and Fertility. Raven Press. New York 1983, pp. 183–192
28. Swerdloff RS, Grover PK, Jacobs HS: Search for a substance which selectively inhibits FSH. Effects of steroids and protaglandins on serum FSH and LH levels. Steroids 21:703, 1973
29. Takihara H, Sakatoku J, Fujii M, Nasu T, Cosentino MJ, Cockett ATK: Significance of testicular size measurement in andrology. I. A new orchiometer and its clinical applications. Fertil Steril 39:836, 1983
30. Traub AI: An evaluation of the HCG stimulation tests in the investigation of male infertility. Brit J Urol 53:274, 1981
31. Verhoeven G, Franchimont P: Regulation of inhibin secretion by Sertoli-cell-enriched cultures. Acta Endocrinol (Copenh) 102:136, 1983
32. Zipf WB, Wukie JJ: Role of prolactin and growth hormone in maintenance of normal Leydig cell function. In Negro-Vilar A, (ed) Male Reproduction and Fertility. Raven Press. New York 1983, pp. 65–76
33. Van der Molen HJ, Van Beurden WMO, Blankenstein MA, De Boer W, Cooke BA, Grootegoed JA, Janszen FHA, De Jong FH, Mulder E, Rommerts FFG: The testis: biochemical actions of trophic hormones and steroids on steroid production and spermatogenesis. J Steroid Biochem 11:13, 1979

6

CONGENITAL ANOMALIES OF THE TESTIS AND THE EPIDIDYMIS

PRESENCE OF REMNANT EMBRYONIC STRUCTURES

The testicular spermatic duct systems, that is, the epididymis, the ductus deferens, the seminal vesicles, and the ejaculatory ducts, are formed from the Wolffian duct. The remaining mesonephric ducts atrophy early. However, some mesonephric ducts as well as the ends of the Müllerian ducts may persist, even in adulthood, and attain a certain degree of development, giving rise to different remnant embryonic structures (Fig. 6–1).

Appendix of the Epididymis (Pedunculated Hydatid of Morgagni)

The appendix of the epididymis is a cystic, pedunculated structure, lying on the caput epididymis. It is found in 25 percent of adult human testes, and corresponds to a blind remnant of the cephalic portion of the mesonephric duct (Wolffian duct) (Fig. 6–2**A**).

The wall of the cystic formation possesses an outer mesothelial lining, a middle layer of connective tissue, and an inner epithelial lining, consisting of tall columnar cells with vacuolated cytoplasm.

The appendix epididymis may undergo pathological alterations, such as torsion or tumoral transformations.

Appendix of the Testis (Sessile Hydatid of Morgagni)

The appendix of the testis is a pedunculated structure located on the anterior and superior testicular pole, near the insertion of the caput epididymis. Its diameter varies from a few millimeters to several centimeters. The testicular appendix is a blind remnant of the proximal portion of the Müllerian duct (Fig. 6–2**B**, **C**, and **D**).

The outer surface of the testicular appendix is sinuous. Its epithelial lining is made up of tall columnar cells, and they are flattened at the borders. The epithelium is continuous with the mesothelial cells lining the neighboring structures. The stroma of the testicular appendix consists of loose connective tissue, containing glandlike formations that are analogous to the epithelial folds of the Fallopian tube. Discontinuous rings of smooth muscle cells incompletely surround the glandlike structures, the lumen of which can contain mummified cells as well as calcifications.

The appendix of the testis is present in more than 90 percent of adult testes. The pathological alterations most frequently observed in the appendix of the testis are:

1. Cystic transformation.
2. Torsion, which is clinically manifested as a localized pain that begins suddenly and may urgently require surgical intervention. Hydrocele or hematocele may accompany the torsion. The highest incidence of this lesion occurs between 10 and 13 years of age (Skoglund and others, 1970). It is relatively frequent during infancy and less common in adulthood (Altaffer and Steele, 1980). At times it is difficult to distinguish this disorder from torsion of the spermatic cord.
3. Detached appendix pedicle. The tes-

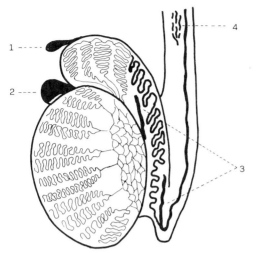

FIGURE 6–1. *Embryonic remnants in the testis, epididymis, and spermatic cord. 1: appendix of the epididymis; 2: appendix of the testis; 3: aberrant ducts; 4: paradidymis.*

ticular appendix is free within the tunica vaginalis testis and can undergo calcification (Fig. 6–2E).

Aberrant Ducts (Haller's Organ)

Aberrant ducts correspond to remnants of the mesonephric ducts, located at different levels along the length of the epididymis. Both superior and inferior aberrant ducts are distinguishable (Fig. 6–1). The superior ducts are blind, occasionally multiple ducts located in the caput epididymis and correspond to remnants of the most cranial mesonephric ducts. The inferior ducts are located in the corpus or cauda epididymis and show a tortuous course parallel in some degree to the epididymal axis. The superior end is

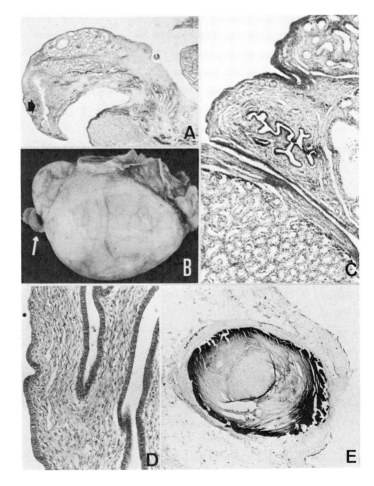

FIGURE 6–2. *A, Appendix of the epididymis (arrow) (H&E, x10). B–E, Appendix of the testis. B, Anatomical location (arrow). C, Epithelial folds within the testicular appendix (H & E, x25). D, Higher magnification of the columnar outer epithelium continuous with the mesothelium (asterisk) (H & E, x125). E, Calcified appendix of the testis. (H & E, x10).*

blind and the inferior opens into the ductus of the epididymis in the cauda epididymis.

Histologically, the two ducts consist of a tall or low columnar epithelium surrounded by rings of smooth muscle cells.

Paradidymis (Giraldés' Organ or Henle's Paraepididymis)

The paradidymis is a group of small, blind, tortuous ducts located in the anterior and inferior portion of the spermatic cord. They derive from the most caudal portion of the mesonephric ducts and are not related to the lumen of the ductus deferens. Their histological features are identical to those of the aberrant ducts (Fig. 6–1).

CHORISTOMA AND HAMARTOMA

Adrenal Cortex Choristoma

Adrenal cortex choristoma is a frequent finding in autopsies of newborn infants or in males operated on for inguinal hernia or cryptorchidism. In a study of 360 males whose ages ranged from 13 days to 13 years, and who had been operated on because of some scrotal-inguinal disorder, 12 (3.8 percent) showed aberrant adrenocortical tissue along the spermatic cord (Mares and co-workers, 1980). In a series of infants with cryptorchid testes on whom an extensive dissection of the spermatic cord was performed, a higher frequency (9.3 percent) of ectopic adrenal cortex tissue was found. According to Dahl and Bahn (1962), 15 percent of autopsies of infants reveal adrenal cortical tissue in the paratesticular structures.

Adrenal choristomas appear as isolated or multiple yellowish nodules along the length of the spermatic cord, epididymis, the tunica albuginea testis or within the testis itself. Their size varies from microscopic to several millimeter nodules (Fig. 6–3 **A**). They are most frequent on the right side.

Histologically, adrenal choristomas are exclusively formed by adrenal cortical cells. In the newborn, the fetal adrenal cortex predominates and undergoes the same transformation as that of the adrenal glands. During infancy, the ectopic adrenal tissues consist mainly of *zona fasciculata* and a peripherally placed ring of *zona glomerulosa*. From 9 years of age onward, the *zona reticularis* appears.

The presence of ectopic adrenal cortical tissue along the length of the spermatic cord, in the epididymis or in the testis is related to the common embryonic origin of both testes and adrenal glands.

Adrenal nodules may show cytological features suggesting secretory activity, and it is easy to observe cytomegalic cells

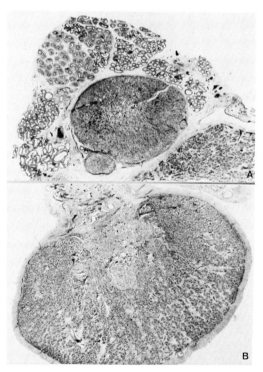

FIGURE 6–3. *Adrenal choristoma. A, An adrenal choristoma in the caput epididymis (H&E, x25). B, Multiple adrenal choristomas on the periphery of the rete testis (H&E, x10).*

in males with adrenal cytomegalia. Compensatory hyperplasia of adrenal cortex tissue has been reported in Addison's disease and in the adrenogenital syndrome secondary to congenital adrenal hyperplasia.

The presence of ectopic adrenal cortical tissue within the testis is particularly interesting. Sometimes, this occurs in normal-sized testes, in which case the ectopic adrenal tissue is an autopsy finding. Other times the intratesticular adrenal tissue is part of a congenital adrenal hyperplasia. Patients with intratesticular adrenal tissue usually are seen because of testicular tumor or infertility (Fig. 6–3B).

In the testicular biopsy one or several nodules consisting of adrenal tissue are found, which are located under the tunica albuginea or surrounded by atrophic tubules. It is not easy to recognize this tissue when only histological parameters are used. The differential diagnosis is with Leydig cell tumors (Johnson and Scheitauer, 1982). In these cases, the observation of bilateral lesions with a multilayered cellular disposition and absence of Reinke's crystals suggests the presence of adrenal tissue rather than a Leydig cell tumor.

A diagnostic test in addition to biochemical studies, is the dexamethasone treatment. The testicular size in congenital adrenal hyperplasia decreases during treatment and increases when the drug is stopped.

Splenic Choristoma

The presence of splenic tissue near the testis or in the paratesticular structures was first described by Pommer (1887). It is less frequent than the presence of adrenal tissue and may appear attached to the testis (splenic-gonadal fusion) or included within either the epididymis or the spermatic cord. It always appears on the left side.

This ectopic splenic tissue is believed to occur because of the close proximity of the left gonad to the spleen during embryonic development.

The splenic-gonadal fusion may appear with two different anatomical patterns: continuous or discontinuous. In the continuous form, the testicular parenchyma and the splenic tissue are only separated by connective tissue, resulting from the fusion of the capsules of the two organs. In the discontinuous form, a fibrous band, supplied with abundant blood vessels, joins both organs. Complete fusion is observed in 30 percent of cases (Putschar and Manion, 1956).

Patients with splenic-gonadal fusion frequently show other associated abnormalities, either local, such as hernia and cryptorchidism, or general, such as multiple congenital malformations (Quinn-Hill, 1969).

Cartilaginous Choristoma

Cartilaginous nodules in both epididymides of two infants have been found in a study of 2000 consecutive autopsies. Each nodule consisted of poorly differentiated cartilaginous cells surrounded by the perichondrium. The cartilage was located in the caput epididymis. The mechanism leading to the cartilage formation might be a metaplasia similar to that observed in different renal lesions, such as renal dysplasia and polycystosis. The significance remains unknown (Fig. 6–12E).

Paraganglia

The paraganglia as well as the adrenal medulla and the sympathetic ganglia are structures that have a neural crest origin and catecholamine storage in common. The paraganglia are ovoid or lobulated formations covered by a fibrous capsule. They are symmetrically and segmentally distributed on both sides of the sagittal plane of the body. They are found in the neck, trunk, and following the branches of the autonomic nervous system.

Histologically, they comprise two cell types: chief cells and sustentacular cells. Chief cells possess cytoplasmic secretory granules containing epinephrine. The sustentacular, or supporting, cells are similar to Schwann cells. Both cell types are grouped and form cords or nests separated from each other by abundant capillaries. Among these are numerous nerve fibers.

Paraganglia are, during fetal life, the first catecholamine reservoir, since the adrenal medulla is at a primitive stage of development. For many years it was thought that the paraganglia undergo involution after birth. However, the observation of paraganglia in several locations in adult males, such as the gallbladder, prostatic capsule, basal portion of the seminal vesicle (Hervonen and others, 1976) indicate that paraganglion involution may not necessarily occur and that paraganglia may constitute an important catecholamine source in the adult.

Epididymal paraganglia are not observed frequently, having been reported in two newborns (Nistal, 1977). In both cases the paraganglia were bilateral and were found among the ductuli efferentes in one case and in the connective tissue located between the testis and the epididymis in the other (Fig. 6–4).

Ectopic Testicular Parenchyma

The presence of seminiferous tubules within the tunica albuginea is often found in testicular serial sections obtained from autopsies of infant. The tubular pattern is not identical to that of seminiferous tu-

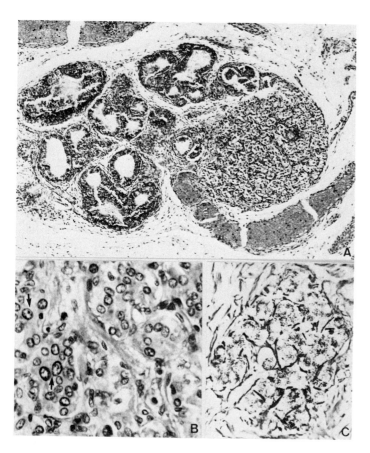

FIGURE 6–4. *Paraganglia of the epididymis.* A, Nodular paraganglion, located among the ductuli efferentes (H&E, x60). B, The chief cells of the paraganglion form small accumulations and exhibit a voluminous nucleus and an eosinophilic granular cytoplasm (arrows). The supporting cells are fusiform and show an elongated nucleus (H&E, x250). C, Argyrophilic granulations in the cytoplasm of the chief cells (Laidlaw, x250).

bules located within the testis; however, both Sertoli cells and spermatogonia may be recognized. In some cases, serial sections show continuity between the seminiferous tubules present in the tunica albuginea and those of the true testicular parenchyma (Fig. 6–5).

Testes with ectopic seminiferous tubules in the albuginea should be distinguished from testicular dysgenesis, in which tubules are also seen in the albuginea. Characteristic features that differentiate ectopic tubules from testicular dysgenesis are that, in the testes with ectopic tubules, the albuginea shows normal thickness except for the area containing the tubules, is well-collagenized, and is separated from the testicular parenchyma by a precise borderline. In addition, Müllerian duct remnants are not observed, and the external genitalia are normal (see Chapter 17).

Simple Cysts of the Testis and the Tunica Albuginea

A cystic formation develops within either the testicular parenchyma (simple cyst of the testis), or the tunica albuginea (cysts of the tunica albuginea) (Figs. 6–6A, B, C, and D).

These cysts are rare and most com-

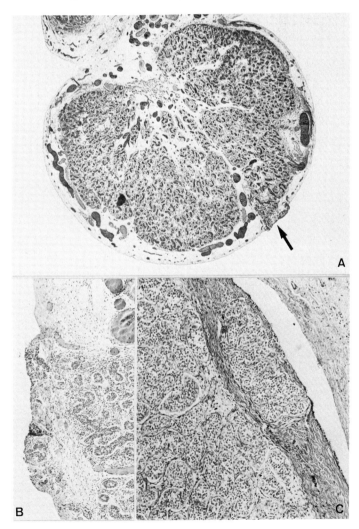

FIGURE 6–5. *Ectopic seminiferous tubules. A, Cross-sectioned testis of a newborn infant showing seminiferous tubules within the tunica albuginea. The tubules connect with the testicular parenchyma (arrow) (H&E, x10). B, Higher magnification of seminiferous tubules located in the tunica albuginea (H&E, x60). C, Group of seminiferous tubules located in a division of the tunica albuginea, in a 6-month-old infant (H&E, x60).*

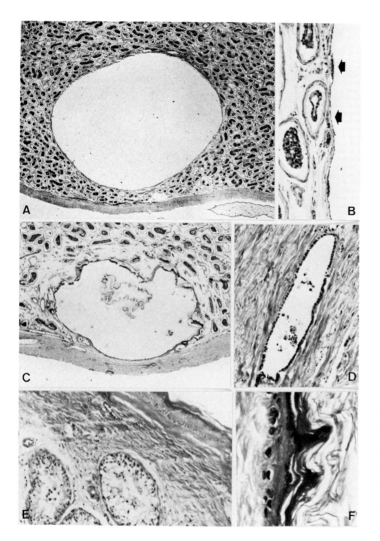

FIGURE 6–6. *A, Simple cyst of the testis (H & E, x25). B, Epithelial lining of the cyst, displaying zones with flattened cells alternating with others and with cuboidal cells (arrow) (H & E, x125). C, Simple cyst of the tunica albuginea (H & E, x40). D, Cystic formation within the tunica albuginea containing cellular debris and several spermatozoa (H & E, x125). E, Epidermoid cyst in the testis of a 12-year-old boy (H & E, x125). F, The epithelial lining of the epidermoid cyst is squamous stratified with abundant keratin layers (H & E, x250).*

monly observed in the fifth and sixth decades of life. By light microscopy, they are seen as isolated or multiple, uni- or multilocular, small and containing serous material (Rifkin and Jacobs, 1983). They are lined by a cuboidal or squamous epithelium that is stained with alcian-blue for acid mucopolysaccharides. The cysts are surrounded by a fibrous capsule, in the border of which atrophic seminiferous tubules or Leydig cell clusters can be found.

The simple cysts probably originate from mesothelial inclusions embedded in the testis during embryonic development. This hypothesis is maintained by most investigators and is supported by the high incidence of other urogenital system malformations, principally renal anomalies, such as renal dysplasia. It is possible that some of these cysts are histogenetically related to the cystic dysplasia of the testis, since they are a minimal morphological expression of dysplasia. In a testis studied by us, testicular dysplasia and tunica albuginea cysts were observed together (Nistal and Solas, 1977).

Epidermoid Cyst

Epidermoid cysts are keratin-filled cystic formations that are commonly found in the skin and, less frequently, in other locations. These cysts can appear in the testis as well as in the epididymis, although their frequency is low. Price (1969) found 69 in 5845 cases of testicular tumors studied in the Testicular Tumor Registry from the Armed Forces Institute of Pathology.

The diagnostic criteria are strict. The cyst wall is made up of three- or four-layered squamous epithelium that produces keratin. A connective tissue capsule surrounds the cyst and separates it from the tunica albuginea or the seminiferous tubules. The encapsulated cyst is easily removed. Neither scars nor teratoid elements are encountered in these cysts. Bilateral epidermoid cysts (Stahlberg and Brown, 1973) and cysts associated to Gardner's syndrome (Jalota and co-workers, 1974) have been described.

The diagnosis is usually made during the third and fourth decades of life, although most cysts develop in infancy and their size remains stable until puberty (Nistal and Santamaría, 1977).

With regard to its histogenesis, some investigators assume that the epidermoid cyst has a teratoid origin, which might be from the unilateral teratogenic development of an ectodermal structure. Others have suggested that the cyst develops from tunica vaginalis inclusions through a metaplastic process (Kihl and Magnusson, 1977) (Fig. 6–6E and F).

Congenital Testicular Lymphangiectasis

Congenital lymphangiectasis is responsible for different clinicopathological conditions. Patients with a generalized abnormal development of lymphatic vessels display body hemihypertrophy, malabsorption, and respiratory insufficiency. More frequently, only one organ is affected and this produces characteristic clinical symptoms that are related to the organ affected. Thus, a loss of albumin occurs in intestinal lymphangiectasis and respiratory distress in pulmonary lymphangiectasis (Nistal and co-authors, 1973).

Congenital testicular lymphangiectasis has been reported in a 7-year-old child with bilateral inguinal cryptorchidism. Lymphangiectasis was observed in both testes. The testicular size was slightly diminished and its consistency was spongy. By light microscopy, numerous irregularly dilated lymphatic ducts were observed in the tunica vasculosa and interlobular septa, as well as among the seminiferous tubules. Many of the ducts contained an eosinophilic, acellular material, whereas others appeared to be empty. The mean tubular diameter and the tubular fertility index were slightly diminished. Lymphangiectasis does not seem to be related to cryptorchidism. Rather it is more probable that the pressure caused by the dilated lymphatic vessels is responsible for the decrease in seminiferous tubule development (Nistal and Paniagua, 1977) (Fig. 6–7). A second case of testicular lymphangiectasis has been reported in a child with Noonan's syndrome (Nistal and others, 1984).

CONGENITAL ABNORMALITIES OF TUBULAR DEVELOPMENT

Both the testis and the epididymis are closely related with regard to their embryology, anatomy, and function. This interrelationship is the end product of the differentiation of two embryologically different structures: (1) the mesonephric duct that gives rise to both the ductuli efferentes and the ductus of the epididymis, and (2) the sex cords that differentiate into the seminiferous tubules, tubuli recti, and rete testis (see Chapter 1).

A constellation of morphological abnormalities in this tubular system have been observed in the study of testicular specimens obtained from autopsy, orchidectomy, and explorations to investigate male infertility. The abnormalities described in this and in the following chapters usually are not found in isolation, but are associated with other malformations

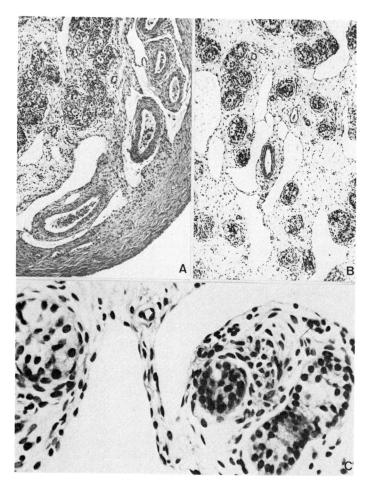

FIGURE 6–7. *Congenital testicular lymphangiectasis.* **A**, Dilated lymphatic vessels in the tunica vasculosa testis (H&E, x60). **B**, Cystic transformation of lymphatic vessels in the testicular interstitium. Some vessels surround seminiferous tubules (H&E, x60). **C**, Detail of the endothelium of a dilated lymphatic vessel (H&E, x250).

of the genitourinary system. Thus, the finding of one abnormality leads to the investigation of whether there are other associated conditions.

Testis

Deficiency in the Rete Testis and Ductuli Efferentes Connection

When an azoospermic male has spermatozoa in a testicular biopsy and the epididymography reveals that all tubular structures of the epididymis are completely filled with the contrast medium, it is probable that the rete testis and ductuli efferentes are not connected. Macroscopically, the patients have large, soft testes, which persist in that state for many years. They are probably caused by a lack of testicular fluid reabsorption by the epithelial cells lining the ductuli efferentes. Histologically, a cystic transformation of the rete testis is observed. Some zones of the rete testis protrude into the epididymis. Within the cysts there are spermatozoon accumulations and numerous macrophages.

The testicular parenchyma shows a moderate degree of atrophy. The seminiferous tubules appear somewhat dilated in some lobules, with reduced height of the seminiferous epithelium and a slightly thickened basement membrane. The testicular interstitium shows a marked edema.

The connection between the rete testis and the ductuli efferentes is probably more often incompletely than completely closed.

Adenomatous hyperplasia of the Rete Testis

The term "adenomatous hyperplasia of the rete testis" has been used to designate a testicular malformation consisting of an excessive development of tubular structures in the testicular mediastinum reported in a child, who had, in addition, bilateral renal dysplasia (Fig. 6–8). The tubular formations observed in the mediastinum showed a sinuous course, were lined by a low or tall columnar epithelium, and were connected to the ductuli efferentes by their distal segment and to the seminiferous tubules by their proximal segment. The testicular parenchyma occupied a peripheral crescent. The development of both seminiferous tubules and interstitium was in keeping with the age. The epididymis was normal (Nistal and others, 1976).

Cystic Dysplasia of the Testis

The pathological entity of cystic dysplasia of the testis is characterized by the presence of multiple cystic formations in the testicular mediastinum and the neighboring testicular parenchyma. They are separated by thin connective tissue septa and bordered by cuboidal epithelium (Fisher and co-workers, 1982; Leissring and Oppenheimer, 1973).

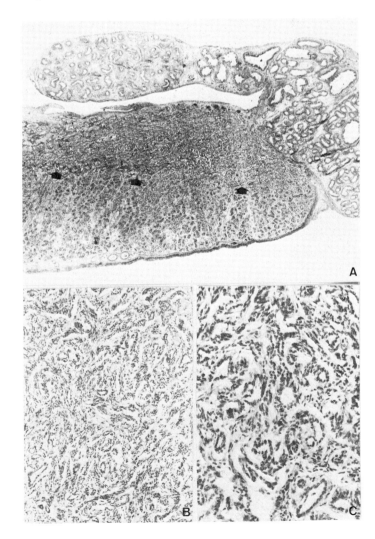

FIGURE 6–8. *Adenomatous hyperplasia of the rete testis. A, The surface occupied by the rete testis, in this logitudinally sectioned testis (arrows), is more than a third of the whole testicular surface (H&E, x20). B and C, Anastomosed tubular formations that form the hyperplastic rete testis (H&E, x2).*

Two forms of cystic dysplasia have been observed: diffuse and segmentary. The diffuse form was present in both testes of a child with Potter's syndrome. The testes were enlarged and located intra-abdominally. On section, they showed a spongy yellowish surface. Light microscopy examination revealed only sparse testicular parenchyma, located under the tunica albuginea (Fig. 6–9). The remaining testicular tissue was occupied by interconnected, thin-walled cystic formations. Peripheral cysts reached and extended into the tunica albuginea. Other cysts continued along the normal seminiferous tubules through short, funnel-shaped channels. Serial sections performed did not show continuity between cystic formations and ductuli efferentes. The epididymides were normal (Nistal and co-workers, in press).

The segmentary form of testicular cystic dysplasia has been observed in a surgical specimen obtained from an adult male with cancer of the penis (Fig. 6–10). Cross examination revealed an enlarged testis with a 1.5 cm diameter cyst in the anterior pole. On section, a wedge-shaped cystic formation extended from the rete testis to the tunica albuginea. The dilated rete testis formed multiple small cysts that protrude into the epididymis. Many of the cysts contained spermatozoa. The remaining testicular parenchyma showed moderate atrophy of the seminiferous tubule, although spermatogenesis was seen in some tubules.

Both the adenomatous hyperplasia of the rete testis and the cystic dysplasia of the testis might be considered as testicular parenchyma anomalies caused by a deficiency in the connection between the extratesticular spermatic ducts, derived from the mesonephric ducts, and the intratesticular spermatic ducts, developed from the sex cords. A permeable connection, which is also anomalous, would prevent the cystic transformation of the ad-

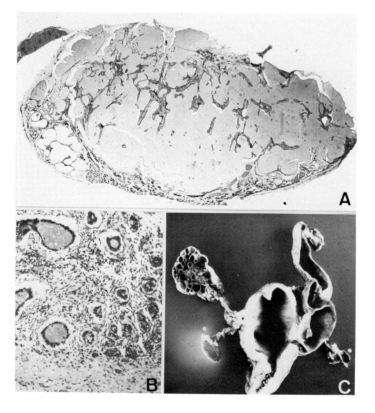

FIGURE 6–9. *Cystic dysplasia of the testis. A, Diffuse cystic transformation of the rete testis. The remaining testicular parenchyma forms a peripheral crescent (H&E, x10). B, Normal seminiferous tubules alternating with dilated tubules under the tunica albuginea (H&E, x125). C, Malformations of the urogenital system associated with the cystic dysplasia of the testis: renal dysplasia, megaloureters, megalobladder, and cryptorchidism. Cryptorchid testes are indicated by asterisks.*

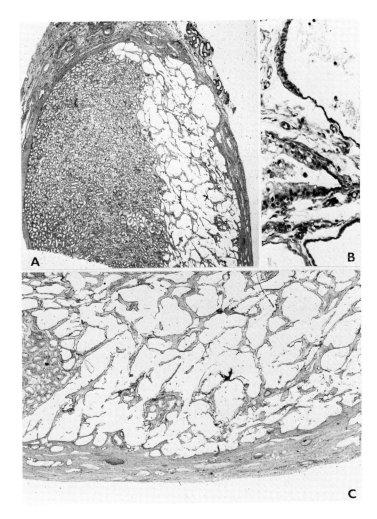

FIGURE 6–10. Segmental cystic dysplasia of the testis. A, Cystic transformation of several testicular lobules (H & E, x10). B, The epithelial lining of cystic formation is similar to that of the rete testis, with alternating zones of flattened and columnar cells (H&E, x125). C, Anomalous development of the tunica albuginea, which contains cystic formation associated with cystic dysplasia of the testis. Some of the albuginea cysts contain spermatozoa (H&E, x20).

enomatous rete testis hyperplasia. This etiology, failure in the connection of the mesonephric ducts and sex cord derivatives, is similar to that of renal dysplasia, caused by a lack of connection between mesonephric and metanephric derivatives. The reported cases of both diffuse rete testis hyperplasia and testicular cystic dysplasia were accompanied by renal dysplasia.

Epididymis

Congenital epididymal abnormalities occur during the first 6 weeks of embryonic life, since this is when the connections between the mesonephric ducts and the sex cords take place.

At the end of the second month of pregnancy, the undifferentiated gonad is transformed into a testis, the Müllerian ducts become atrophied, and the Wolffian ducts develop into the extratesticular spermatic duct system. The mesonephric ducts, in connection with the rete testis, give rise to the ductuli efferentes. Once the ductuli efferentes connects with the ductus of the epididymis, testicular descent occurs (see Chapter 1).

The anomalies in the implantation of the epididymis on the testis may be due to two different mechanisms: Either an excessive regression of the medial mesonephric ducts, or a defect in the connection between the mesonephric ducts and the genital ridge. In the latter, the inguinal ligament, which is developed in the inferior portion of the Wolffian duct, cannot be attached to the superior testicular pole, remaining attached to the epididymis. Later, the ligament attracts the epididymis toward the scrotum, whereas the testis remains undescended or in a high location.

Abnormalities in Epididymal Configuration

Anatomical variations of epididymal morphology are common in cryptorchid testes and less frequent in scrotal testes. The most frequent defects are as follows (Fig. 6–11).

Elongated epididymis. An elongated epididymis is the most common abnormality. The epididymis can be several times longer than the longest testicular axis. In some abdominal cryptorchid testes, the epididymis can extend as far as the external inguinal orifice (Fig. 6–12 D).

Free epididymis. The whole epididymis, or only a part of it, is not in continuity with the testis. Numerous variations have been found, the most common being the free cauda epididymis, and the most interesting being the epididymis lodged in the scrotal pouch while the testis remains in the abdomen. Therefore, if this malformation is found at exploration, the abdominal cavity must also be explored before a diagnosis of unilateral anorchism can be made.

Angulated epididymis. When angulation occurs, the angle is generally at the level of the corpus epididymis, which is usually thin.

Epididymis with mesorchium. There is a group of epididymides with a high insertion of the vaginalis. Thus, testis and epididymis appear suspended by a long mesorchium. This malformation occurs in 10 percent of patients with cryptorchidism, which would contribute toward explaining the high incidence of spermatic cord torsions in cryptorchidism.

The abnormalities in epididymal configuration may be associated with tubular development abnormalities.

Deficiency in the Ductuli Efferentes and Epididymal Duct Connection

The ductuli efferentes may end in a blind sac, and thus no continuity with the ductus of the epididymis is established (Fig. 6–12A and B). In the normal epididymis, using microdissection techniques, it has been shown that some of the 5 to 30 ductuli efferentes found in each epididymis are short with a blind end. When most of the ductuli efferentes are not connected with the epididymis, the epididymis remains separated from the testis, and the testicular parenchyma undergoes a slow, progressive atrophy (Mourot and others, 1975).

Anomalies effecting only one or two ductuli efferentes are more frequent than a complete failure in the ductuli efferentes and epididymal duct connection. This leads to the development of one or several cysts in the caput epididymis. In the adult, the cysts are designated under the term "spermatocele." They possess an inner epithelial lining similar to, but lower than, that of the ductuli efferentes and contain a clear fluid with numerous spermatozoa

ABNORMAL CONFIGURATION OF THE EPIDIDYMIS

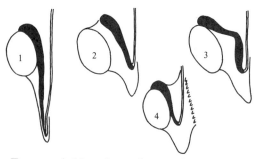

FIGURE 6–11. *Anomalies in the epididymal configuration. 1: elongated epididymis; 2: free epididymis; 3: angulated epididymis; and 4: epididymis with mesorchium.*

Congenital Anomalies of the Testis and the Epididymis

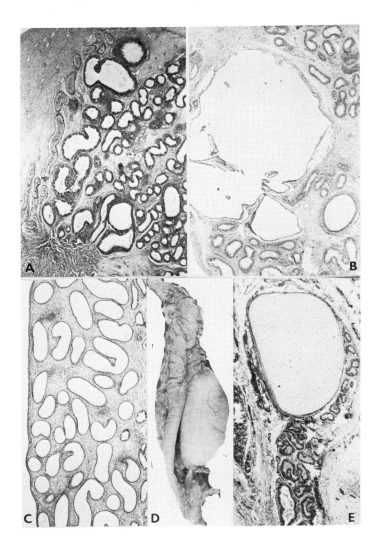

FIGURE 6–12. *A and B: Failure in the ductuli-efferentas-ductus of the epididymis connection. A, Dilated ductuli efferentes in an infant testis (H & E, x60). B, Simple cyst of the epididymis (H & E, x60). C, Dilation of the ductus of the epididymis because of cauda epididymis absence. D, Elongated epididymis. E, Cartilaginous choristoma of the epididymis (H & E, x60).*

(see Chapter 18). The cysts of infants and children, as well as those of the adult lacking spermatozoa, may be termed "simple cysts of the epididymis."

Absence of the Epididymis

The absence of the epididymis may be complete or segmentary, an isolated event or associated with anomalies of the ductus deferens (Amelar and Hotchkiss, 1963) (Fig. 6–13). The complete absence of the epididymis is a frequent anomaly in anorchism and monorchism. The region corresponding to the epididymis consists of loose connective tissue with abundant blood vessels and nerve fibers. The blind ductus deferens ends at this level. The absence of the epididymis has been reported in association with apparently normal testes in infants with cystic fibrosis (Landing and co-authors, 1969).

The absence of only one portion of the epididymis is more frequent. Absence of the corpus epididymis gives rise to a lobulated epididymis. All intermediate stages from simple strangling to complete separation between caput and cauda epididymis have been observed. The lack of both corpus and cauda, as well as the lack of only the cauda, are the most frequent anomalies. The association of these anomalies with the absence of ductus deferens is frequent (Fig. 6–12 C).

ABSENCE OF A SEGMENT OF EPIDIDYMIS
OR DUCTUS DEFERENS

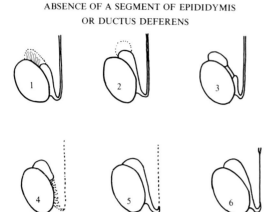

FIGURE 6–13. *Absence of an epididymal or ductus deferens segment. 1 and 2: anomalies in the caput epididymis; 3: absence of the corpus epididymis; 4: absence of ductus deferens, corpus, and cauda epididymis; 5: absence of the ductus deferens,; and 6: atresia of the ductus deferens.*

Hypoplasia of the Epididymis

The epididymis is an androgen-dependent structure, and, thus, its development is susceptible to involution in all those situations in which the testicular endocrine function is deficient. Rudimentary epididymides are observed in anorchism, most monorchism, hypogonadotropic hypogonadism, testicular dysgenesis, and some cryptorchidisms (Marshall and Shermeta, 1979).

The histological pattern varies between two extreme conditions: (1) a few convoluted ducts with dilated lumen and formed by a low columnar epithelium surrounded by poorly developed muscular layers; or (2) one or a few remains of small ducts with reduced lumen, lined by cuboidal epithelium, and lacking a muscular coat (Fig. 6–14A and B).

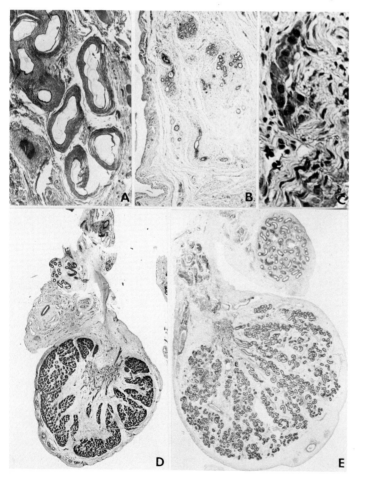

FIGURE 6–14. *Hypoplasia of the epididymis. A, Postpubertal epididymis. The ductus sections show dilation of the lumen and poor development of the muscular coat (H&E x10). B, Epididymis of newborn infant reduced to smaller tubular formations (H&E, x10). C, Anorchism. Leydig cells in the vicinity of a nerve in the spermatic cord (H&E, x250). D and E, Severe testicular hypoplasia in cryptorchid infants. D shows an increase in connective tissue (H&E, x8). E shows a decrease in the number of seminiferous tubules (H&E, x10).*

Hyperplasia of the Epididymis

Hyperplasia of the epididymis is observed in newborn infants with multiple malformations, primarily anencephaly. The epididymides are large, not only in comparison with the small testes of anencephalic newborns, but also with the normal epididymides. The cause of this anomaly is unknown (Fig. 6–15).

Absence of the Ductus Deferens

Morphological abnormalities of the ductus deferens may be either completely or segmentally absent. Complete absence is usually bilateral and has been found in 2 percent of males evaluated for infertility. It is generally associated with the lack of ejaculatory ducts, and, in many subjects, but not in all, to the lack of seminal vesicles. The ejaculate is scarse because of the absence of seminal vesicles, does not contain fructose, and does not coagulate immediately after ejaculation. In 60 percent of males with bilateral absence of ductus deferens high levels of sperm-agglutinating antibodies occur. This percentage is similar to that found in vasectomized males.

The absence of a ductus deferens segment is more frequent. The affected segment can be completely absent, hypoplastic, or replaced by a fibrous cord. The segment of the ductus deferens most commonly affected is the initial epididymal portion (Fig. 6–13).

Light microscopic examination reveals that the epididymides are enlarged in the absence of the ductus deferens, and the ductus of the epididymis as well as the ductuli efferentes appear dilated. The tubular system contains numerous spermatozoa, free or in the macrophage cytoplasm. On occasion, the rupture of some duct gives raise to spermatic granuloma (see Chapter 18).

ABNORMALITIES IN THE NUMBER, SIZE, AND LOCATION OF THE TESTES

Anorchism

Anorchism includes the absence of one (monorchism) or both (true anorchism) testes (Overzier and Linden, 1956). The incidence of unilateral anorchism is about 3.5 percent of males with cryptorchid testes, and one in 5000 males in the general population. The incidence of bilateral testicular absence is 1 in 20,000 males. Before the diagnosis can be made, the complete absence of testicular parenchyma must be verified. Exploration of the inguinal canal and the observation of a ductus deferens ending either in a blind sac or in a hypoplastic epididymis are not sufficient for a diagnosis of anorchism. It is also necessary to perform an intra-abdominal exploration, since the initial de-

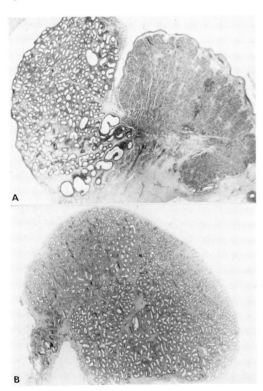

FIGURE 6–15. *Hyperplasia of the epididymis. A*, Longitudinal section of the testis and epididymis of a newborn infant showing a more developed epididymis than testis (H&E, x10). *B*, Caput epididymis of a newborn showing numerous sectioned ductuli efferentes (H&E, x20).

velopment of the testis and spermatic ducts begins separately, and a failure in the fusion of both tubular systems can determine epididymal and ductus deferens descent while the testis remains in a high position (Gracia and co-workers, 1973). Abdominal exploration and removal of testicular tissue can prevent the development of tumors in patients with undescended testes who were previously misdiagnosed as having anorchism (Brothers and others, 1978).

Testicular absence requires the presence of a male gonad developing a normal function during the fetal period in order to inhibit the Müllerian ducts and to develop the external male sex characteristics of the fetus. Anorchism is produced after the first 16 weeks of embryonic life. An earlier disappearance of the testis would give rise to clinical intersex conditions (Federman, 1967).

The causes of anorchism are varied and difficult to establish in each case. The most commonly stated causes are: (1) a not well-defined intrinsic gonadal disorder responsible for its precocious involution; (2) pre- or postnatal gonadal atrophy caused by infection, trauma, or torsion; and (3) prenatal gonadal atrophy induced by hormones, when either an increase in androgen production occurs during gestation (arrhenoblastoma) or hormones are administered during gestation (synthetic progestagens). Intrauterine testicular atrophy or absence of testis development has been observed associated with the clinical syndrome known as "cystic seminal vesicle with ipsilateral renal dysgenesis." (Das and Amar, 1980).

If the testes disappears between the 16th week and the seventh month, the spermatic cord components are retroperitoneal in location but not as yet in the inguinal canal. If there is an epididymis in the blind initial portion of the ductus deferens, located either in the inguinal canal or high in the scrotum, the testicular atrophy has probably been produced after the seventh month. This latter condition is known as "the vanishing testis syndrome" (Tosi and Morin, 1976).

The histological study of the ductus deferens epididymal portion in anorchism reveals that this portion is either hypoplastic (50 percent of cases) or absent (10 percent). The epididymis can also be hypoplastic (75 percent of cases) or absent (25 percent). An intensely collagenized tissue, with or without calcifications, which might correspond to a testis with regard to its shape, is observed in 20 percent of the cases. In 15 percent of cases, adrenal cortical tissue nodules occur, and 10 percent of cases have calcification of one or several blood vessel walls.

Hormonal assays performed in monorchism do not reveal abnormalities. Increased follicle-stimulating hormone and luteinizing hormone levels and decreased testosterone levels are usually found in true anorchism. In addition, a lack of testosterone response to human chorionic gonadotropin administration has been encountered (Aynsley-Greer and others, 1976).

In order to avoid repeated injections of depo-testosterone in adult patients with anorchism, transplantation of human testis by means of microsurgical techniques has been successfully carried out (Silber, 1978).

Leydig-cell-only syndrome is seen in a group of males with normal male phenotype and well-differentiated external genitalia, in whom a detailed surgical exploration fails to find testicular remnants. Serial sections of ductus deferens epididymal portions reveal Leydig cell clusters in these males with "agonadism without eunuchoidism" (Amelar, 1956). Testosterone levels measured in the spermatic veins are high enough for one to assume that they are produced by the Leydig cells (Fig. 6–14C). The testosterone secreted by these cells is sufficient to obtain a male phenotype differentiation, but insufficient to obtain a complete development of the male secondary sex characteristics in most cases.

True agonadism (46,XY gonadal agenesis syndrome), is a variety of male pseudohermaphroditism with gonadal agenesis associated with a 46,XY karyotype, and variable underdevelopment of the gonadal ducts and external genitalia. Most of the patients show female phenotype, and structures derived from the Müllerian duct or the Wolffian ducts are not seen. (Wu and others, 1976).

Polyorchism

Polyorchism is a rare anomaly consisting of three, four, or even five testes. Gross observations of more than three testes have not been histologically confirmed. Polyorchism is a possibility to be considered when a mass that does not correspond to spermatocele, Morgagni's hydatid cyst, testicular tumor, or aberrant epididymis is found during surgical exploration of the scrotum.

The first report of polyorchism was by Ashfeld in 1880 as an autopsy finding. Five years later, Lane (1895) reported the first histologically confirmed case. Since then, 37 cases have been reported; two-thirds of them show left side testicular duplication (Butz and Croushore, 1978). Spermatogenesis has been observed in eight cases.

The testicular anomaly may be due to either a duplication or a transverse division of the genital ridge (Fig. 6–16). With duplication the testis that is located medially is not connected to the mesonephric ducts, and rarely develops spermatogenesis. The transverse division of the genital ridge may occur at two different levels: (1) caudal to mesonephric ducts; the testis that remains unconnected to the excretory ducts reaches neither normal size nor adequate spermatogenesis; (2) at the level of the genital mesonephric ducts; the two resulting testes have a similar size and can have complete spermatogenesis (Nocks, 1978).

The epididymis may be single or double. The single epididymis originates at the

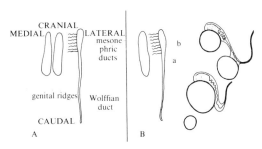

FIGURE 6–16. *Polyorchism. A, Longitudinal division of the genital ridge that determines the appearance of two testes. The medially located testis is not connected to the mesonephric ducts. B, Transverse division of the genital ridge at the level "a" determines that only one testis remains connected to the mesonephric ducts. Division at level "b" may result in two testes of similar size, both connected to the mesonephric ducts.*

inferior testis, extends to the superior one, and continues in one ductus deferens. With double epididymides, each testis possesses its own epididymis and ductus deferens. Both ducti deferentes, after a relatively long independent course, join to form a single duct. Atresia and hypoplasia of the ductus deferens are frequent in both cases (Wescott and Dykhuizen, 1967).

The maldescended testes in polyorchism can bear testicular tumors (Grechi and others, 1980; Scott, 1980) or torsion (Feldman and Droch, 1983).

Testicular Fusion

Testicular fusion is a rare anomaly. The fused testes may be lodged at midline, forming a single anatomical structure. Each testis or testicular lobule possesses its own epididymis and ductus deferens. Other malformations, such as adrenal gland fusion and horseshoe-shaped kidney, have been reported in males with testicular fusion.

Testicular Hypoplasia

Testicular hypoplasia is a term frequently used to designate small, soft testes, without reference to location or a determinate clinico-pathological syndrome. In all the cases, a genetic, histological, and hormonal study is required to determine the exact characteristics of the lesion, which can include positive or negative sex chromatin tubular dysgenesis, hypogonadotropic hypogonadism, testicular atrophy secondary to other etiologies, and rudimentary testis syndrome. The histological patterns of these lesions are described elsewhere.

Bilateral testicular hypoplasia is usually associated with external genital hypoplasia, which can be included in numerous malformation syndromes. In unilateral testicular hypoplasia, the testis can be so small that it becomes a histological discovery encountered during the study of the epididymal end of the spermatic cord, removed in a surgical intervention for cryptorchidism. The histological pattern is nonspecific. Decrease in the number of testicular lobules, increase in the amount of inter- and intralobular connective tissue, and decrease in the mean tubular diameter and tubular fertility index are the most frequent findings (Fig. 6–14 **D** and **E**).

Bilateral testicular hypoplasia may evolve toward a complete testicular parenchymal atrophy, giving rise to the "vanishing testis syndrome." We examined three children with bilateral cryptorchidism, on whom orchiopexy had been performed without difficulties 1 to 3 years before, those testes could not be palpated. Orchidectomy specimens showed small groups of seminiferous tubules in only one of these children.

Most testicular hypoplasias are associated to hypoplastic epididymides.

Testicular Hyperplasia

Bilateral testicular hyperplasia (macro-orchidism) may appear isolated (Breen and others, 1981; Nisula, 1974; Padrón and co-workers, 1979), associated with X chromosome linked mental retardation (Cantu and co-workers, 1978; Hecht and others, 1981; Howard Peebles and Stoddard, 1980; Ruvalcaba and others, 1977; Sutherland and Ashford, 1979; Turner and co-authors, 1980) or obesity. The diagnosis of testicular hyperplasia may only be made when the following syndromes have been eliminated: precocious puberty, juvenile hypothyrodism, congenital adrenal hyperplasia, and bilateral testicular tumors.

The histological study reveals an apparent increase in the number of seminiferous tubules with slight hypospermatogenesis. The mean tubular diameter is normal. The Sertoli cells usually show retraction of apical cytoplasm, and the spermatogonia exhibit cytoplasmic vacuolation.

FSH, LH and testosterone levels are normal. The cause of macro-orchidism remains unknown.

Unilateral testicular hyperplasia is frequent in the contralateral testis of pubertal males with unilateral cryptorchidism. This hypertrophy is due to a compensatory effect.

Unilateral testicular hypertrophy in pubertal boys without cryptorchidism also exists. This has been considered as the morphological expression of a peculiar hormonal receptivity by the testicular parenchyma (Lee and co-workers, 1982).

Ectopic Testis

A testis is considered to be ectopic if it occupies a location outside its normal path of descent. The incidence is estimated at about 20 percent of all undescended testes. Contrasting with the cryptorchid testis, the ectopic testis is accompanied by a spermatic cord of normal, or even longer than normal, length. Macroscopically, this testis has a normal size, as does the scrotum, contrasting with the sparsely developed scrotum of most cryptorchid testes (Campbell, 1970). Histological studies are rare and the results are not in agreement. Whether or not these testes bear lesions other than those due to their location requires further histological study.

The different kinds of ectopic testis, mentioned in order of frequency, are interstitial, femoral, perineal, transverse, pubic-penile, and pelvic (Fig. 6-17).

Interstitial or Superficial Inguinal

The testis, after descent through the external inguinal orifice, ascends to the anterosuperior iliac crest and locates on the aponeurosis of the major oblique muscle.

Femoral or Crural

The testis is lodged in Scarpa's triangle, after passing through the inguinal canal.

Perineal

The testis finds a subcutaneous location between the scrotum and the anus, on one or the other side. Because of its location, the testis is highly susceptible to trauma in cyclists and horsemen (Páramo and co-workers, 1971).

Transverse or Crossed Testicular Ectopia

Both testes descend through the same inguinal canal and become lodged within the same scrotal pouch. Each testis possesses its own vascular supply, epididymis, and ductus deferens. Hernia is a frequent finding in this testicular ectopia (Rao and Kaper, 1980).

Pubic-penile

The ectopic testis is in the dorsal region of penis, near the base or on the pubic symphysis (Middleton and others, 1976).

Pelvic

The testis is located deep in the pelvis, frequently in the Douglas cul-de-sac.

The mechanisms leading to testicular ectopia are not yet well-known. The following hypotheses have been put forth.

1. Multiple insertions of the gubernaculum testis (Lockwood, 1887). Six insertions of the gubernaculum testis are formed: into the scrotum, perineum, external oblique aponeurosis, base of the penis, pubis, and Scarpa's triangle. The predominating normal scrotal insertion is not effective in these cases and the testis slides along other insertions.
2. Failure in the gubernaculum contraction. Sonneland (1924), did not find either an embryological or anatomical basis to support the aforementioned hypothesis and proposed another explanation. Once the testis has descended through the inguinal canal, the gubernaculum testis contraction introduces it into the scrotum. In the ectopic testes, the gubernaculum would be fragmented and its fibers would be inefficient. However, many

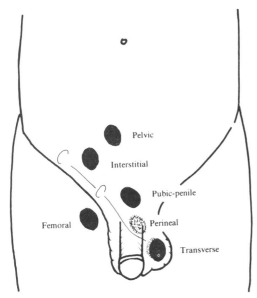

FIGURE 6-17. *Ectopic testes. Different locations adopted by the ectopic testis. Modified from Middleton et al.*[30]

investigators find no histological basis to support this hypothesis.
3. The third inguinal ring (McGregor, 1929). In this hypothesis it is assumed that there is a tightening of the scrotal neck. This stenosis would be responsible for testicular ectopia and would be caused by perineal or scrotal duplication of Colles' fascia.

Today, the three hypotheses: intrabdominal pressure, failure in the gubernaculum, and stenosis of the scrotal neck are in current favor.

The incidence of testicular torsion is higher in ectopic than in scrotal testes.

Cryptorchidism. See Chapter 9.

REFERENCES

1. Altaffer LF, Steele SM: Torsion of testicular appendages in men. J Urol 124:56, 1980
2. Amelar RD: Anorchism without eunuchoidism. J Urol 76:174, 1956
3. Amelar RD, Hotchkiss RS: Congenital aplasia of the epididymis and vasa deferentia: Effects on semen. Fertil Steril 14:44, 1963
4. Ashfeld F: Die Nissbildungen des Menschen. Grunow, Leipzig, 1880
5. Aynsley-Greer A, Zachmann M, Illig R, Rampini S, Prader A: Congenital bilateral anorchia in childhood: A clinical, endocrine and therapeutic evaluation of twenty-one cases. Clin Endocrinol 5:381, 1976
6. Breen DH, Braunstein GD, Neufeld N, Kudish H: Benign macro-orchidism in a pubescent boy. J Urol 125:589, 1981
7. Brothers LR, Weber CH, Ball TP: Anorchismus versus cryptorchidism; the importance of a diligent search for intra-abdominal testes. J Urol 119:707, 1978
8. Butz RE, Croushore JH: Polyorchism. J Urol 119:289, 1978
9. Campbell MF: Anomalies of the testicle. In Campbell MF, Harrison JH (eds); Urology, 3th ed. Philadelphia: W.B. Saunders, 1970, p. 1632
10. Cantu JM, Scaglia HE, González-Diddi M, Hernández-Jauregui P, Morato T, Moreno ME, Giner J, Alcantar A, Herrera D, Pérez-Palacios, G: Inherited congenital normofunctional testicular hyperplasia and mental deficiency. Hum Genet 41:331, 1978
11. Dahl EV, Bahn RC: Aberrant adrenal cortical tissue near the testis in human infants. Am J Pathol 40:587, 1962
12. Das S, Amar AD: Ureteral ectopia into cystic seminal vesicle with ipsilateral renal dysgenesis and monorchia. J Urol 124:574, 1980
13. Federman DD: Abnormal sexual development: A genetic and endocrine approach to differential diagnosis. Philadelphia: W.B. Saunders, 1967, p. 87
14. Feldman S, Drach GW: Polyorchidism discovered as testicular torsion. J Urol 130:976, 1983
15. Fisher JE, Jewett TC, Nelson SJ, Jockin H: Ectasia of the rete testis with ipsilateral renal agenesis. J Urol 128:1040–1043, 1982
16. Gracia R, Nistal M, Jara P, Lledó G, Jover J: Dos casos de síndrome de Hanhart. Uno de ellos con anorquia. An Esp Pediatr 6:333, 1973
17. Grechi G, Zampi GC, Selli C, Carini M, Ucci M: Polyorchidism and seminoma in a child. J Urol 123:291, 1980
18. Hecht JT, Moore CM, Scott CI: A recognizable syndrome of sex-liked mental retardation, large testes, and marker X chromosome. South Med J. 74:1493, 1981
19. Hervonen A, Vaalasti A, Vaalasti T, Partanen M, Kanerva L: Paraganglia in the urogenital tract of man. Histochemistry 48:307, 1976
20. Howard-Peebles PN, Stoddard GR: Familial X-linked mental retardation with a marker X chromosome and its relationship to macro-orchidism. Clin Genot 17:125, 1980
21. Jalota R, Middleton RG, McDivitt RW: Epidermoid cyst of the testis in Gardner's syndrome. Cancer 34:464, 1974
22. Johnson RE, Scheitauer B: Massive hyperplasia of testicular adrenal rests in a patient with Nelson's syndrome. Am J Clin Pathol 77:501, 1982
23. Kihl B, Magnusson PH: Epidermoid cyst of the testis. Scand J Urol Nephrol 11:73, 1977
24. Landing BH, Wells TR, Wang CI: Abnormality of the epididymis and vas deferens in cystic fibrosis. Arch Pathol 88:569, 1969
25. Lane WA: A case of supernumerary testis. Trans Clin Soc Lond 28:59, 1895
26. Lee PA, Marshall FF, Greco JM, Jeffs RD: Unilateral testicular hypertrophy: An apparently benign occurrence without cryptorchidism. J Urol 127:329, 1982
27. Leissring JC, Oppenheimer ROF: Cystic dysplasia of the testis: A unique congenital anom-

aly studied by microdissection. J Urol 110:362, 1973
28. Lockwood CB: Development and transition of testicles normal and abnormal. Br Med J 1:444, 1887
29. Mares AJ, Shkolnick A, Sacks M, Fleuchtwanger M: Aberrant (ectopic) adrenocortical tissue along the spermatic cord. J Pediatr Surg 15:289, 1980
30. Marshall FF, Shermeta DW: Epididymal abnormalities associated with undescended testis. J Urol 121:341, 1979
31. McGregor AL: The third inguinal ring. Surg Gynecol Obst 49:273, 1929
32. Middleton GW, Beamon CR, Gillenwater JY: Two rare cases of ectopic testes. J Urol 115:445, 1976
33. Mourot M, Aubert D, Sava P, Gille P: L'independence épididymo-testiculaire totale: A propos de deux observations. Ann Chir 16:189, 1975
34. Nistal M, Belaustegui A, Quero J, Garcia-Sánchez P, Pérez-Martínez V: Las linfangiectasias pulmonares congénitas como causa de distress respiratorio letal en el recién nacido. Med Clin (Barc) 61:616, 1973
35. Nistal M, Paniagua R, Bravo MP: Testicular lymphangiectasis in Noonan's syndrome. J Urol 131:759, 1984.
36. Nistal M, García-Villanueva M, Sánchez J: Displasia quística del testículo. Anomalía en la diferenciación del parénquima testicular por probable fallo de la conexión entre los conductos de origen mesonéfrico y los cordones testiculares. Arch Esp Urol 29:431, 1976
37. Nistal M: Paraganglios del epidídimo humano. An Anat [suppl] 25:307, 1977
38. Nistal M, Paniagua R: Congenital testicular lymphangiectasis. Virchows Arch [Pathol Anat] 377:79, 1977
39. Nistal M, Solas IM: Quistes testiculares. Quiste simple del testículo y quiste de la albugínea. Arch Esp Urol 30:53, 1977
40. Nistal M, Santamaría L: Quiste epidermoide del testículo. Arch Esp Urol 30:131, 1977
41. Nistal M, Regadera J, Paniagua R: Cystic dysplasia of the testis: Light and electron microscope study of three cases. Arch Pathol Lab Med. (In press)
42. Nisula BC, Coriaux DL, Sherins RJ, Kulin HE: Benign bilateral testicular enlargement. J Clin Endocrinol Metab 38:440, 1974
43. Nocks BN: Polyorchidism with normal spermatogenesis and equal sized testes: A theory of embryological development. J Urol 120:638, 1978
44. Overzier C, Linden H: Echter agonadismus (anorchismus) bei Geschwistern. Gynecol Invest 142:215, 1956
45. Padrón RS, Hung S, Licea M, Pérez-Plaza M, Arce B: Bilateral macro-orchidism in otherwise normal men. Int J Androl 2:1, 1979
46. Páramo PG, Nacarino L, Polo G: Ectopia didimoperineal. Arch Esp Urol 24:61, 1971
47. Pommer G: Verwachsung des linken Kryptorchischen Hodens und Nebenhodens mit der Milz in einer Missgeburt mit Zahlreichen Bildungsdefecten. Ber Naturw Med Ver Innsbruck 17:144, 1887
48. Price EB: Epidermoid cyst of the testis: A clinical and pathological analysis of 69 cases from the testicular tumor registry. J Urol 102:708, 1969
49. Putschar WGJ, Manion WC: Splenic-gonadal fusion. Am J Pathol 32:15, 1976
50. Quinn-Hill M: Ectopic splenic tissue in the gonad: A case report. Can J Surg 12:457, 1969
51. Rao BK, Kapur MM: Transverse testicular ectopia: A case report. J Urol 124:149, 1980
52. Rifkin M, Jacobs JA: Simple testicular cyst diagnosed preoperatively by ultrasound. J. Urol 129:982, 1983
53. Ruvalcaba RH, Myhre SA, Roosen-Runge EC, Beckwith JB: X-linked mental deficiency megalotestes syndrome. JAMA 238:1646, 1977
54. Scott KW: A case of polyorchidism with testicular teratoma. J Urol 124:930, 1980
55. Silber SJ: Transplantation of a human testis for anorchia. Fertil Steril 30:181, 1978
56. Skoglund RW, McRoberts JW, Radge H: Torsion of testicular appendages: Presentation of 43 new cases and a collective review. J Urol 104:598, 1970
57. Sonneland SE: Congenital perineal testicle. Ann Surg 80:176, 1924
58. Strahlberg M, Brown JS: Concomitant bilateral epidermoid cysts of the testes. J Urol 109:434, 1973
59. Sutherland GR, Ashforth PL: X-linked mental retardation with macroorchidism and the fragile site at X_q27 or 28. Hum Genet 48:117, 1979
60. Tosi SE, Morin LS: The vanishing testis syndrome: Indications for conservative therapy. J Urol 115:758, 1976
61. Turner G, Daniel A, Frost M: X-linked mental retardation, macro-orchidism, and the X_q27 fragile site. J Pediatr 96:837, 1980
62. Wescott J, Dykhuizen RF: Polyorchism. J Urol 98:497, 1967
63. Wu RH, Boyar RM, Knight R, Hellman L, Finkelstein JW: Endocrine studies in a phenotypic girl and XY gonadal agenesis. J Clin Endocrinol Metab 43:506, 1976

7

TESTICULAR BIOPSY. BASIC TESTICULAR LESIONS

Testicular Biopsy

The systematic practice of a biopsy as a precise method for evaluating testicular function in infertile patients was first introduced by Charny (1940) and Hotchkiss (1942). Nowadays, the widespread application of this diagnostic technique may be mainly attributed to the great importance that male infertility has attained. Nevertheless, this diagnostic practice has become indispensable in other clinical areas, such as in the determination of intersex stages, the precise evaluation of cryptorchid testes, or the classification of hypogonadism. In all these cases, the testicular biopsy, aside from its diagnostic value, provides the basis for the selection of adequate therapeutic measures.

Gonadal biopsies performed on intersex stages help to determine the exact nature of the gonads—ovary, ovotestis, or gonadal dysgenesis—and to evaluate the degree of gonadal development and fertility.

In patients with cryptorchidism, the testicular biopsy supplies the most appropriate information relative to testicular abnormality and permit the physician to make a prognosis with respect to testicular function. A testicular biopsy during the first years of life has revealed the congenital nature of a great number of lesions that in the past were attributed exclusively to the noxious effect of temperature. Although the cryptorchidism may be unilateral, testicular biopsy of both testes is advisable, because it is well-known that the contralateral scrotal testis may bear congenital abnormalities.

In 40 percent of infertile couples, the infertility is caused by the man. A bilateral testicular biopsy is advisable in all patients with azoospermia or severe oligospermia without excessively increased FSH values. In some cases, decreases in spermatozoon number have been reported following biopsy, but the oligospermia is transitory and, after a few weeks, the spermatozoon number returns to prebiopsy levels. In addition, testicular biopsy provides information that is useful in investigating the cause of the infertility from other than the purely histological point of view. It is useful in cytogenetic studies, which have led to the understanding of other structural alterations besides chromosomal anomalies, such as defective chiasma formation.

Testicular biopsy is also recommendable in other pathological conditions, for which it can provide sufficient information to obtain a precise diagnosis. This is the case in periarteritis nodosa; studies carried out on this disease indicate that two-thirds of the patients have characteristic lesions in the branches of the testicular artery.

Testicular Biopsy Techniques

Obtaining testicular specimens for microscopic study can be accomplished by several procedures. Simple puncture (Posner and Cohn) is a technique by which a sufficient sample to ascertain spermatozoon presence is obtained. With puncture-aspiration, (Obrant and Persson, 1965) all testicular cell types are obtained. This provides material for the diagnosis of several processes and is as useful as the histological sections (Persson and co-authors, 1971). Flow cytometric DNA measurements permit the performance of quantitative studies on spermatogenesis (Clausen and others, 1978). For a needle biopsy (Hendricks and co-workers, 1969; Palmer,

1944), cylinders of testicular parenchyma with satisfactory preservation of testicular architecture are obtained.

Testicular biopsy by surgical procedure is by far the most common method. According to Rowley and Heller (1956), the testes are approached through one incision along the center of the interscrotal septum. The tunica vaginalis is separated from the testis and incised to expose the testis. The least vascularized area of the tunica albuginea is then chosen for the biopsy. With a scalpel, an incision no longer than 0.5 cm is made through the albuginea. Enough testicular parenchyma protrudes to be removed with a slicing motion of the scalpel. A three-cornered section including the albuginea is advisable for a better preservation of the testicular tissue. Both a qualitative and a quantitative study can be carried out when the testicular architecture is preserved. The presence of albuginea is necessary in order to establish a diagnosis in most intersex stages and is required for the adequate evaluation of the Leydig cells, which are more abundant beneath the albuginea.

If only light microscopy is to be done, testicular specimens may be fixed with formalin solution (testes of infants or children) or with Bouin's, Helly's or Steve's fixatives (postpubertal testes). For adult testes, the use of formalin is not recommended, since it causes loss of mature spermatids as well as nuclear hyperchromatism and the swelling of Leydig cells. Fixation with Zenker's fixative is also to be avoided inasmuch as it is responsible for an erroneous picture of seminiferous epithelium cell sloughing.

It is advisable that testicular biopsies fixed with Bouin's fluid be washed several times with a 50 percent alcohol solution in order to eliminate the excess of picric acid. Sections are usually stained with hematoxylin and eosin (H & E), periodic acid-Schiff and Masson trichrome techniques. Besides these techniques, the van Gieson method or orcein for elastic tissue must be used in biopsies of postpubertal testes. In some special cases, the Laidlaw technique and methods for amyloid demonstration must be utilized.

For electron microscopy, testicular specimens are fixed in a 4 percent glutaraldehyde solution. If meiotic studies are to be carried out, the unfixed testicular tissue may be processed according to the Evans and others (1964) method and its variants. (Hsu and others, 1979) If histochemistry or immunofluorescence techniques are desired, the recently removed specimens must be frozen in liquid nitrogen.

Complications of testicular biopsy are rare. In only 2 percent of cases, scrotal pain or hematomas have been reported. Usually, the hematomas do not require any treatment. In some cases, synechia of the tunica vaginalis are formed, but they heal without causing any symptoms.

PREPUBERTAL TESTIS

Prepubertal and adult testicular lesions are considered separately. The reactive capacity of a prepubertal testis is expressed in a rather restricted way compared with that of the adult testis. Following are the most interesting connections between prepubertal lesions and those found in the adult, and special reference is made to the development of these lesions.

Tubular Alterations

Tubular alterations occur from (1) a decrease in the tubular diameter, (2) a decrease in the tubular fertility index (TFI), and (3) changes in Sertoli cell number.

Decrease in Tubular Diameter

Mean tubular diameter (MTD) may be evaluated by calculating the mean value of transverse tubular section measurements. For a correct evaluation of each testis in relation to this parameter, the mean value obtained must be compared with the corresponding values for each age.

A decrease in tubular diameter is the most common alteration observed in prepubertal testes, and it occurs in scrotal testes as well as undescended testes. In the latter it is the most frequent lesion. According to the MTD, different degrees of tubular hypoplasia can be distinguished.

In slight tubular hypoplasia testes the seminiferous tubules have only a slightly reduced diameter (up to 10 percent reduction). In marked tubular hypoplasia seminiferous tubules have a 10 to 30 percent MTD decrease. In severe tubular hypoplasia seminiferous tubules have greater than 30 percent MTD decrease. The decrease in MTD may be the expression of either tubular dysgenesis or hypogonadotropic hypogonadism (Fig. 7–1A).

Decrease in Tubular Fertility Index

TFI indicates the percentage of seminiferous tubules containing germ cells (Mack and co-workers, 1961). This index varies during infancy; the variations are, in many cases, parallel to those of the MTD (Fig. 7–1B and C). The different

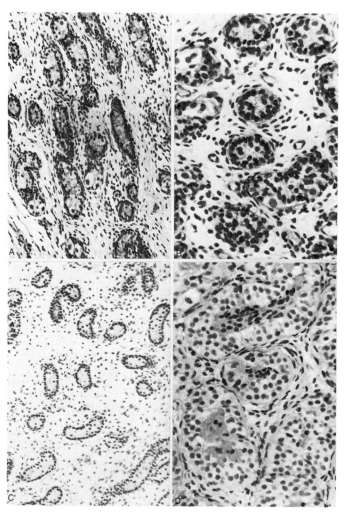

FIGURE 7–1. *A, Seminiferous tubules in a 4-year-old infant, affected by a granulomatous hypothalamic lesion, showing marked tubular hypoplasia and adequate preservation of the tubular fertility index (H&E, x125). B, Seminiferous tubules showing slight tubular hypoplasia and marked germinal hypoplasia, in a 3-year-old infant with inguinal cryptorchidism (H&E, x250). C, Testicular parenchyma with severe tubular hypoplasia associated with reduced TFI in a 6-year-old child with inguinal cryptorchidism (H&E, x125). D, Immature Sertoli cell hyperplasia in a 2-year-old infant with intraabdominal cyrptorchidism (H&E, x250).*

degrees of TFI decrease or germinal hypoplasia are the following: (1) slight germinal hypoplasia, TFI above 50 percent; (2) marked germinal hypoplasia, TFI between 30 and 50 percent; (3) severe germinal hypoplasia, TFI below 30 percent. Marked and severe germinal hypoplasias are frequently associated with a decrease in MTD, and they usually represent tubular dysgenesis.

Variations in Sertoli Cell Index

The number of Sertoli cells per transverse tubular section, or Sertoli cell index (SCI), progressively decreases from birth (24 $\pm$2) to adulthood (10 $\pm$1) (Hadziselimovic and Seguchi, 1974; Nistal and others, 1982a). According to this SCI, a distinction must be made between diffuse Sertoli cell hypoplasia (testes with seminiferous tubules in which the SCI is less than two-thirds of that corresponding to their age) and diffuse Sertoli cell hyperplasia (testes with seminiferous tubules in which the SCI is higher than one-third of that corresponding to their age). Both alterations of the SCI are an expression of tubular dysgenesis, whether isolated, a characteristic of Klinefelter's syndrome (Nistal and others, 1982b) or cryptorchidism, or in different intersex syndromes (Fig. 7–1C and D).

Tubular Malformations: Megatubules, Ring-Shaped Tubules, Calcospherites

The most frequent tubular malformations are megatubules. These very large tubules contain immature Sertoli cells. Ring-shaped tubules are a variant of megatubules in which the Sertoli cells are disposed in such a way that they form two concentric layers; the inner layer usually surrounds an eosinophilic acellular material, similar to that forming the basement membrane. Both megatubules and ring-shaped tubules can contain laminated, eosinophilic, silver-stained, Feulgen positive structures, called calcospherites. These can undergo calcification, as occurs in testicular microlithiasis (Fig. 7–2A and B).

Association of Different Patterns of Tubular Alterations

Different diffuse testicular alterations tend to be related to each other. Four basic association patterns are most frequently found. Most prepubertal testes undergoing tubular alteration can be classified in one of these four groups. Terminology refers to the most characteristic lesion.

Type I: Testes with Minimal Alterations. The TFI is normal or similar to that corresponding to slight germinal hypoplasia. The MTD is normal or similar to that in slight tubular hypoplasia. The SCI is normal.

Type II: Testes with Marked Germinal Hypoplasia. The TFI corresponds to that of marked germinal hypoplasia. The MTD is similar to that of slight tubular hypoplasia. The SCI is normal.

Type III: Testes with Diffuse Tubular Hypoplasia. The TFI reflects severe germinal hypoplasia. The MTD indicates severe tubular hypoplasia. The SCI reflects diffuse Sertoli cell hypoplasia.

Type IV: Testes with Diffuse Sertoli Cell Hyperplasia. The TFI is variable, often similar to that of either severe or marked germinal hypoplasia. The MTD is also variable and indicates slight marked, or severe tubular hypoplasia. The SCI reflects diffuse Sertoli cell hyperplasia (Nistal and co-workers, 1980).

Leydig Cell Alterations

Leydig cells undergo regression just after birth. However, fetal Leydig cells have also been observed in the testes of 2-year-old infants. The alterations most often found in these cells are the following.

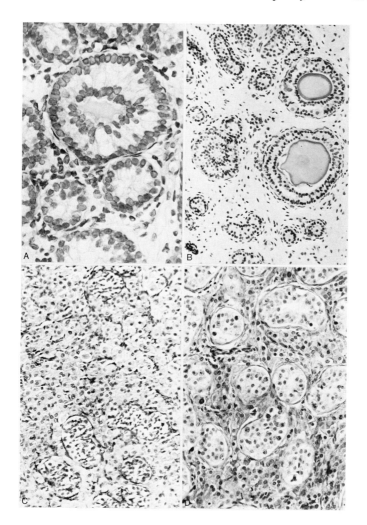

FIGURE 7–2. *A*, Ring-shaped tubules in a cryptorchid testis of a 4-year-old boy (H&E, x250). *B*, Megatubules containing concentric laminated concretions in the testis of a 7-year-old boy (H&E, x250). *C*, Congenital Leydig cell hyperplasia in a newborn with Beckwith-Wiedemann syndrome (H&E, x60). *D*, Acquired Leydig cell hyperplasia in an 8-year-old child showing a choriocarcinoma in the contralateral testis (H&E, x200).

Variations in Newborn Leydig Cell Physiological Involution

A rapid Leydig cell involution often occurs in cryptorchid testes (Hayaski and Harrison, 1971). A delay in Leydig cell physiological involution can be observed in the undescended testes of some male pseudohermaphrodites. Whether or not the higher temperature affecting these cells is responsible for their delayed involution is uncertain.

Leydig Cell Hyperplasia

Diffuse fetal Leydig cell hyperplasia in the testes of infants with complex malformations, such as leprechaunism, is a rather common finding. This feature is generally found in relation to enlarged external genitalia. Adenomatous Leydig cell hyperplasia seems to represent a hyperfunctional stage. These cells may show hyperplasia as well as hypertrophy. This condition can be observed associated with adrenal cytomegaly, either isolated or included in Beckwith-Wiedermann syndrome (Nistal and Ríos, 1973), or in triploid liveborn fetuses (Doshi and others, 1983) (Fig. 7–2C).

A diffuse Leydig cell hyperplasia, with or without association with tubular maturation, is present in some patients with pseudo-precocious puberty with familial presentation (Schedewie and others,

1981) and in testicular tumors with a choriocarcinoma component (Fig. 7-2**D**). Hyperplasia of immature Leydig cells is sometimes found in cryptorchid testes. This histological pattern is difficult to evaluate, since testicular biopsy is very often performed some time after initiating hormonal treatment.

Leydig Cell Absence

The absence of Leydig cells in infants is difficult to evaluate. The absence of these cells after puberty causes eunuchoidism or male pseudohermaphroditism.

Precocious Testicular Maturation

Two variants of precocious testicular maturation are known: tubular and tubulointerstitial.

Tubular Maturation

Tubular maturation is characterized by the precocious maturation of seminiferous tubules while the interstitium remains immature. Diffuse tubular maturation is observed in some children with hypothyroidism; focal tubular maturation is present in androgen-producing Leydig cell tumors in the seminiferous tubules near the tumor cells (Chemes and others, 1982).

Tubulointerstitial Maturation

Maturation occurs in the seminiferous tubules as well as in the interstitium. The cause and pathogenesis of this precocious testicular development are studied in Chapter 8.

Testicular Atrophy

During infancy, testicular atrophy is synonymous with tubular atrophy, which later leads to hyalinization and tubular sclerosis. Testicular atrophy is an infrequent lesion that can affect the testis in different ways.

Diffuse atrophy is observed in patients with destructive lesions of the anterior hypothalamus or hypothalamic-hypophyseal lesions, such as brain malformations, microcephaly, hydrocephaly hemorrhages, histiocytosis X. The seminiferous tubules decrease in diameter until they are reduced to epithelial cords surrounded by a thickened basement membrane.

Peripheral atrophy is probably secondary to vascular disease. Tubular atrophy is greater at the periphery of the lobules, beneath the tunica albuginea, and later affects deeper zones (Fig. 7-3**A**).

Lobular atrophy is a group or groups of fully sclerosed seminiferous tubules that probably belong to the same lobule. Lobular atrophy is observed in children with Klinefelter's syndrome and cryptorchidism, who were treated with gonadotropins before the diagnosis of Klinefelter's syndrome was established (Fig. 7-3**B**).

ADULT TESTIS

For the precise evaluation of the variety of lesions observed in adult testes, the quantitative methods described by Roosen-Runge (1956) Clermont (1963), Steinberger and Tjioe (1968), and Van Dop et al (1980), recommended mainly for investigation, may be useful for diagnostic purposes. The evaluation of a sole parameter, germ cell development, may be carried out by the methods of Johnsen (1970), Skakkebaek and Heller (1973), and De Kretser et al (1974). According to Nelson (1953), an evaluation of the seminiferous tubules, sufficient for routine diagnosis, may be carried out by evaluating the MTD, the thickness of the tunica propria, and the development of the seminiferous epithelium and interstitial tissue. Determinations of hormone levels in serum are as important as the histological study in order to arrive at an adequate

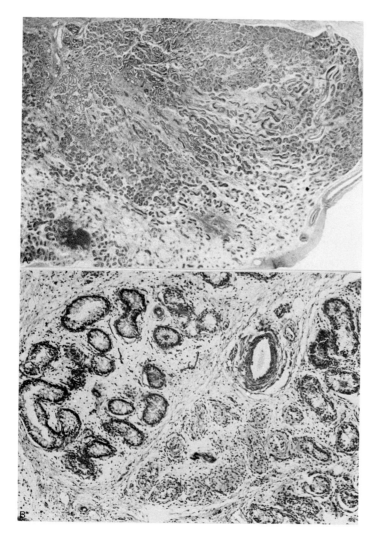

FIGURE 7–3. *Tubular atrophy.* A, Tubular atrophy, more severe beneath the tunica albuginea, in a 9-year-old child with bilateral cryptorchidism (H&E, x10). B, Seminiferous tubules showing tubular hyalinization. The seminiferous epithelium is absent. Child with Klinefelter's syndrome treated with gonadotropins (H&E, x60).

determination of the types of abnormalities (Yoshida and others, 1982).

In the following paragraphs we analyze separately the pathologic state that is most frequently observed in each of the testicular components. However, we must consider that such alterations are usually not isolated but are in relation to each other.

Tubular Development Failure

The examination of tubular diameter is in itself a good index of tubular development. The growth and maturation of the seminiferous tubules in an adult male may have been arrested during infancy or puberty. Two types—diffuse and focal—of tubular hypoplasia can be observed in the adult testis.

Diffuse Tubular Hypoplasia

The testes that have diffuse tubular hypoplasia can present either a prepubertal or pubertal pattern. If it is prepubertal, the seminiferous tubules show a diameter ranging from 60 to 80 microns. The seminiferous epithelium exhibits only two cell types: immature Sertoli cells and spermatogonia. The TFI is generally low but can also be normal. If it is pubertal, maturation of the seminiferous tubules does not progress further than that of the first or second pubertal stages, and the MTD can reach 150 microns. Both variants of diffuse tubular hypoplasia are the morphological expression of a hypogonadotropic hypogonadism. (Kretser and Burger, 1972)

Focal Tubular Hypoplasia

Focal tubular hypoplasia is characterized by the presence of groups of seminiferous tubules containing only one cell type: columnar cells showing a round to elongated nucleus with dense chromatin and a small nucleolus, all characteristic features of immature Sertoli cells (Hedinger and co-authors, 1967). This tubular hypoplasia is often observed in cryptorchid testes and has multiple names, such as hypoplastic zones, dysgenetic areas, focal Sertoli cell hyperplasia, Sertoli cell tumor, tubular adenoma. The alteration is less frequently found in scrotal testes.

The distinction can be made between hypoplastic tubules and hypoplastic zones, according to the extension of the malformation. Hypoplastic tubules are variable in diameter. They are lined with columnar cells showing a pseudostratified nuclear distribution. The relevant nuclear features are the following: small size, radial disposition, and dense heterochromatin masking the nucleoli. Laminar concentric concretions, densely stained by hematoxylin, can be observed within the seminiferous tubules as well as in the tunica propria and interstitium. Sloughed Sertoli cells also appear within the tubular lumen (Fig. 7–4A).

Hypoplastic zones are lesions that are more widespread and affect enough testicular parenchyma to be considered significant. They are formed by groups of hypoplastic tubules. Their most relevant characteristics are Sertoli cell immaturity and germ cell absence (Figs. 7–4B, C, and D).

The frequency of these two forms is in an inverse proportion to their extension. Hypoplastic tubules may be found in 20 percent of specimens not previously selected, whereas hypoplastic zones only appear in 2 percent. In both cases bilateral lesions are not observed in a proportion higher than 30 percent. The frequency distribution of these lesions according to patient age can be equated to a parabola, which levels off at approximately 40 years of age.

Both hypoplastic tubules and hypoplastic zones mostly represent a primary dysgenetic testicular lesion that is incapable of evolving toward normal testicular parenchyma. A variant of the alteration with hypoplastic zones is frequent in male pseudohermaphroditism (Neubecker and Theiss, 1962). This variant is multiple and bilateral and has been misinterpreted as a Sertoli cell tumor or a well-differentiated arrhenoblastoma. However, it must be emphasized that no relation exists between these two lesions.

The question as to whether hypoplastic zones can be easily identified in prepubertal testes or, whether, on the contrary, they are only apparent after puberty, coinciding with tubular development, is still subject to discussion. The latter hypothesis is supported by numerous reports and by the high incidence of cases found just after puberty. It would be worthwhile investigating the presence of these hypoplastic zones in prepubertal undescended testes since they are more frequent in cryptorchid than in normal testes. Although hypoplastic zones have been observed in testes that later develop normally, they indicate an unfavorable prognosis.

Tunica Propria Alterations

The tunica propria of the seminiferous tubules includes both an inner basement membrane that contains glycoproteins and collagen fibers and an outer layer

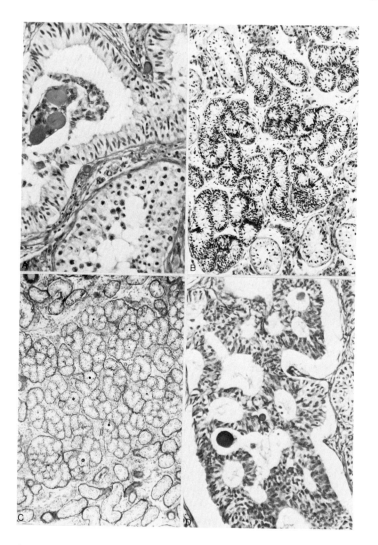

FIGURE 7–4. *Focal tubular hypoplasia. A, Hypoplastic seminiferous tubule, showing a pseudostratified epithelium with immature Sertoli cells. In the tubular lumen as well as in the tunica propria, eosinophilic laminar concretions are observed. This is in contrast to that of a normal seminiferous tubule located in its vicinity (H&E, x125). B, C, D: Groups of hypoplastic seminiferous tubules surrounded by normal seminiferous tubules. B, The seminiferous epithelium shows marked nuclear pseudostratification (H&E, x125). C, Concretions within the seminiferous tubules (PAS, x60). D, Testicular areas showing a trabecular pattern of Sertoli cells (H&E, x125).*

formed by myofibroblasts, collagen, and elastic fibers. Alterations in the tunica propria can affect both structures.

Basement Membrane Hyalinization

Basement membrane hyalinization refers to a thickening of the inner basement membrane that does not affect the outer myofibroblast layer. The alteration consists of an accumulation of a hyaline, eosinophilic, and PAS positive material showing a laminar structure.

Hyalinization of the basement membrane can be either a diffuse or focal process. The degree of hyalinization is variable, from a slight thickening only demonstrable by silver methenamine or PAS stains to the transformation of the entire seminiferous tubule into a small hyalinized nodule with complete loss of the seminiferous epithelium.

Slight diffuse hyalinization may be the onset of tubular atrophy that has multiple etiologies (obstructive, dysgenetic, caused by toxins or by heating). In the initial stage, the seminiferous tubules can have a normal diameter and a well-developed seminiferous epithelium. If the lesion advances, a progressively thickened barrier is interposed between the peritubular capillaries and the seminiferous epithelium, leading to the rapid atrophy of the germ cells.

Diffuse hyalinization (tubular sclerosis) is usually induced by a hormonal mechanism and can present in two forms: The first form is hypogonadotropic hypogonadism that is secondary to destructive processes of the pituitary (adenomas) or hypothalamus, originating during adulthood, and to complex neurogenic diseases, such as olivopontocerebellar degeneration.

The second form is hypergonadotropic hypogonadism in which the hyalinization of the basement membrane is the expression of tubular dysgenesis. This lesion can be observed in Klinefelter's syndrome, Werner's syndrome, and some cryptorchid testes.

In hypogonadotropic hypogonadism, the outer myofibroblast layer is usually normal; in contrast, testes with hypergonadotropic hypogonadism have a thin myofibroblast layer with sparse, or absent, elastic fibers.

Focal hyalinization is only significant if it produces tubular sclerosis. The observation of isolated, fully sclerosed seminiferous tubules in adult testes is a frequent finding, and it probably represents the evolution of dysgenetic tubules. However, the finding of focal testicular sclerosis, isolated or in a mosaic pattern, is more significant. When this focal sclerosis occurs, the following etiologies should be considered: orchitis due to mumps virus, arterial lesions, obstruction of the initial portion of the spermatic ducts, and dysgenetic lesions (Hatakeyama and others, 1979).

Peritubular Fibrosis

The thickening of the outer myofibroblast layer of the tunica propria is a lesion secondary to injury caused by toxins or alcohol or by inflammatory diseases of the interstitium. This thickening results in an increase in the number of myofibroblast layers as well as in the amount of collagen fibers intermingled with the myofibroblasts. Diffuse peritubular fibrosis, although less intense, has been observed in chronic varicocele, as well as following treatment with immunosuppressants, estrogens, and androgens.

The increase in the amount of collagen fibers is usually more marked in the vicinity of the basement membrane, in accordance with the normal distribution of collagen fibers in normal seminiferous tubules (Hermo, 1977); however, in one-third of the cases, large collagen fiber bundles appear among the myofibroblasts.

Diffuse Alterations of the Seminiferous Epithelium

Alterations of the seminiferous epithelium are variable and difficult to classify. This is not surprising if both the multiple causes of testicular lesions and the different sensitivity of the different cell types to noxious agents is considered. In addition, the alterations become more prominent with increase in age. The classification of the different seminiferous epithelial alterations that we have considered follows: germ cell hypoplasia, maturation arrest, germ cell absence, immature germ cell sloughing, anomalies in spermatozoon maturation, and tubular atrophic mosaicism.

Germ Cell Hypoplasia (Hypospermatogenesis)

Germ cell hypoplasia is characterized by a decrease of both seminiferous epithelial height and spermatocyte, spermatid, and spermatozoon numbers; the spermatogonium number may be only slightly decreased (Narbaitz and co-authors, 1978).

Tubular diameter is generally well preserved in the cases presenting only slight germinal hypoplasia, whereas it can appear diminished when marked or severe germinal hypoplasia exists. The basement membrane is normal in slight germinal hypoplasia and thickened in other hypoplasias (Fig. 7–5A, B, and C).

Germ cell hypoplasia is the most frequent pattern of germ cell atrophy, and it can present as slight, marked, or severe.
Slight Germ Cell Hypoplasia (Slight Hypospermatogenesis). Slight germ cell hypoplasia may appear in adults showing well-developed secondary sex characteristics and normally sized testes. The tubular diameter and the thickness of the tunica propria are normal. Zones of tubular sclerosis are not observed. The height of the seminiferous epithelium is slightly diminished. The number of tubular sections showing spermatozoa is about 50 percent. The interstitium exhibits a normal number of Leydig cells. Most of the patients studied for infertility had oligospermia (spermatozoa counts from 10 to 20 million/ml).

Marked Germ Cell Hypoplasia (Marked Hypospermatogenesis). The pattern of marked germinal cell hypoplasia atrophy is usually related to alterations in testicular size (most often in the form of a decrease) as well as to a decrease in tubular diameter or to a slight hyalinization of the basement membrane. There are cases in which some of these characteristics are lacking.

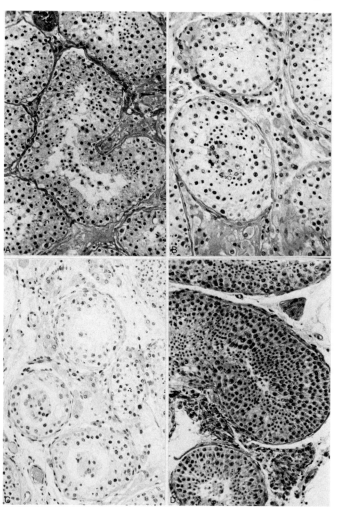

FIGURE 7–5. *A, B, C,* Germinal hypoplasia: slight *(A)*, marked *(B)*, and severe *(C)*. *(A and B: H&E, x200; C: PAS x250). D,* Incomplete maturation arrest at spermatid level *(H&E, x250)*.

The most interesting findings are both the low height of the seminiferous epithelium, with a proportionate reduction of the different stages of maturation, and the sparsity of spermatozoa, which are only present in 25 percent of tubular sections. Leydig cell number is slightly increased in some cases. Patients show oligospermia (spermatozoon counts from 2 to 10 million/ml).

Severe Germ Cell Hypoplasia (Severe Hypospermatogenesis). Severe germ cell hypoplasia most often appears in small testes. The tubular diameter varies from tubule to tubule (from 180 to 280 microns). Most testes show a minimally thickened basement membrane, in some cases associated with slight peritubular fibrosis. Germ cells are present in most tubules, but the number of tubules containing spermatogonia is less than 10 percent, and they are completely lacking in some testicular biopsies specimens. Tubules containing spermatogonia and primary spermatocyte are numerous. In addition, there are tubules with only Sertoli cells and that are fully hyalinized. Semen analysis in all patients with severe germinal hypoplasia shows the spermatozoa count to be less than two million/ml.

Maturation Arrest

Maturation arrest means the stopping of germ cell differentiation at the level of a specific cell type. This involves the intratubular accumulation of a cell population corresponding to those cell types preceding the arrested cell type. Azoospermia or severe oligospermia is subsequent to the arrest. The arrested cell type is relatively constant for each patient, but varies from patient to patient. Maturation arrest can result from spermatid, primary spermatocyte, or spermatogonium arrest.

The testes of patients with *spermatid arrest* show normal or increased size. The tubular diameter is normal. There are no alterations of the basement membrane or of the myofibroblast layer. The height of the seminiferous epithelium is normal but in some areas appears increased. Most of the tubules contain spermatids, but in their immature forms. Spermatozoa are sparse. The interstitium is normal (Fig. 7–5D).

Primary spermatocyte arrest is the most common form of maturation arrest. The testes are small. The patients can exhibit some features of hypogonadism, such as a small penis and incomplete descent of the contralateral testis. The tubular diameter is slightly reduced. The basement membrane shows no alterations. The seminiferous epithelium is comprised of spermatogonia, primary spermatocytes, and mature Sertoli cells. The tubular lumen contains numerous primary spermatocyte stages arrested during meiotic division. The spermatogonium number is normal. The interstitium shows slight Leydig cell hypoplasia (Fig. 7–6A).

The testes of patients with *spermatogonium arrest* are small. The tubular diameter appears decreased. Alterations of the tunica propria are sparse. Only a few spermatogonia can be observed. In some tubules, isolated primary spermatocytes can be distinguished. The interstitium can exhibit an increase in Leydig cell number (Fig. 7–6B).

Hypospermatogenesis and maturation arrest are the most frequent findings observed in infertile males and represent about 55 percent of testicular biopsy findings in infertility (Wong and co-workers, 1973). The causes of hypospermatogenesis and maturation arrest are not always well understood. In some patients the cause is congenital but in most it is secondary to various physicochemical agents or to the dysfunction of other organs or glands. These alterations are observed in chronic degenerative processes, tumors of the pituitary, and in different avitaminoses (Söderström and Suominem, 1982).

It has been emphasized that the cause

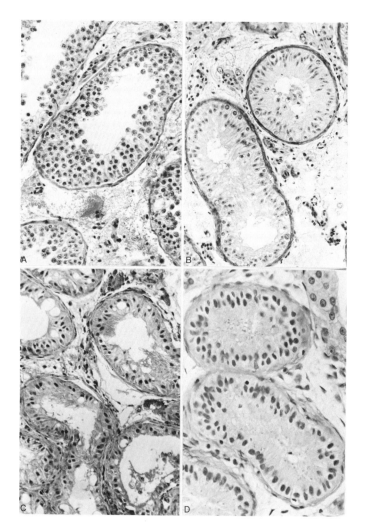

FIGURE 7-6. *A*, Maturation arrest at primary spermatocyte level (H&E, x250). *B*, Maturation of the germ cell line is arrested at spermatogonia level (H&E, x125). *C*, Germ cell absence and mature Sertoli cells in testis of a male with Del Castillo's syndrome (H&E, x125). *D*, Germ cell absence and Sertoli cell hyperplasia in a cryptorchid testis (H&E, x250).

of hypospermatogenesis is a spermatogonium deficiency. This has been attributed to either a decreased number of these cells or a difficulty in spermatogonium mitosis. Nevertheless, more recent studies suggest that the failure in many cases of hypospermatogenesis lies in the Sertoli cells. In idiopathic as well as in prolactin deficiency hypospermatogenesis, the glycogen content of the Sertoli cells appears increased (Arzac, 1950; Maseki 1979), whereas the lipid content decreases (Chemes and others, 1977). It has been shown that the greater the germ cell hypoplasia, the higher the acid phosphatase activity in the Sertoli cells (Goslar and coauthors, 1982). Ultrastructural studies on Sertoli cells in oligospermic males have revealed alterations in the size and shape of the nucleus as well as the presence of osmiophilic substances in the cytoplasm (Schulze, 1976).

Hypospermatogenesis is a frequent finding in all alterations that affect scrotal thermoregulation (close-fitting underwear, varicocele, exposure to high environmental temperature, endogenous hyperthermia such as typhoid fever and influenza, and induced hyperthermia).

Maturation arrest has been reported in patients working with lead or different toxics, such as benzine derivates, and after the administration of drugs. Maturation arrest is a frequent observation in congenital adrenal hyperplasia. It has also been observed to be associated with low follicle-stimulating hormone (FSH)-levels in a family in which the females has polycystic ovaries. Most of our cases showed normal or elevated FSH levels. A postmeiotic maturation arrest, at the spermatid level, has been reported in patients bearing a balanced autosomal translocation (8:15).

Germ Cell Absence. Sertoli-Cell-Only

Two different testicular patterns show germ cell absence: one with mature Sertoli cells and one with immature Sertoli cells.

The Sertoli cells of normal adult testis show a deeply indented nucleus, irregular in outline, with a prominent tripartite nucleolus. This is the only cell type present in this variant of seminiferous tubules with only adult Sertoli cells. The tubular diameter is slightly decreased and the basement membrane can be somewhat thickened. The interstitium can be normal, but slight Leydig cell hyperplasia is also frequent. Testicular size is slightly less than normal (Fig. 7–6C). The causes of germ cell absence are examined in Chapter 11.

The other variant of this lesion is found in small testes, cryptorchid testes of high location, and in the testes of male pseudohermaphrodites. The seminiferous tubules are small in diameter and contain Sertoli cells with a spheric to elongated nucleus and small nucleolus. The nuclei are distributed so that they form a pseudostratified epithelium (Nistal and others, 1982b). The basement membrane shows some thickening. The interstitium contains normal Leydig cell numbers. In undescended testes the Leydig cells usually show a vacuolated cytoplasm (Nistal and others, 1981) (Fig. 9–2D). This alteration is examined in the chapters dealing with cryptorchidism (Chapter 9), pseudohermaphroditism (Chapter 17), and Klinefelter's syndrome (Chapter 11).

Immature Germ Cell Sloughing

The sloughing of immature germ cells from the seminiferous epithelium is one of the most frequent artifacts in testicular biopsies. It may be attributed to manipulations of the testicular parenchyma, trauma occurring during excision, inadequate fixation, among others. However, if the specimen has been well-preserved, sloughing of germ cells may have a pathological significance. Sloughing represents a constant finding in testes with varicocele, although the exact cause remains unknown (Fig. 7–5A and B).

Anomalies in Spermatozoon Maturation

The examination of testicular biopsies only provides sufficient information about spermatozoon nuclear anomalies, although the evaluation is partial, in as much as spermatozoa are sectioned. In Chapter 16 the most constant morphological alterations of spermatozoa are discussed. Maturation anomalies of the spermatozoon head can be: (1) secondary to other pathological processes, such as the apparition of elongated heads in spermatozoa of patients with varicocele or retractile testes; or (2) primary, such as round-headed spermatozoa lacking acrosomes. The anomalies secondary to other pathological processes disappear as soon as their cause is removed; the primary anomalies are not alleviated by any treatment.

Tubular Atrophic Mosaicism

Tubular atrophic mosaicism results from the juxtaposition of several lesions: germinal hypoplasia, maturation arrest, germ cell absence, and sclerosed tubules, although the presence of all these lesions is not required. This mosaicism is frequent in retractile testes, varicocele, giant Y chromosome, and male pseudohermaphroditism.

Seminiferous Epithelium Focal Alterations

Seminiferous epithelium focal lesions are located in a reduced zone of the testicular parenchyma. The special distribution of impaired seminiferous tubules suggests that this lesion affects only one or a limited group of seminiferous tubules, probably included in the same lobule. The localization of these lesions is peripheral in spermatocele, spermatic granuloma, and Sertoli cell oncocytic transformation. The localization is variable in focal germinal hypoplasia, athrocytosis, and Sertoli cell vacuolation.

The pathogenic mechanism is more likely to be obstructive, and the different alterations observed may be subsequent to the same process. In the spermatocele, spermatic granuloma, and the Sertoli cell oncocytic transformation, the obstruction is intratesticular and probably results in the atrophy of only one tubule; in the other processes mentioned the obstruction occurs in both the testis and the epididymis.

Focal Germinal Hypoplasia

Seminiferous tubules affected are similar to those of slight, marked, or severe germinal hypoplasia and have been described in the diffuse lesions.

Spermatocele

In contrast to what occurs in the epididymis, spermatoceles do not form true cysts in the testis. The appearance is that of a seminiferous tubule, with a normal or even reduced diameter, full of spermatozoa. The seminiferous epithelium remains reduced to several low cuboidal Sertoli cells. Spermatozoa can be seen either free within the lumen, within the Sertoli cell cytoplasm, or phagocytosed by macrophages (Fig. 7–7A).

Spermatic Granuloma

Testicular spermatic granuloma responds to the same pathogenic mechanism as the epididymis. It does not reach a great size. In the central zone, debris of seminiferous tubules associated with numerous spermatozoa are recognizable. Very often it is difficult to establish whether or not a true breakdown of the tubular wall occurs. In the most advanced lesions only a focal infiltrate of lymphocytes, macrophages, and plasma cells is observed (Fig. 7–7A).

Sertoli Cell Athrocytosis

Athrocytosis is the result of an elevated ingestion of liquid with high protein content by the Sertoli cells. These cells display several eosinophilic granules in their cytoplasm (lysosomes). Sertoli cells usually phagocytose a variety of materials present in both the seminiferous epithelium and the tubular lumen. The cytoplasmic granules observed in some tubules (athrocytosis) probably represent the result of an increase in this phagocytic activity (Fig. 7–7B).

Sertoli Cell Vacuolation

The vacuolated appearance of the Sertoli cell cytoplasm is not usually related to lipid droplets. Both histochemical and ultrastructural studies suggest that the vacuoles correspond to a liquid with little protein content. The Sertoli cell cytoplasm contains abundant smooth endoplasmic reticulum cisternae involved in the fluid transport necessary for spermatogenesis. This fluid will later become the tubular fluid. A blockage of the fluid elimination, due to an increased intratubular pressure, would explain several cases of vacuolated Sertoli cells (Fig. 7–7C).

Sertoli cell vacuolation is responsible

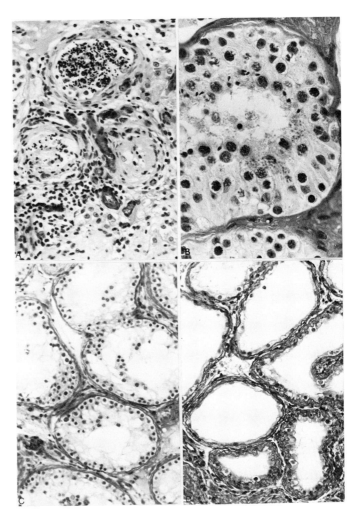

FIGURE 7–7. *A, Accumulations of spermatozoa within a seminiferous tubule. Granulomatous inflammatory process around a destroyed seminiferous tubule (H&E, x125). B, Eosinophilic granular deposits near the lumen of the Sertoli cell cytoplasm (H&E, x400). C, Seminiferous tubules showing only spermatogonia and vacuolated Sertoli cells (Masson trichrome, x250). D, Widened seminiferous tubules lined with both cuboidal eosinophilic Sertoli cells and isolated spermatogonia (Masson trichrome, x250).*

for the sloughing of immature germ cells lodged within the Sertoli cell cytoplasm, with the exception of spermatogonia, which are usually not affected. Sertoli cell vacuolization is a non-specific lesion that can appear in several different pathological conditions such as Sertoli-cell-only tubules, post-radioactive testicular atrophy, and atrophies caused by drug administration in tumor treatments.

Sertoli Cell Oncocytic Transformation

Oncocytic changes affecting cells are reflected by an eosinophilic granular cytoplasm. Seminiferous tubules with Sertoli cells undergoing this transformation have a low cuboidal epithelium and show a nearly complete loss of germ cells. Frequently, Sertoli cells show vacuolation of the cytoplasm facing the lumen. This suggests a further degree of cell atrophy (Fig. 7–7D).

Leydig Cell Alterations

Leydig cell lesions may be classified as either quantitative or qualitative alterations. The principal quantitative alterations are the absence, decrease in number, and hyperplasia of Leydig cells.

Leydig cell absence may occur in several conditions, such as the following: (1) hypogonadotropic hypogonadism with a deficiency of gonadotropins, associated or unassociated with anosmia (see Chapter 12); (2) hypogonadotropic hypogonadism with low LH levels: fertile eunuch (see Chapter 12); (3) testicular atrophy related to brain lesions: olivopontocerebellar atrophy (see Chapter 12); and (4) male pseudohermaphroditism (see Chapter 17).

A *decrease in Leydig cell number* is observed in different pathological conditions, including: (1) first stages of postpubertal testicular atrophy caused by hypothalamic or hypophyseal lesions (see Chapter 13); (2) hormonal therapy, including androgens and estrogens, and treatments with alkylating agents (see Chapter 14); and (3) testicular atrophy secondary to ischemia. Although Leydig cells are the most resistant cell type present in the testicular parenchyma, they can disappear if the ischemia is prolonged (see Chapter 15).

Leydig cell hyperplasia may adopt the following forms: (1) focal hyperplasia. This is difficult to evaluate, since a distinction must be made between pseudohyperplasia and true Leydig cell hyperplasia. The first condition is observed in severe tubular atrophy and is due to the decrease in tubular diameter. The second is found in both diffuse tubular sclerosis of cryptorchid testes and sclerosis postmumps-orchitis (see Chapter 18); (2) diffuse hyperplasia. The Leydig cells form streaks among the seminiferous tubules, thereby separating them. This lesion is frequent in Del Castillo's syndrome and Klinefelter's syndrome, in maturation arrest at the level of primary spermatocytes, in testes with lesions secondary to advanced stages of varicocele, and in some cryptorchid testes; and (3) adenomatous hyperplasia. The Leydig cells form accumulations or nodules occupying most of the testicular parenchyma. This lesion is usually associated with tubular atrophy of the tubular sclerosis type. The Leydig cells are so numerous that they infiltrate sclerosed seminiferous tubules. This alteration is a pathognomonic pattern of chromatin positive tubular dysgenesis (47,XXY Klinefelter's syndrome) (see Chapter 11).

Qualitative alterations are generally accompanied by quantitative alterations (Fig. 7–8). The main alterations are pyknosis, lipofuscinosis, cytoplasmic vacuolation, Leydig cell hypertrophy, multiple paracrystalline inclusions.

Leydig cells with small hyperchromatic nuclei are common at advanced ages. On the other hand, these cells are also observed in cryptorchid testes, changes due to ischemia, and in patients treated with estrogens.

The presence of lipofuscin pigment granules in Leydig cell cytoplasm, in addition to Reinke's crystals and mitochondria with tubular cristae, has been interpreted as an expression of proper steroid function. In tubular dysgenesis and in most hypergonadotropic hypogonadism there is a marked decrease in lipofuscin granules. Lipofuscin granules usually increase with age (Fig. 7–8A).

Most of the vacuoles present in the Leydig cell cytoplasm represent lipid storage. In some patients the size and number of these vacuoles decrease, due to a previous hyperfunction that exhausts the lipid deposits. In patients treated with human chorionic gonadotropin and in most hypergonadotropic hypogonadisms, a decrease in lipid reserves occurs. However, in other conditions, Leydig cells increase their lipid storage, conferring a vacuolated appearance to the cytoplasm. This is a common finding in elderly men, but it is also observed in cryptorchidism (Nistal and co-workers, 1981), several primary testicular disorders (Paniagua and others, 1984), and after exposure to heat (Damber and others, 1980) (Fig. 9–2D).

The polymorphism of normal Leydig cells is a well-known feature. However, this polymorphism is more evident in testes subjected to prolonged gonadotropin administration. Leydig cell hypertrophy is manifested through different forms: cytomegaly, bizarre cells, oncocytic cells,

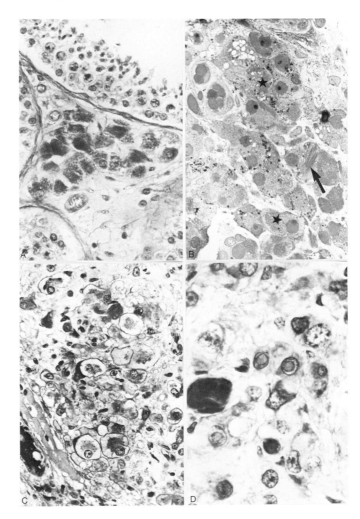

FIGURE 7–8. Leydig cell alterations. A, Increase in the number of lipofuscin pigment granules (H&E, x250). B, Intracytoplasmic crystalloid inclusions. Some of them correspond to Reinke's crystals (arrows), characteristic of normal Leydig cells; others are aggregates of paracrystalline inclusions (stars), and their ultrastructure differs from that of Reinke's crystals (see Figs. 3–18A, B, and C; and Fig. 11–7B). One micron section (toluidine blue, x450). C, Hypertrophic Leydig cells (H&E, x250). D, Cytoplasmic protrusions within the nucleus (H&E, x450).

multinucleated cells, or cells possessing a polyploid nucleus. These forms are frequent in Klinefelter's syndrome (Fig. 7–8C and D).

Paracrystalline inclusions, instead of Reinke's crystals, have been described in the Leydig cells of normal men with normal androgenic status (see Chapters 2 and 3), but they are more abundant in oligospermic or azoospermic men, estrogen-treated men, and in some men with primary testicular disorders (Paniagua and others, 1984; Payer, 1980). These inclusions were located in the cytoplasm or in the nucleus. The most common type of paracrystalline inclusion resembles several parallel lamellae that resulted from several foldings of a single lamella (see Fig. 3–18 and Fig. 11–3). Payer (1980) has reported four other types of paracrystalline inclusions in the Leydig cells of both estrogen-treated and nonestrogen-treated prostatic carcinoma patients. Several hypotheses have been proposed to explain the significance of these inclusions, which have been considered as Reinke's crystal precursors, the result of some modifications in male hormone metabolism, or as a response to drug administration. Although the significance of the paracrystalline inclusions remains unknown, their abundance may be considered as a characteristic abnormal feature of many dysgenetic Leydig cells (Fig. 7–8B).

REFERENCES

1. Arzac JP: Glycogen in human testicular biopsy material. J Clin Endocrinol 10:1465, 1950
2. Charny CW: Testicular biopsy, its value in male infertility. JAMA 115:1429, 1940
3. Chemes HE, Dym M, Fawcett DW, Javadpour N, Sherins RS: Pathophysiological observations of Sertoli cells in patients with germinal aplasia or severe germ cell depletion. Ultrastructural findings and hormone levels. Biol Reprod 17:108, 1977
4. Chemes HE, Pasqualini T, Rivarola MA, Bergadá C: Is testosterone involved in the initiation of spermatogenesis in humans? A clinicopathological presentation and physiological considerations in four patients with Leydig cell tumors of the testis or secondary Leydig cell hyperplasia. Int J Androl 5:229, 1982
5. Clausen OPF, Purvis K, Mansson V: Quantitation of spermatogenesis by flow cytometric DNA measurements. Int J Androl [Suppl] 2:513, 1978
6. Clermont Y: The cycle of the seminiferous epithelium in man. Am J Anat 112:35, 1963
7. Damber JE, Berg A, Jonson PU: Leydig cell function and morphology in rat testis after exposure to heat. Andrologia 12:12, 1980
8. Doshi N, Surti U, Szulman AE: Morphologic anomalies in triploid liveborn fetuses. Hum Pathol 14:716, 1983
9. Evans EP, Breckon G, Ford CE: An air-drying method for meiotic preparations from mammalian testes. Cytogenetics 3:289, 1964
10. Goslar HG, Hilscher B, Haider SG, Hofmann N, Passia D, Hilscher W: Enzyme histochemical studies on the pathological changes in human Sertoli cells. J Histochem Cytochem 30:1268, 1982
11. Hadziselimovic F, Seguchi H: Ultramikroskopische Untersuchungen an Tubulus Seminiferous bei Kinder von der Geburt bis zur Pubertät. II. Entwicklung und Morphologie der Sertolizellen. Verh Anat Ges 68:149, 1974
12. Hatakeyama S, Takizawa T, Kawahara Y: Focal atrophy of the seminiferous tubule in the human testis. Acta Pathol Jpn 29:901, 1979
13. Hayashi H, Harrison RG: The development of the interstitial tissue of the human testis. Fertil Steril 22:351, 1971
14. Hedinger CE, Huber R, Weber E: Frequency of so-called hypoplastic or dysgenetic zones in scrotal and otherwise normal testes. Virchows Arch [Pathol Anat] 342:165, 1967
15. Hendricks FB, Lambird PA, Murphy GP: Percutaneous needle biopsy of the testis. Fertil Steril 20:478, 1969
16. Hermo L, Lalli M, Clermont Y: Arrangement of connective tissue components in the walls of seminiferous tubules of man and monkey. Am J Anat 148:433, 1977
17. Hotchkiss RS: Testicular biopsy in the diagnosis and treatment of sterility in the male. Bull NY Acad Med 18:600, 1942
18. Hsu TC, Elder E, Pathak S: Method for improving the yield of permatogonial and meiotic metaphase in mammalian testicular preparations. Environ Mutagen 1:291, 1979
19. Johnsen, SJ: Testicular biopsy score count. A method for registration of spermatogenesis in human testis: Normal values and results in 355 hypogonadal males. Hormones 1:2, 1970
20. Kretser DM de, Burger HG: Ultrastructural studies of the human Sertoli cell in normal men and males with hypogonadotropic hypogonadism before and after gonadotropic treatment. In Saxen BB, Berlin CG, Gandy HM (eds): Gonadotropins. New York: Wiley-Interscience, 1972, p. 640
21. Kretser DM de, Burger HG, Hudson B: The relationship between germinal cells and serum FSH levels in males with infertility. J Clin Endocrinol Metab 38:787, 1974
22. Mack WS, Scott LS, Ferguson-Smith MA, Lennox B: Ectopic testis and true undescended testis: A histological comparison. J Pathol Bacteriol 82:439, 1961
23. Maseki Y: The histochemistry of complex carbohydrates in the testes of patients of idiopathic male infertility. Histochemistry 64:223, 1979
24. Narbaitz R, Tolnai G, Jolly EE, Brawin N, McKay DE: Ultrastructural studies on testicular biopsies from eighteen cases of hypospermatogenesis. Fertil Steril 30:679, 1978
25. Nelson W: Interpretation of testicular biopsy. JAMA 151:449, 1953
26. Neubecker RP, Theiss EA: Sertoli cell adenomas in patients with testicular feminization. Am J Clin Pathol 38:52, 1962
27. Nistal M, Ríos MJ: Citomegalia adrenal. Estudio postmortem de once casos. Patología 6:171, 1973
28. Nistal M, Paniagua R, Díez-Pardo JA: Histologic classification of undescended testes. Hum Pathol 11:666, 1980
29. Nistal M, Paniagua R, Abaurrea MA: Multivacuolated Leydig cells in human adult cryptorchid testes. Andrologia 13:436, 1981
30. Nistal M, Abaurrea MA, Paniagua R: Morphological and histometric study on the human Sertoli cell from birth to the onset of puberty. J Anat 134:351, 1982a
31. Nistal M, Paniagua R, Abaurrea MA, San-

tamaría L: Hyperplasia and the immature appearance of Sertoli cells in primary testicular disorders. Hum Pathol 13:3, 1982b
32. Obrant KO, Persson PS: Zytologische Untersuchung des Hodens durch Aspirationsbiopsie zur Beurteilung der Fertilität. Urol Int 20:176, 1965
33. Palmer R: Biopsie ambulante du testicule. Ann Endorcrinol 5:84, 1944
34. Paniagua R, Nistal M, Bravo MP: Leydig cell types in primary testicular disorders. Hum Pathol. 15:181, 1984
35. Payer AF: Ultrastructural classification of paracrystalline inclusions in untreated and estrogen treated human Leydig cells. Anat Rec 198:175, 1980
36. Persson PS, Ahren C, Obrant KO: Aspiration biopsy smear of testis in azoospermia. Scand J Urol Nephrol 5:22, 1971
37. Posner C, Cohn J: Cited by Obrant and Persson.[32]
38. Roosen-Runge EC: Quantitative investigations on human testicular biopsies. I. Normal testis. Fertil Steril 7:251, 1956
39. Rowley MH, Heller EG: The testicular biopsy: Surgical procedure, fixation and staining techniques. Fertil Steril 7:251, 1956
40. Schedewie HK, Reiter EO, Beitins IZ, Seyed S, Wooten VD, Jiminez FJ, Aiman EJ, DeVane GW, Redman JF, Elders MJ: Testicular Leydig cell hyperplasia as a cause of familial sexual precocity, J Clin Endocrinol Metab 52:271, 1981
41. Schulze C, Holstein AF, Schirren C, Körner F: On the morphology of the human Sertoli cells under normal conditions and in patients with impaired fertility. Andrologia 8:167, 1976
42. Skakkebaek NE, Heller CG: Quantification of human seminiferous epithelium. I. Histological studies in twenty-one fertile men with normal chromosome complements. J Reprod Fertil 32:379, 1973
43. Söderström KO, Suominen J: Human hypospermatogenesis. Histopathology and ultrastructure. Arch Pathol Lab Med 106:231, 1982
44. Steinberger E, Tjioe DY: A method for quantitative analysis of human seminiferous epithelium. Fertil Steril 19:960, 1968
45. Van Dop PA, Scholtmeijer RJ, Kurver PHJ, Baak JPA, Oort J, Stolte LAM: A quantitative structural model of the testis of fertile males with normal sperm counts. Int J Androl 3:153, 1980
46. Wong T, Straus FH, Warner NE: Testicular biopsy in the study of male infertility. I. Testicular causes of infertility. Arch Pathol Lab Med 95:151, 1973
47. Yoshida KI, Lanasa JA, Takahashi J, Winters SJ, Oshima H, Troen P: Studies of the human testis. XVI Evaluation of multiple indexes of testicular function in relation to advanced age, idiopathic oligospermia or varicocele. Fertil Steril 38:712, 1982

8

PRECOCIOUS TESTICULAR MATURATION (PRECOCIOUS PUBERTY)

The appearance of some of the morphological changes characteristic of puberty before 10 years of age defines male precocious puberty.

Two types of male precocious puberty are distinguishable: true and pseudoprecocious. The hypothalamic-hypophyseal-gonadal system is responsible for true precocious puberty, and the clinical events characteristic of puberty appear in the same sequence as in normal puberty. Pseudoprecocious puberty includes several conditions, such as adrenal and testicular alterations, with pathogenic mechanisms that are not directly related to the hypothalamic-hypophyseal-gonadal system (Sigurjonsdottir and Hayles, 1968; Wilkins, 1965).

True Precocious Puberty

The causes of precocious puberty are only known in 60 percent of the cases. Primarily, they are lesions affecting the central nervous system, the McCune-Albright syndrome, hypothyroidism, and Silver's syndrome. Precocious puberty is idiopathic in the remaining 40 percent of cases. The first symptom is testicular enlargement, followed by axillary and pubic hair growth, increase in penis size, and so on (Bacon and co-authors, 1982).

Lesions Affecting the Central Nervous System (Neurogenic Form)

Nervous system lesions are responsible for more than 50 percent of cases of male precocious puberty. The cause of these lesions is variable, but they all have in common the ability selectively to affect a delimited zone of the posterior hypothalamus: the median eminence (including the tuber cinereum), the corpus mamillare, the third ventricle floor, or the pineal gland (Bierich, 1975; Cloutier and Hayes, 1970).

According to Barnes and associated (1974), the most frequent lesions are: (1) central nervous system tumors, including hypothalamus tumors (astrocytomas, ependymonas, craniopharyngiomas, ganglioneuromas, gangliogliomas, and third ventricle cysts), tuber cinereum and corpus mamillare hamartomas (gangliocytomas) (Judge and co-workers, 1977), pineal tumors (teratomas, pinealomas) (Kitay, 1954), optic nerve tumors (gliomas), and cerebral or cerebellar astrocytomas (Herranz and Ley-Gracia, 1959) (Fig. 8–1); (2) infections, including meningitis, encephalitis, toxoplasmosis, and syphilis; (3) hereditary diseases, including neurofibromatosis and sclerosis tuberosa; (4) cerebral malformations, includingaqueductal stenosis, microcephaly, and craniostosis; and (5) trauma, including postpartum or accidental trauma (Bovier-Lapierre, 1972; Bovier-Lapierre and others, 1972).

Precocious puberty due to brain tumors appears in advanced stages and the clinical symptoms are preceded by other cerebral symptoms, such as hydrocephaly, papillary edema, psychic alterations. Precocious puberty caused by infections or malformations have similar clinical manifestations.

Gangliocytomas consist of abnormally located neurons and glial cells. They are multiple, small-sized tumors located in the hypothalamus between the anterior portion of the corpus mamillare and the posterior region of the tuber cinereum. The mechanisms through which ganglio-

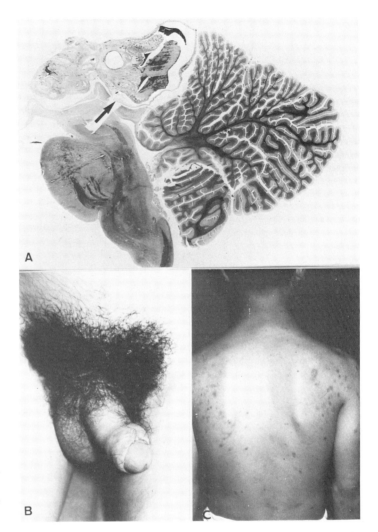

FIGURE 8–1. *True precocious puberty produced by a pineal teratoma in a 5-year-old boy. A, Pineal teratoma (arrow) (Spielmeyer, x4). B, External genitalia showing advanced pubertal maturation. C, Advanced muscular development and acne.*

cytomas causes precocious puberty are as yet unknown.

Pineal tumors are rare in children, and 30 percent of them give rise to precocious puberty, primarily in males. Two pathogenic mechanisms have been considered: (1) a deficiency in the pineal hormone gonadotropin secreting inhibitory mechanisms; and (2) hypothalamic destruction caused by the tumor itself.

McCune-Albright Syndrome

The McCune-Albright syndrome includes skin lesions with hyperpigmented, café au lait spots, osseous lesions (polyostotic fibrous dysplasia), and precocious puberty. Cases are infrequently reported in males. Since this syndrome is usually associated with other endocrinological disorders, such as hyperthyrodism, Cushing's syndrome, and acromegaly, it has been suggested that the etiology of precocious puberty in this syndrome is a failure in neuroendocrine control, with the subsequent hypothalamic hyperproduction of one or several pituitary hormone releasing factors (Hall and Warrick, 1972; Lightner and others, 1975).

Juvenile Hypothyroidism

The association between hypothyroidism and precocious testicular maturation is well-known, and it is mediated through the hypothalamus (Franks and

Stempfel, 1963, Laron and others, 1970). Patients with this disease show a gonadotropin level increase. As a pathogenic hypothesis, it has been suggested that pituitary gonadotropic cells are intensely stimulated by the high levels of the hypothalamic hormone thyrotropin-releasing hormone, which is frequently elevated in these patients (Hopwood and co-authors, 1971).

Microscopic observation reveals that the testes show advanced precocious maturation, primarily in the seminiferous tubules. Tubular diameter increase, Sertoli cell pubertal maturation, and a slight increase in germ cell number are features that are usually observed.

The only germ cells present in the patient we studied were spermatogonia. The testicular interstitium did not show pubertal changes and was at a stage of development corresponding to the patient's age (Cordero and others, 1972) (Fig. 8–2**A** and **B**). After supplementary thyroid treatment to block the hypothalamic-hypophyseal testicular axis, an involution of pubertal characteristics took place. In addition, a decrease of testicular size, in keeping with a decrease of the tubular diameter, was observed. The seminiferous tubules were transformed into epithelial cords surrounded by thickened basement membranes.

Idiopathic Precocious Puberty

Forty percent of patients with precocious puberty in males and 80 percent in females is idiopathic, and this sex difference might be attributable to the female gonadotropic cells' higher sensitivity to luteinizing hormone-releasing hormone (LH-RH) stimulation.

Idiopathic precocious puberty is usually an isolated condition and is familial in 10 percent of the cases. It seems to be due to a dominant autosomal trait in some cases, or to a sex-linked gene with variable penetrance in others (Ferrier, 1961). Hormonal assays usually reveal elevated gonadotropin and testosterone levels in keeping with the patients' somatic development (Fig. 8–2**C**).

PSEUDOPRECOCIOUS PUBERTY

Pseudoprecocious puberty is the clinical manifestation of steroid hormone hyperproduction without hypothalamic-hypophyseal-gonadal axis involvement. The resulting clinical symptoms include the development of secondary sexual characteristics, either in accordance with the patient's own sex (isosexual) or with the opposite sex (heterosexual).

Isosexual Pseudoprecocious Puberty

The most frequent causes of isosexual pseudoprecocious puberty in the male are: congenital adrenal hyperplasia, Leydig cell hyperplasia, Leydig cell tumors, gonadotropin-producing tumors, and long-term gonadotropin or androgen administration. Both complete and incomplete forms have been described.

Congenital adrenal hyperplasia leads to precocious virilization with nearly complete development of the secondary sexual characteristics, in contrast to the infantile testicular appearance (Fig. 8–2**D**).

Another adrenal gland alteration causing pseudoprecocious puberty is Cushing's syndrome. In this syndrome, excessive glucocorticoid secretion is added to the precocious puberty symptoms. Androgen-secreting adrenal tumors (adenomas or carcinomas) also cause pseudoprecocious puberty (Costin and others, 1977).

Leydig cell hyperplasia has been recently described associated with pseudoprecocious puberty (Schedewie and co-authors, 1981). Hormone assays reveal normal serum FSH and LH levels and elevated testosterone levels. The levels of adrenal androgens and their metabolites are increased with respect to the chronological age, but in accordance with the

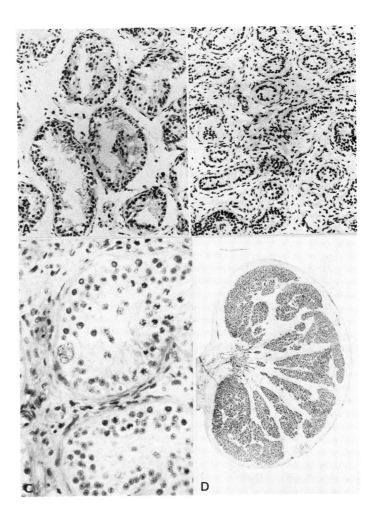

FIGURE 8–2. *A and B. Testis of a boy with hypothyroidism and precocious puberty. The seminiferous tubules show a marked increase in the tubular diameter (A). After a supplementary thyroid treatment (B), a decrease in tubular diameter and basement membrane hyalinization are observed (A and B: H&E, x125). C, Testis of a 6-year-old boy with idiopathic precocious puberty. The seminiferous tubules show primary spermatocytes (H&E, x250). D, Virilizing congenital adrenal hyperplasia. The testis shows a connective tissue enlargement secondary to tubular atrophy (H&E, x10).*

pubertal development reached by these patients. Testicular biopsy studies show, in addition to Leydig cell hyperplasia, a certain diffuse development of seminiferous tubules. This has been attributed to the effect of the high intratesticular concentration of testosterone. (Wilson and Netzloff, 1983).

Leydig cell tumors are usually benign and nonfunctional. If they are functional, they cause, besides precocious pubertal development, testicular parenchyma maturation in the vicinity of the tumors so that spermatogenesis in the tubules surrounding the tumor is frequent (see Chapter 21) (Chemes and co-workers, 1982).

Besides choriocarcinomas and teratomas of the gonads, pineal gland, and mediastinum, hepatoblastomas are the most frequent gonadotropin-producing tumors observed during childhood. Some hepatoblastomas cause virilization through the production of human chorionic gonadotropin (HCG) substances with either follicle-stimulating hormone or LH, or HCG beta-subunit activity. This leads to bilateral increase in testicular size with Leydig cell hyperplasia. These manifestations disappear after the removal of the tumor and reappear if the tumor metastasizes. Cytological studies have shown that, in spite of the hormones produced, the tumor cells are different from those of choriocarcinomas (Ferrier and co-authors, 1961; Murthy and others, 1980).

Long-term HCG administration causes pseudoprecocious puberty with enlargement of testes and penis, pubic hair development, and gynecomastia.

Among the forms of pseudoprecocious puberty, premature adrenarche stands out. This is characterized by the precocious appearance (7 to 10 years of age) of axillary and pubic hair, with normal testis and penis, slightly advanced osseous age, and increased stature. These clinical symptoms are considered to be subsequent to a precocious maturation of the adrenal cortex androgenic zone (Sizonenko, 1975).

Heterosexual Pseudoprecocious Puberty

The most frequent causes of heterosexual precocious puberty in the male are estrogen-producing adenomas or carcinomas (Mosier and Goodwin, 1961).

REFERENCES

1. Bacon GE, Spencer ML, Hopwood NJ, Kelch RP: Isosexual precocious development. In Bacon GE, Spencer ML, Hopwood NJ, Kelch RP, (eds) Pediatric Endocrinology. Year Book Medical Publishers. Chicago 1982, pp. 193–201
2. Barnes ND, Cloutier MD, Hayles AB: In Grumbach MM, Grave GD, Mayer FE, (eds) The Control of the Onset of Puberty, John Wiley and Co., New York 1974. p. 212
3. Bierich JR: Sexual precocity. J Clin Endocrinol Metab 4:107, 1975
4. Bovier-Lapierre M: Aspects particuliers des pubertés précoces neurogènes. Pediatrie 27:611, 1972
5. Bovier-Lapierre M, Sempe M, David M: Aspects etiologiques cliniques et biologiques des pubertés précoces d'origéne centrale. Pediatrie 27:587, 1972
6. Chemes HE, Pasqualini T, Rivarola MA, Bergadá C: Is testosterone involved in the initiation of spermatogenesis in humans? A clinicopathological presentation and physiological considerations in four patients with Leydig cell tumors of the testis or secondary Leydig cell hyperplasia. Int J Androl 5:229, 1982
7. Cloutier MD, Hayes AB: Precocious puberty. Adv Pediatr 17:125, 1970
8. Cordero GL, Gracia R, Nistal M, Lledó G, Peralta A: Hipotiroidismo y maduración testicular precoz. Presentación de un caso y revisión de la literatura. Rev Clin Esp 128:83, 1972
9. Costin G, Goebelsmann U, Kogut MD: Sexual precocity due to a testosterone-producing adrenal tumor. J Clin Endocrinol Metabol 45:912, 1977
10. Ferrier RP, Shepard TM, Smith EH: Growth disturbances and values for hormone excretion in various forms of precocious sexual development. Pediatrics 28:258, 1961
11. Franks RC, Stempfel RS: Juvenile hypothyroidism and precocious testicular maturation. J Clin Endocrinol Metabol 23:805, 1963
12. Hall R, Warrick C: Hypersecretion of hypothalamic releasing hormones: A possible explanation of the endocrine manifestations of polyostolic fibrous dysplasia (Albright's syndrome). Lancet 1:1313, 1972
13. Herranz G, Ley-Gracia A: Teratoma de la región pineal asociado a un cuadro de macrogenitosomía precoz. Rev Med EG Navarra 3:164, 1959
14. Hopwood NJ, Lockhart LH, Bryan GT: Acquired hypothyroidism with muscular hypertrophy and precocious testicular enlargement. J Pediatrics 85:233, 1974
15. Judge DM, Kulin HE, Page R, Santen R, Trapukdi S: Hypothalamic hamartoma. A source of luteinizing hormone-releasing factor in precocious puberty. N Engl J Med 296:7, 1977
16. Kitay JI: Pineal lesions and precocious puberty, a review. J Clin Endocrinol Metab 14:622, 1954
17. Laron Z, Karp M, Dolberg L: Juvenile hypothyroidism with testicular enlargement. Acta Paediatr Scand 59:317, 1970
18. Lightner ES, Penny R, Frasier SD: Growth hormone excess and sexual precocity in polyostotic fibrous dysplasia (McCune-Albright's syndrome). Evidence for abnormal hypothalamic function. J Pediatr 87:922, 1975
19. Mosier HD, Goodwin WE: Feminizing adrenal adenoma in a seven-year-old boy. Pediatrics 27:1016, 1961
20. Murthy SSK, Vawter GF, Lee ABH, Jockin H, Filler RM: Hormonal bioassay of gonadotropin-producing hepatoblastoma. Arch Pathol Lab Med 104:513, 1980
21. Schedewie HK, Reitter EO, Beitins IZ, Seyed S, Wooten VD, Jiminez FJ, Aiman EJ, DeVane GW, Redman JF, Elders MJ: Testicular Ley-

dig cell hyperplasia as a cause of familial sexual precocity. J Clin Endocrinol Metab 52:271, 1981
22. Sigurjonsdottir TS, Hayles AB: Precocious puberty. Report of 96 cases. Am J Dis Child 115:309, 1968
23. Sizonenko PC: Endocrine laboratory findings in pubertal disturbances. J Clin Endocrinol Metabol 4:173, 1975
24. Wilkins L: The diagnosis and treatment of endocrine disorders in childhood and adolescence, 8th ed. Springfield, Ill.: Charles C Thomas, 1965
25. Wilson BE, Netzloff ML: Primary testicular abnormalities causing precocious puberty Leydig cell tumor, Leydig cell hyperplasia, and adrenal rest tumor. Annals of Clin Sci 13:315, 1983

9

CRYPTORCHIDISM

Finding an empty scrotum at the time of physical examination leads to differential diagnosis among the following types of undescended testes (Schoorl, 1982): (1) retractile testes, which are not located within the scrotum but can easily be manipulated into it (see Chapter 10); (2) cryptorchid testes, which have followed the normal testicular descent pathway but have not reached the scrotum and remain arrested at different levels: abdominal cavity, inguinal canal or in the higher portion of the scrotal pouch; and (3) ectopic testes, which are located outside the normal pathway of testicular descent, including superficial inguinal ectopic testes or Scorer's obstructed testes, besides femoral and perineal testes (Mack and co-authors, 1961).

The present chapter is primarily concerned with the study of cryptorchid testes, but also includes some references to obstructed testes. Although the latter represent a different problem from true cryptorchid testes, they may present similar histological lesions. The next chapter will be devoted to retractile testes, which bear different lesions.

Cryptorchidism may appear as an isolated finding or associated with other pathological conditions. As an isolated finding, it constitutes the disease known as "cryptorchidism." In the second circumstance, it is only one of several symptoms of many syndromes. The results mentioned in this chapter have been obtained in children and adults only evaluated for cryptorchidism. At the end of this chapter, the principal syndromes in which cryptorchidism occurs are mentioned.

INCIDENCE

The incidence of cryptorchidism varies slightly with age. In newborns it is related to body weight. Newborns weighing 1 kg show undescended testes; 3.4 percent of newborns weighing 3 kg have cryptorchidism, whereas only 0.8 percent of newborns weighing 3.5 kg have undescended testes. Many testes descend during the first months of life. If a testis has not descended during the first year of life, it will never descend, and the frequency of cryptorchidism after the first year of life does not change. This frequency has been estimated at between 0.7 and 0.8 of adults who were examined for military service.

Among the undescended testes that cannot be introduced into the lower portion of the scrotal pouch through manipulation, 70 percent are high scrotal or obstructed testes, 20 percent are located in the inguinal canal, and the remaining 10 percent are abdominal.

ETIOLOGICAL FACTORS

Although the causes of cryptorchidism are multiple and probably differ from one case to another, the following are considered to be the most decisive.

Hormonal Factors

Testicular descent occurs late. It is well-known that testicular descent does not take place in hypophysectomized mammals. In addition, the effectiveness of gonadotropin administration in the treatment of cryptorchidism, observed in animals as well as in humans, has led to the suggestion that cryptorchidism is caused by a deficiency in gonadotropin secretion (Canlorbe and co-authors, 1974; Hadziselimovic and others, 1976). A congenital absence of gonadotropins has been found in association with undescended testes, hypogonadism, and hypogenitalism (Battin and Colle, 1977; Bierich and others, 1977). Short ovarian cycles plus late menarche observed in mothers of cryptorchid males support the hypothesis that a certain degree of hypogonadotropic hypogonadism is responsible for testicular maldescent. (Czeizel and co-authors, 1981b)

The results of hormonal assays differ in uni- and bilateral cryptorchidism. Basal testosterone levels, before and after human chorionic gonadotropin (HCG) stimulation, are normal in unilateral cryptorchidism. This suggests that testicular descent failure is not caused by an androgen secretion deficiency in these cases. However, in some bilateral cryptorchidisms, both before and after HCG stimulation, testosterone levels are lower than in unilateral cryptorchidism and in the control group. This suggests a functional anomaly of the Leydig cells.

There is no agreement between the results obtained by different investigators who have studied the hypothalamic-hypophyseal-testicular axis. Whereas some (Gendrel and others, 1977; Job and others, 1977) have found low levels of basal luteinizing hormone (LH) and reduced response to luteinizing hormone-releasing hormone (LH-RH) administration, others (Cacciari and co-workers, 1976; Van Vliet and co-authors, 1980) have recorded normal LH levels, before and after LH-RH stimulation. Most of these researchers have reported an increase in the basal follicle-stimulating hormone (FSH) levels and a marked increase of FSH levels after LH-RH administration in both bilateral and unilateral cryptorchidism. These findings suggest that testicular lesions are bilateral, affecting the cryptorchid testis as well as the contralateral scrotal testis.

Local Anatomical Anomalies

A great number of anatomical anomalies associated with cryptorchidism have been observed. The most relevant are short spermatic cords, and thin, short spermatic arteries that do not permit testicular descent further than the external inguinal ring. In some the ductus deferens is the shortest structure. Other anatomical malformations are an abnormal insertion of the gubernaculum testis and a lack of intrascrotal extension. The most frequent abnormalities of the inguinal canal are absence of the external inguinal ring, absence of inguinal canal, and closure of the processus vaginalis with an empty vaginal cavity. (Cendron, and others, 1966)

Dysgenetic Testis

Histological studies have shown that, at birth, a great number of lesions in undescended testes are present (Bergada, 1974; Canlorbe, 1974; Charny, 1960; Farrington, 1969; Numanoglu and others, 1969; Robinson and Engle, 1954; Sniffer, 1952; Sohval, 1954). As yet, none of the basic histological testicular lesions (see Chapter 7) may be considered specific of cryptorchidism.

Genetic Factors

Cryptorchidism is included among the symptoms of numerous malformation syndromes—associated with or without chromosomal anomalies—that are well-known to be hereditary. The reported cases of familial incidence of cryptorchidism support the hereditary character of this disease. (Pardo-Mindán, and co-authors, 1975)

HISTOPATHOLOGY

The following data have been obtained from 203 cryptorchid patients in whom testicular biopsy or orchidectomy was performed (Nistal and others, 1980 and 1982). Seventy percent presented with unilateral cryptorchidism, and the remaining 30 percent were bilateral. Cryptorchidism affected the right testis more frequently (60 percent), than the left (40 percent).

Lesion Types in Prepubertal, Pubertal, and Adult Cryptorchid Testes

Prepubertal Testes

Undescended testes may be classified according to the type of histological lesion observed. However, these lesions are not diffuse in all the testes studied, since in some cases a mosaic pattern is observed, in which impaired areas interrupted nearly normal ones.

Twenty-six percent of prepubertal cryptorchid testes have a nearly normal histological pattern (type I: testes with slight alterations; see Chapter 7). The testicular size is normal or slightly decreased. Histologically they show a slightly reduced mean tubular diameter (MTD), a tubular fertility index (Lipshultz and others, 1976) (TFI) higher than 50 percent, and a normal Sertoli cell index (SCI: number of Sertoli cells per transverse tubular section; see Chapter 7). The basement membrane is slightly thickened after the second year of life. The testicular biopsies performed from 4 years of age onward do not show a significant germ cell increase. The MTD as well as the TFI does not vary during infancy. Some basic testicular lesions, such as megatubules and calcospherites, are focally observed. Of the testes examined, 63.5 percent were obstructed, 15.5 percent being high scrotal, 19 percent funicular, and 2 percent abdominal (Fig. 9–1A and 9–2).

In 24 percent of prepubertal undescended testes type II histological lesions (testes with marked germinal hypoplasia) are present. In 7.5 percent of obstructed testes, 30 percent are high scrotal, 58.5 percent are funicular, and 4 percent are abdominal. All the testes were small and some had a short spermatic cord. Histologically, the MTD is reduced during the infancy period, and only increases slightly during puberty (Figs. 7–1A and 9–3A). Testicular biopsies performed 4 to 5 years after the first biopsy revealed an insignificant increase in germ cells. The appearance of the testicular interstitium is ample, edematous, and nearly acellular. Some biopsies have shown ring-shaped tubules and calcospherites.

In 33 percent of prepubertal undescended testes type III histological lesions (testes with diffuse tubular hypoplasia) are present. Of these 57.5 percent are funicular, 33 percent are scrotal, 5.5 percent are superficial inguinal, and 4 percent are abdominal. All are usually small, in some cases with a short spermatic cord. Histologically, besides the marked or severe germinal hypoplasia and the severe tubular hypoplasia, there is also a SCI decrease. Most of these testes show TFI lower than 10 percent and some of them completely lack germ cells. Megatubules and calcospherites are frequent. The testicular interstitium is loose and abundant (Fig. 9–1B).

Finally, 17 percent of prepubertal undescended testes are type IV lesions (diffuse Sertoli cell hyperplasia). Of these 67 percent are abdominal, 22 percent are funicular, and 11 percent are high scrotal. Thirty-one percent are normal sized, 22 percent have a slightly reduced size, and 47 percent are small. Histologically, the MTD are only slightly reduced. The seminiferous tubules do not have a lumen, or it is only just apparent, even during puberty. The Sertoli cells adopt a marked pseudostratified distribution. The SCI is markedly elevated. According to the TFI,

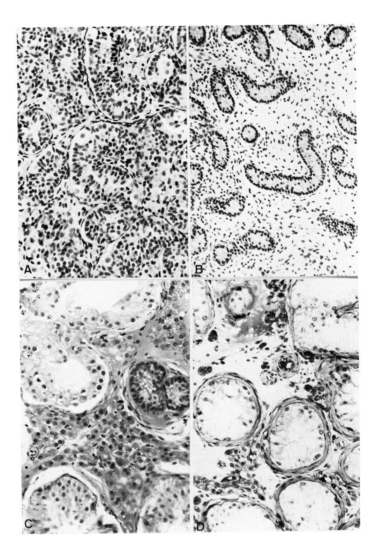

FIGURE 9–1. *A, Obstructed testis of a 2-year-old-infant with slight alterations (slight TFI decrease) (H&E, x125). B, Inguinal testis of a 4-year-old infant showing diffuse tubular hypoplasia and marked decrease of the TFI (H&E, x60). C, Testicular biopsy of a 16-year-old male whose inguinal testis was surgically repaired at 5 years of age. The seminiferous tubules show spermatogonia and primary spermatocytes. Two hypoplastic tubules are seen. The interstitium has apparent Leydig cell hyperplasia. D, Second biopsy, performed at 22 years of age, of a cryptorchid testis descended at 4 years of age. The seminiferous tubules show thickening of the basement membrane, isolated spermatogonia, and some primary spermatocytes. The interstitium exhibits vacuolated Leydig cells (H&E, x125).*

14 percent of these testes have slight germinal hypoplasia, 33 percent, marked, and 53 percent, severe. In 25 percent of these testes there are zones with hypoplastic tubules. Occasionally, ring-shaped tubules and calcospherites are seen (Fig. 7–2**A** and **B**). Vacuolated Leydig cells are frequently observed during the first year of life (9–3**B**).

In relation to the tunica propria, most undescended testes show a progressive increase in collagen fibers and acid mucopolysaccharides, followed by variable thickening of the basement membrane, disorganization of the collagen fiber bundles, as well as poor myofibroblast differentiation (Cotelli and co-authors, 1979).

Pubertal Testes

Testicular biopsies performed during puberty reveal variable lesions. In 42 percent of testes, a marked delay occurs in seminiferous epithelial maturation, in 25 percent only Sertoli cells lacked germ cells, and in 33 percent only initial spermatogenesis or maturation was arrested at the level of spermatogonia (Schindler and others, 1982).

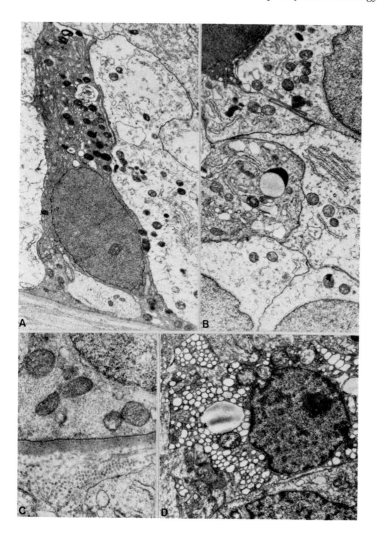

FIGURE 9–2. *Cryptorchid testis with slight alterations (7-year-old-boy). A, Degenerated Sertoli cells showing a dark cytoplasm and nucleus between normal lighter Sertoli cells (x10,000). B, Supranuclear Sertoli cell cytoplasm showing abundant rough endoplasmic reticulum besides the other cell components of immature Sertoli cells (x22,000). C, Moderate thickening of the basal lamina (x40,000). D, Semi-differentiating Leydig cells (x25,000).*

Adult Testes

The most frequently observed lesions in postpubertal undescended testes are the following: testes with only adult Sertoli cells and isolated spermatogonia (29 percent), most of which are located in the inguinal canal; testes with immature Sertoli cells with or without isolated spermatogonia (21 percent), most of which are abdominal and the others are funicular; testes with maturation arrest (12.5 percent), which are usually obstructed; and testes with germinal hypoplasia (37.5 percent), which may be obstructed, scrotal, or located in the inguinal canal.

Testes with complete germ cell differentiation show some morphological abnormalities (Sohval, 1954). The spermatids may be binucleate, with abnormal chromatin condensation or abnormal acrosomal configuration. Degeneration of pachytene primary spermatocytes is also seen. The interstitial Leydig cells can show a normal appearance, or a vacuolated appearance due to lipid accumulation (Nistal and others, 1981). Leydig cells containing filamentous intracytoplasmic inclusions similar to those described by Yamada (1965) in normal adults have also been observed in cryptorchid testes (Gotoh and co-workers, 1983).

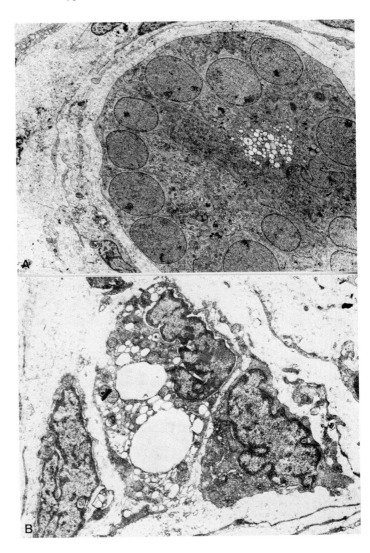

FIGURE 9–3. *A, Cross-section of a seminiferous tubule from an inguinal cryptorchid testis in a 2-year-old infant. The tunica propria appears enlarged. The seminiferous epithelium shows only immature Sertoli cells and lack germ cells (x25,000). B, Inguinal cryptorchid testis of a 1-year-old infant showing fetal Leydig cells that contain large lipid inclusions (x13,000).*

Bilateral Maldescent

The histological lesions observed in bilateral maldescent do not differ from those found in unilateral maldescent. In 79 percent of patients the same lesion type occurs in both testes; the remaining 21 percent present different lesions in each testis, so that all the possible combinations of the four lesion types described can be found.

Fetal Leydig cells persist usually until the end of the second year of life in normal scrotal testes. In many cryptorchid testes that were surgically descended during the first year of life, fetal Leydig cells were either absent or not fully developed.

These latter are usually small and fusiform. Their nucleus is eliptical or irregular in shape, having deep infoldings. There are abundant peripherally placed heterochromatin and one or two nucleoli. The cytoplasm has a dark appearance and contains more lipids and lipofuscin pigment bodies than normal. However, the smooth endoplasmic reticulum and the Golgi complex are scarcely developed. The mitochondria form clumps. During the first year, the Leydig cells form numerous cytolysosomes and, at the end of the first year, fetal Leydig cells are not observed in most of the biopsies studied.

Evolution of the Testicular Histological Pattern After Orchiopexy

Comparison between the first biopsy of a cryptorchid testis and the second biopsy performed years after the orchiopexy reveals the following:

1. High scrotal testes, which showed marked germinal hypoplasia in the first biopsy, in the second biopsy show a complete maturation arrest at the level of the primary spermatocyte or severe hypospermatogenesis.
2. Testes located in the inguinal canal, which showed severe germinal hypoplasia in the first biopsy, in the second biopsy exhibit only adult Sertoli cells and usually lack germ cells.
3. Testes with the same location but showing marked germinal hypoplasia in the first biopsy, in the second biopsy demonstrate seminiferous tubules with Sertoli-cell-only or Sertoli cells and some isolated spermatogonia and spermatocytes.
4. Testes located in the inguinal canal or in the intraperitoneal cavity and with Sertoli cell hyperplasia before orchiopexy show seminiferous tubules with immature Sertoli cells only in the second biopsy (Figs. 9–1**C** and **D**, and 9–4).

All rebiopsied testes usually have variable enlargement of the tunica propria. The spermatozoa found in the second biopsy frequently show several morphological abnormalities in both the nucleus and the acrosome, such as small, irregular acrosomes separated from the nucleus, and a little condensed nuclear chromatin.

Contralateral Testis

In some patients, the scrotal contralateral testis was biopsied at the same time as the undescended testis. Comparison of the two biopsies revealed that the contralateral testis was histologically normal in 25 percent of patients. The remaining 75 percent of contralateral testes showed the four lesion types described in the cryptorchid testis, types I and II being the most frequent.

The lesions are usually the same in both the undescended and the contralateral testes, except for patients with type I lesion in the undescended testis, who exhibit type II lesion in the contralateral testis. When the same lesion type is observed in both testes, the MTD appears less reduced in the scrotal testis. This is principally true in types I and II lesions; whereas in types III and IV both testes show a similar MTD. In 5 percent of cases the scrotal testis shows types II or III lesions, and the undescended testis only exhibits minimal changes.

During puberty, limited maturation of the tunica propria, Sertoli cells, and Leydig cells occurs in the contralateral scrotal testis. If spermatogenesis takes place in these testes, the spermatozoa present the same morphological abnormalities described in the cryptorchid testes (Vegni-Talluri and co-authors, 1978).

Relationship Between the Lesions and the Testis Location

Although the four lesion types may be found in undescended testes situated in all the possible locations, there is a certain correlation between the location and the lesion type. Type I lesions (testes with slight alterations) are principally found in obstructed testes. Testes with either types I or II lesions are high scrotal or funicular, and testes with type IV lesions are preferentially located in the ab-

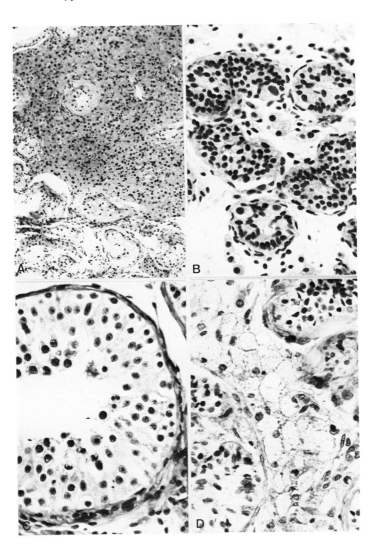

FIGURE 9–4. *A,* Orchidectomy specimen obtained from a 26-year-old man whose cryptorchid testis was descended at 7 years of age. Sclerosed seminiferous tubules and adenomatous Leydig cell hyperplasia are observed (H&E, x60). *B,* Second biopsy, from a 13-year-old male, of a cryptorchid testis descended at 4 years of age. Leydig cell maturation contrasts with seminiferous tubules showing immature Sertoli cells and isolated spermatogonia (H&E, x125). *C,* Seminiferous tubule at 16 years of age, from a testis that was descended at 4 years of age. Sertoli cell hyperplasia is notable. Among these cells, isolated developing germ cells are observed (H&E, x250). *D,* Vacuolated appearance of Leydig cells in the abdominal testis of a 20-year-old man (x250).

dominal cavity (Scorer and Farrington, 1971).

Prognosis for the Different Histological Testicular Lesions

Testes showing type I lesions have no more morphological alterations than a minimal decrease in both MTD and TFI. They are the sole group of human cryptorchid testes comparable to other mammalian testes in experimental cryptorchidism. The case reported by Comhaire et al (1978) is probably representative of this group. The patient had both testes located in the inguinal duct and underwent orchiopexy at 25 years of age. Previous semen analysis revealed azoospermia. Semen analysis performed after testicular descent showed spermatozoon numbers at about 22 million/ml, although their motility was low and their morphology was abnormal.

The noxious effects of temperature upon these prepubertal testes are probably a disruption in tubular growth, a slight decrease of germ cell number, absence of germ cell development at about 4 years of age, and incomplete maturation arrest with abnormal spermatids and spermatozoa at adulthood.

The remaining undescended testes probably bear congenital lesions onto which temperature lesions are superimposed. These testes may be considered to bear tubular dysgenesis (Farrington, 1969; Salle and co-workers, 1968). The tubular dysgenesis is morphologically expressed as germinal hypoplasia, Sertoli cell hypo or hyperplasia, or combined alterations of both germ and Sertoli cells.

Testes with type II lesions show a markedly decreased germ cell number, probably from birth on, but the Sertoli cell number is usually normal. In the testes with type III lesions, the tubular dysgenesis is complete, and the severe decrease, or even absence, of germ cells is usually associated with a low SCI. In the testes showing type IV lesions, the tubular dysgenesis causes diffuse Sertoli cell hyperplasia in addition to the low TFI.

The testicular biopsies performed at postpubertal ages confirm the prognostic value of this histological classification, in accordance to the four lesion types. Testes with type II lesions develop several lesions at adulthood. These lesions, listed in order of frequency, are: seminiferous tubules with adult Sertoli cells and some isolated spermatogonia, seminiferous tubules with maturation arrest at the level of the primary spermatocyte, and tubules with severe hypospermatogenesis. Testes with type III lesions give rise to seminiferous tubules with only adult Sertoli cells. Testes with type IV lesions show a failure in Sertoli cell maturation; these cells maintain an infantile pseudostratified distribution, sparse nucleolar development, and absence of nuclear foldings. In the tubules with germ cells at the time of the first biopsy, the pubertal maturation does not progress further than the primary spermatocyte. These findings reveal that testes orchiopexy do not exhibit a great increase in germ cell number, although the orchiopexy does improve the tubular diameter (Canlorbe and others, 1974; Kiesewetter and co-workers, 1969).

As far as fertility is concerned, the prognosis of testes with type I lesions is better than that of the testes with the other lesion types. However, the high incidence of epididymal abnormalities in cryptorchid testes as well as the possibility that testes with normal TFI at infancy develop maturation arrest at adulthood worsens this prognosis.

The development of the contralateral scrotal testis varies from one case to another. Since 75 percent of prepubertal patients show similar lesions in both scrotal and undescended testis, the postpubertal development of the contralateral testis will be parallel to that of the undescended one. Isolated cases showing either precocious testicular maturation (Hedinger, 1971) or compensatory testicular hypertrophy (Farrington, 1969; Laron and Zilka, 1969) have been reported. Testes developing a compensatory hypertrophy during infancy (12 percent) further increase in size during puberty; at the end of this period, growth stops and the definitive testicular size is not greater than normal. The compensatory hypertrophy is considered to be secondary to gonadotropin hypersecretion, mainly FSH. Long-term studies carried out by Laron and others (1980) have revealed that this hypertrophy, which is effective in order to develop a normal puberty, gives rise to azoospermia or oligospermia. In several cryptorchid conditions, it has been noted that lesions are more severe in the contralateral scrotal testis than in the undescended one. Hormonal assays have indicated that the cryptorchidism is heterogeneous. Unilateral cryptorchid patients show no correlation between hormonal patterns and histological lesions. Some cryptorchid patients with low spermatozoon count have low testosterone levels, high FSH levels, and low LH levels after LH-RH administration.

Epididymal Anomalies Associated with Cryptorchidism

The epididymis normally lays on the testis. The caput epididymis is on the superior testicular pole, the corpus epididymis is along the posteroexternal testicular border, and the cauda epididymis is joined to the inferior pole of the testis. Changes in epididymal configuration (the epididymis may be elongated, angulated or with atresia) occur in 25 to 40 percent of cryptorchid conditions (Mack and coauthors, 1961; Marshall and Shermeta, 1979). These macroscopic anomalies are only expressions of the histological alterations in the spermatic ducts. These include either single or multiple, uni- or bilateral stenosis of a particular segment, or even its absence. The presence of these lesions is relevant, since bilateral lesions are responsible for infertility, even if the germ cell line of both testes has no alterations (See Chapter 6).

Urological Anomalies Associated with Cryptorchidism

Inasmuch as the urogenital ridge and the mesonephros are embryologically closely related, a high incidence of urinary system alterations should be expected in cryptorchid patients (Johnston, 1965). The first studies indicated a higher incidence (Felton, 1959); however, the frequent practice of urography in the last years suggests that the true incidence of malformations is about 2 percent. Most urological malformations may be classified as "minor," including ureteral duplication, posterior urethral valves (Krueger and others, 1980), renal malrotation, and horseshoe-shaped kidney. Only 2 to 3 percent of renal anomalies in cryptorchid patients may be considered as "major." The term "major urological malformations" designates those resulting in significant loss of renal substance or requiring surgical correction for conservation of the renal substance (Donohue and others, 1973). These include renal hypoplasia, pyeloureteral stenosis, hydronephrosis. If one realizes that the incidence of urological malformation in the general population is near 2 percent, the levels found in cryptorchidism are only slightly increased, and therefore the practice of urography, although advisable, need not be systematic (Noe and Patterson, 1978).

A frequent malformation associated with cryptorchidism is inguinal hernia. Clinically, it is present in 15 percent of cryptorchidism cases. Anatomically, 90 percent of cryptorchid patients show a small hernial pouch, which is usually too small to contain intestinal loops.

Familial Cryptorchidism

The study of ample series of cryptorchid patients permits the observation of cryptorchidism with familial presentation (Jones and Young, 1982), which is attributed to an inherited multifactorial mechanism. Cryptorchid testes are found in 1.5 to 4 percent of the fathers and 6.2 percent of the brothers of cryptorchid patients (Czeizel and others, 1981a). In 203 cryptorchid patients studied by us, 5 percent had a familial history of unilateral cryptorchidism. A semen analysis was performed in two cases, which was normal in one case and showed slight oligospermia and 65 percent anomalous spermatozoa in the other.

Complications of Cryptorchidism

Some complications of cryptorchidism are directly related to the undescended testis, such as infertility, testicular torsion, malignant transformation, and psychological problems. Other complications are iatrogenetic or secondary to orchiopexy, such as lesions of the ductus deferens (1 to 2 percent), arterial lesions (2 percent) and their consequence: testicular atrophy (Gross and Replogle, 1963). Recidival hernia or testicular retraction toward the external inguinal ring have also been observed in some cases after orchiopexy.

Infertility

Even though the surgical correction of cryptorchidism presents no technical problems, the functional capacity of the descended testes can only be evaluated years after the orchiopexy (Lipshultz and others, 1976). Interesting data for prognosis are the patients' age at the time of the surgical intervention, the presence of uni- or bilateral cryptorchidism, epididymal anomalies associated with cryptorchidism, and the histological type of the testicular lesion.

If the testes are not descended before puberty, even the less altered testes, they will have a germinal hypoplasia resulting in hypospermatogenesis. Of testes descended at puberty 30 percent develop acceptable spermatogenesis, compared with only 13.5 percent of those descended after puberty.

The relationship between fertility and cryptorchidism, estimated from the semen analysis and paternity rates, depends on whether the cryptorchidism was uni- or bilateral, and on whether orchiopexy was performed. In patients with unilateral cryptorchidism, 90 percent of those whose testis are descended, and 35 percent who are unoperated, are fertile. Among the patients with bilateral cryptorchidism, only 20 to 30 percent of those operated are fertile, and all of the nonoperated are infertile. These results raise the question of whether orchiopexy contributes in a significant measure to fertility. The studies of Eldrup and Steven (1982) and Alpert and Klein (1983) have contributed toward defining this question. These authors studied the semen analysis results of patients with unilateral cryptorchidism, whose testes were descended during infancy or puberty, and later underwent contralateral vasectomy. The semen analyses performed after vasectomy did not show spermatozoa in more than half of the patients, and marked or severe oligospermia was present in the remaining patients. These results lead to the suggestion that the treatment of cryptorchidism should be revised. Orchiopexy might be ineffective in the small testes and in those presenting difficulties in descent, and therefore orchiectomy would be advisable in such cases.

The semen analyses performed in cryptorchid patients after orchiopexy show a variable number of spermatozoa with more than 60 percent abnormal forms, mainly alterations in the acrosome, nuclear shape, and chromatin condensation.

Cancer

The undescended testis has a high malignancy risk, which has been well-known for more than a century. Testicular tumors are infrequent, being responsible for 2 of every 100,000 deaths, and 0.6 percent of all deaths due to cancer. Eight to 15 percent of patients with testicular tumors have a history of cryptorchidism. This means that the cryptorchid testis possesses a malignancy risk 48 times higher than the normal scrotal testis (Debre and others, 1979; Fonkalsrud, 1970; Gilbert and Hamilton, 1940; Krabbe and others, 1979).

Orchiopexy has no preventive effect on testicular cancer. It is also improbable that orchiopexy has any influence on the age at which the tumor appears.

The highest incidence of testicular tumors in cryptorchid testes occurs between the third and fourth decades of life, similar to that of testicular cancer in scrotal testes. Testicular tumors develop approximately 20 years after orchiopexy and without relation to the testicular location (inguinal, abdominal, or scrotal).

When a tumor occurs in bilateral cryptorchidism, it is bilateral in 24 percent of the cases. If the testicular tumor develops in unilateral cryptorchidism, another tumor develops in the contralateral scrotal testis in 4 to 24 percent of cases (Batata and others, 1976).

Tumors developing in both undescended and scrotal testes are germ cell tumors, which may be classified as seminomas (43 percent), embryonal carcinomas, pure or associated with seminoma or choriocarcinoma (28 percent), teratocarcinomas, pure or associated with seminoma or choriocarcinoma (26 percent), and choriocarcinomas (Batata and coworkers, 1980) (4 percent) (see chapter 21).

Testicular cancer prognosis is more related to the histological type and the anatomical stage than to the presence of an existing or corrected cryptorchidism.

Testicular Torsion

There are no definitive studies on the frequency of testicular torsion in cryptorchidism. Its incidence is probably higher than in scrotal testes. Testicular torsions in association with cryptorchidism are usually intravaginal torsions, probably induced by the frequent anomalies of the epididymis-testis junction, as well as the inguinal testis having a higher exposure to trauma than the scrotal one (Leape, 1967). Spermatic cord torsion may also be secondary to a testicular tumor in the undescended testis (Mouiel and others, 1979).

Psychiatric Problems

Psychiatric problems are frequent from childhood on and tend to increase at puberty. They occur when the child compares his body outline with that of other children. Since psychiatric problems may appear at 4 years of age, early orchiopexy may be recommended.

TREATMENT OF CRYPTORCHIDISM

The age at which orchiopexy is advisable has decreased with the increase in knowledge of testicular abnormalities associated with maldescent. The best time for orchiopexy would be as early as possible in order to prevent the development of testicular lesions, provided surgical techniques can be efficiently performed without damaging the spermatic structures. The resulting question is whether earlier orchiopexy can prevent the development of testicular lesions. As has been shown undescended testes may bear two types of lesions, those present since birth and those acquired. Early orchiopexy may only prevent the acquired lesions, and these are only partially known. There are undescended testes of 4- to 8-year-old boys showing only a slight decrease of the MTD and normal TFI. The MTD reduction can probably be prevented by orchiopexy, which improves Sertoli cell nourishment. The MTD is the only testicular parameter that improves with orchiopexy, since neither the TFI nor the SCI do, as has been proved by examination of the second biopsy performed during infancy and after orchiopexy. Therefore the practice of an early orchiopexy immediately after the first year of life, recommended by some investigators (Hadziselimovic and others, 1975) is questionable. It might be more advisable to perform the orchiopexy at about 4 years of age, when the acquired lesions are still reversible and the congenital lesions have not yet worsened. Obviously, the choice of the most appropriate time continues to be controversial.

Hormonal treatment may be done by HCG or LH-RH. HCG can be administered in two different ways: long-term treatment (a total of 10,000 IU, following a program of a 500 IU dose per week), and short-term treatment (two doses of 1,000 IU per week for 6 weeks). The long-term treatment is used in unilateral cryptorchidism, whereas both the long-term and short-term treatments provide similar results in uni- or bilateral cryptorchidism. Other protocols used are those of Bierich-Knorr, Bergada, and Gendrel (Yturriaga, 1982.

The HCG increases the permeability of the capillary wall, rapidly reaching the Leydig cells. The stimulation of these cells causes androgen secretion and enlargement of both the spermatic cord and the scrotum. Bilateral cryptorchidisms are the most benefited with this treatment. According to Ehrlich and others (1969) following HCG administration, 33 percent of patients with bilateral cryptorchidism respond, compared with 16 percent in those with unilateral cryptorchidism.

The most frequently used synthetic LH-RH administration is intranasal. Pirazolli and others (1978), Illig and co-workers (1980), Frick (1980), and Hadziselimovic and others (1982) recommended a daily dose of 1.2 μg over 4 weeks. Between 30 and 60 percent of testes descend following this treatment (Hagber and Westphal, 1982). The age of highest efficiency was 2 to 6 years, and the best results were obtained in testes that were not far from the scrotal pouch. This treatment presented no apparent complications and was not accompanied by significant hormonal changes in plasma testosterone, LH, and FSH levels. Other investigators did not obtain this rate of success believe that statistical studies with these results included retractile testes if the LH-RH treatment is completed with a second treatment at a dose of 1500 IU of HCG per week during three weeks, the testicular descent rate increases 20 percent. If, after 6 months of hormonal treatment, testicular descent does not occur, surgical intervention is recommended.

Besides the classical surgical techniques, other techniques have proliferated, for instance, cordopexy (Saha, 1978 and 1983) and, in the abdominal testes, free transplantation with microvascular anastomosis of the spermatic vascular pedicle to both the spermatic artery and the inferior epigastric vein (Grantzow and Zimmerman, 1983; Silber, 1982) or the ligation and the transection of both the testicular artery and vein (Stephens, 1979; Noordhuizen-Stassen and Wensing, 1983).

If an unilateral cryptorchidism is diagnosed after puberty, orchidectomy is advisable (Martin and Menck, 1975). When the cryptorchidism is bilateral and diagnosed at puberty or adulthood, a bilateral orchiopexy, as far as the spermatic cord permits, followed by clinical control is recommended. If difficulties occur in one of the two bilateral cryptorchid testis, it should be removed (Jiménez and others, 1976).

Sometimes, it is difficult to find either or both cryptorchid testes. In order to plan the surgical intervention better and to avoid the prognostic implications derived from not locating the testis, several other diagnostic studies may be performed (Brothers and co-workers, 1978) including gonadal venography (Glickmann and others, 1977), computed tomography (Wolverson, 1980), arteriography (Khademi and others, 1980; Vitale and others, 1974), and scintigraphy (Lopatkin and co-authors, 1978). Computed tomography scanning (Rajfer and others, 1983) has often replaced arteriography and venography. However, due to the expensive cost, this technique should be reserved for the cases in which other techniques like ultrasound (Bockrath and co-authors, 1983) fail to find the testis.

Although the presence and location of all undescended testes should be corroborated by means of the techniques mentioned above, there is a widespread question as to whether the use of such an elaborate approach is required in the cases of hypoplastic testes (Smolko and associated, 1983). These testes should be removed.

Cryptorchidism Associated with Malformation and Endocrinological Syndromes

Cryptorchidism is a frequent finding in the following syndromes

Carpenter's syndrome is characterized by mental retardation, obesity, acrocephaly, brachysyndactyly of the hands with clinodactyly, polydactyly of feet with syndactyly, cryptorchidism, and hypogonadism.

Fraser's syndrome, or cryptophthalmos, is associated with a defect of the auricle, cryptorchidism, and hypospadias.

Oculocerebrorenal syndrome (Lowe's syndrome) usually is characterized by mental retardation, hypotonia, metabolic acidosis, aminoaciduria, proteinuria, vitamin D resistant rickets, glaucoma, congenital cataracts, and cryptorchidism.

Rubinstein-Taybi's syndrome generally is characterized by broad thumbs with radial angulation and broad toes, mental retardation, and facial anomalies, such as maxillary hypoplasia, epicanthal folds, mongoloid slants, and strabismus. Cryptorchidism is present in 85 percent of the males.

Seckel's syndrome is characterized by mental retardation, microcephaly, intrauterine growth retardation, proportionate dwarfism, bird-headed aspect (malar bone hypoplasia, prominent eyes, and micrognathia). Most of the males have cryptorchidism and hypoplastic external genitalia.

Smith-Lemli-Opitz syndrome was described in 1964 and is characterized by the association of low birth weight, developmental difficulties, peculiar facies with prominent nose, microcephaly, mental retardation, multiple congenital malformations, and incomplete development of the external genitalia. Most of the males have cryptorchidism and/or hypospadias. The adult males studied have hypogonadotropic hypogonadism with a marked deficit in the secondary sex characteristics.

Noonan's syndrome. See Chapter 11. Cryptorchidism is present in 63 percent of males.

XXXXY syndrome (Fraccaro's syndrome). See Chapter 11. Cryptorchidism is present in 28 percent of males.

Trisomy 13 syndrome (trisomy D_1) was described by Patau and others (1960) and Smith (1970), and is characterized by dwarfism, mental retardation, deafness, cleft lip and palate, polydactyly (primarily in the hands), cutaneous angiomas, holoprosencephaly, ocular malformations (anophthalmia, microphthalmia, coloboma of the iris, and retinal dysplasia), cardiac malformations, and cryptorchidism.

Trisomy 18 syndrome (trisomy E) was first described by Edwards and coworkers (1960) and Smith (1970). It is characterized by growth retardation, mental retardation, prominent occiput, genitourinary malformations, and umbilical hernia. Among the principal internal malformations are intestinal malrotation, cardiac malformations, and Meckel's diverticulum. Cryptorchidism is frequent.

Chromosome 4, short-arm deletion syndrome associates hypertelorism, broad or beak-shaped nose, microcephaly, cranial asymmetry, low-set ear, preauricular cleft, cryptorchidism, and hypospadias.

Cryptorchidism is only occasionally observed in the following syndromes.

Cerebrohepatorenal syndrome (Bowen's syndrome, Zellweger's syndrome) is an autosomal recessive lethal syndrome with hypotonia, severe mental retardation, peculiar facies (high forehead with shallow supraorbital ridges, flat facies, and inner epicanthal folds), and multiple congenital anomalies in infants. In addition, a congenital alteration in iron deposits, which probably causes the cerebral and hepatic damage, is usually observed.

Cockayne's syndrome is a rare form of dwarfism associated with premature aging and peculiar facies, mental retardation, microcephaly, deafness, retinal degeneration, cerebral calcifications, and skin atrophy due to photosensitivity. If cryptorchid testes are present, these are hypoplastic. This syndrome is linked to an autosomal recessive trait.

Cri-du-chat syndrome is due to deletion of the short arm of chromosome 5. Infants with this syndrome have low birth weight, slow growth, mental retardation, microcephaly, round face, hypertelorism, inner epicanthal folds, antimongoloid slants, simian crease, and cryptorchidism.

Diastrophic dwarfism is characterized by shortening of the tubular bones, primarily the first metacarpal bone, and a limitation of joint movements with bilateral clubfoot, hypertrophy of articular cartilage, and cryptorchidism.

Down's syndrome. See Chapter 11.

Fanconi's syndrome is characterized by pancytopenia with bone marrow hypoplasia, brownish pigmentation of the skin, short stature, malformation of superior extremities, and other congenital malformations. Fifty percent of males have cryptorchidism and/or small testes, and oligospermia in adulthood. The hypogonadism can be secondary to deficient pituitary development.

Hallermann-Streiff's syndrome is associated with microphthalmia, small parrotlike nose and hypotrichosis, mainly in the scalp, eyelids, and eyebrows. Among other malformations, cryptorchidism can occur.

Hypertelorism-hypospadias syndrome (Opitz's syndrome) also includes mental retardation, inguinal hernia, and, in some cases, cryptorchidism.

Popliteal web syndrome, in which the popliteal web can extend from the heel to the ischium, includes cleft palate and prominent pits at the inferior lip salivary glands.

Prune belly syndrome (triad syndrome) includes the following triad: absence of abdominal wall muscles, dilation of the urinary tract, and cryptorchidism. In some cases, gastrointestinal, orthopedic, cardiovascular, and inferior urinary tract anomalies have been observed (Aaronson, 1983; Kroovand and others, 1982). The triad is attributed to a failure in the development of the first lumbar myotome, which occurs between the sixth and tenth weeks of embryonic life (Williams, 1979).

Prader-Willi's syndrome. See Chapter 12.

Chromosome 21, long-arm delection, is characterized by antimongoloid slant, large and malformed auricles, micrognathia, and, less frequently, renal agenesis and cryptorchidism.

Acrocephalosyndactyly syndrome, as with other craniosynostoses, frequently includes cryptorchidism.

Basal cell nevus syndrome is characterized by multiple basal cell nevus, maxillary cysts, skeletal malformations, and ectopic calcifications. Cryptorchidism is frequently present.

Beckwith-Wiedemann syndrome is characterized by exophthalmos, macroglossia, gigantism and, in some cases, cryptorchidism. Testes show Leydig cell hyperplasia (Nistal and Ríos, 1973).

Cornelia de Lange's syndrome includes severe mental retardation, peculiar facies, micromelia, and cryptorchidism.

Goeminne's syndrome includes congenital muscular torticolis, spontaneous multiple keloids, and uni- or bilateral cryptorchidism.

Lenz's microphtalmia syndrome is an inherited X chromosome linked disease associated with multiple malformations, including skeletal and dental, and renal dysplasia. There is also hypospadias and cryptorchidism. Males are always infertile.

Leopard's syndrome is characterized by lentiginosis, electrocardiographic anomalies, hypertelorism, pulmonary stenosis, genital anomalies, growth delay, and deafness. The principal genital anomalies may be asymmetric gonadal differentiation, hypospadias, cryptorchidism, and delayed puberty. Occasionally, genital development is normal.

Meckel's syndrome is a lethal condition with severe malformations of the central nervous system, such as encephalocele, cerebral or cerebellar dysgenesis, or microcephaly. In addition, it is associated with mental retardation, growth retardation, and renal, genital, and skeletal malformations. Cryptorchidism is observed in some cases, hypospadias or pseudohermaphroditism in others.

Osteochondritis dissecan with associated malformations in many patients affects multiple joints, and such conditions as pectus excavatum, hypertelorism, ptosis palpebral, and cryptorchidism can be associated with this syndrome.

Russell-Silver's syndrome is a type of congenital dwarfism characterized by body asymmetry, low birth weight, elevated gonadotropin levels, precocious sexual development, retarded bone age, café au lait spots or other abnormal skin pigmentation, short fifth fingers, fifth finger clinodactyly, triangular facies, downturned corners of the mouth (shark mouth), and syndactyly of the toes. Genitourinary anomalies include cryptorchidism (42 percent of males), hypospadias, small testes and penis, maldevelopment of scrotal folds, absence of the scrotum, hydrocele, chronic pyelonephritis, ureteral obstruction, kidney ectopia, kidney hypertrophy, and renal lobulation (Marks and Bergeson, 1977).

Van Beuthrem's syndrome is associated with cryptorchidism and testicular agenesis. In addition there are thoracic deformities, muscular hypoplasia, absence of subcutaneous adipose tissue, dolichocephaly, and mental retardation. This syndrome has been reported in three brothers.

Sanctis-Cacchione's xerodermic idiotia occurs in some patients with xeroderma pigmentosum and includes progressive mental retardation, microcephalia, dwarfism, neurological anomalies, such as ataxia and athetosis. Leukemia is frequently observed. In addition, males may have hypogonadism with small testes and cryptorchidism.

Congenital hemihypertrophy is frequently associated with congenital anomalies of the urinary tract, such as sponge kidney (10 percent of cases), hypospadias (1 percent), and cryptorchidism (2 percent). The incidence of malignancies is high, nearly 14 percent of subjects develop Wilm's tumor. One patient developed a seminoma in an undescended testis (Parra and others, 1977).

TESTICULAR MICROLITHIASIS

The presence of calcifications or microliths in the lumen of seminiferous tubules is a frequent finding, observed in males with tubular dysgenesis with or without Klinefelter's syndrome, male pseudohermaphroditism, cryptorchidism, peritumor testicular parenchyma, and even in normal testes.

Diffuse intratubular calcification or testicular microlithiasis is a rare syndrome that was first described by Priebe and Garret in 1970. It is characterized by the presence of spherical laminated concretions (calcospherites), consisting of an acellular basophilic material, totally or partially calcified, showing a laminated structure, and is found in most of the seminiferous tubules (Fig. 9–5A and B). The best-preserved tubules show a decreased MTD and a low TFI during infancy. In adults, there is maturation arrest at the

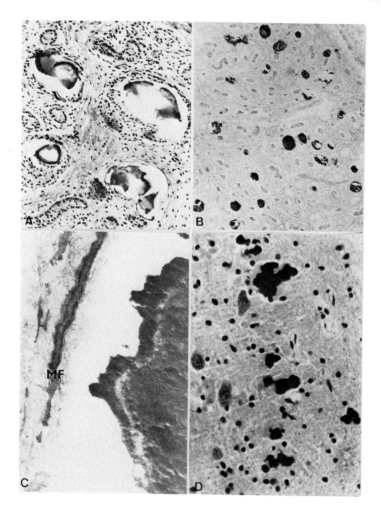

FIGURE 9–5. Testicular microlithiasis. A, Concentric laminated calcifications in the lumen of the seminiferous tubules. Cryptorchid testis located in the inguinal canal in a 6-year-old child (H&E, x60). B, Testicular parenchyma from the same patient showing the mineralization of tubular concretions using Von Kossa's technique for calcium (x25). C, Electron micrograph of a calcospherite near the myofibroblasts of the tunica propria (x4000). D, Microcalcifications in the brain of a patient with testicular microlithiasis. (H&E, x125).

level of the primary spermatocyte (Schantz and Milsten, 1976). The most evolved calcospherites compress the seminiferous epithelium against the basement membrane, which can even disappear (Fig. 9–5C).

Bieger and co-authors (1965) studied the formation of microliths and suggested the following steps in the process. It begins with the accumulation of degenerated cells with a pyknotic nucleus and vacuolated cytoplasm in the lumen of the seminiferous tubules. By electron microscopy, these cells have an irregular nucleus with abundant heterochromatin, ribosome accumulations, several lysosomes, and numerous cytoplasmic vesicles with electron dense content. Calcification occurs in the central core, which is surrounded by a dense matrix which, in the most developed lesions, is in turn surrounded by abundant collagen fibers. In the latter stages, the calcified cells are covered by an amorphous layer that separates them from the peritubular myofibroblasts, the only layer of the seminiferous tubule present at this time (Vegni-Talluri and co-authors, 1980).

Testicular microlithiasis has been found to be associated with pulmonary microlithiasis in some cases. In other cases, calcifications in the nervous system have also been observed (Fig. 9–4D). This has led to the suggestion that microlithiasis may be a systemic disease (Nistal and co-workers, 1979). The relationship between testicular microlithiasis and cryptorchidism does not seem to be fortuitous. The bilateral presence of testicular microlithiasis, as well as the tubular dysgenesis with reduced MTD and TFI, suggests a negative prognosis in relation to fertility.

REFERENCES

1. Aaronson IA: Posterior urethral valve masquerading as the prune belly syndrome. Brit J Urol 55:508, 1983
2. Alpert PF, Klein RS: Spermatogenesis in the unilateral cryptorchid testis after orchiopexy. J Urol 129:301, 1983
3. Batata MA, Whitmore WF, Hilaris BS, Tokita N, Grabstald H: Cancer of the undescended or maldescended testis. Am J Roentgenol 126:302, 1976
4. Batata MA, Whitmore WF, Chu FCH, Hilaris BS, Loh J, Grabstald H, Golbey R: Cryptorchidism and testicular cancer. J Urol 124:382, 1980
5. Battin Y, Colle M: Heterogenité du syndrome "cryptorchide." Arch Fr Pediatr 34:595, 1977
6. Bergada C: Cryptorchidism and fertility. In Mancini RE and Martin L (eds): Male Fertility and Sterility. New York: Academic Press, 1974, p. 311
7. Bieger RC, Passarge E, McAdams AJ: Testicular intratubular bodies. J Clin Endocrinol 25:1240, 1965
8. Bierich JR, Rager K, Ranke MB (eds): Maldescensus Testis. Urban and Schwarzenberg, Munich, 1977, p. 198
9. Bockrath JM, Schaeffer AJ, Kiers MS, Neiman HL: Ultrasound identification of impalpable testicle tumor. J Urol 130:355, 1983
10. Brothers LR, Weber CH, Ball TP: Anorchism versus cryptorchidism: The importance of a diligent research for intra-abdominal testes. J Urol 119:707, 1978
11. Cacciari E, Cicogniani A, Pirazzola F, Tessoni P, Bernardi F, Salardi S: Hypophysiogonadal function in the cryptorchid child: Differences between unilateral and bilateral cryptorchids. Acta endocrinol 83:182, 1976
12. Canlorbe P, Toublanc JE, Job JC, Scholler R, Roger M, Castanier M: Fonction endocrine du testicule dans 125 cas de cryptorchidies. Ann Endocrinol 35:177, 1974
13. Canlorbe P: Problems of cryptorchidism. Helv Pediatr Acta [Suppl] 34:47, 1974
14. Cendron J, Canlorbe P, Lange J: Anatomie macroscopique du testicle cryptorchide. Ann Pediatr 42:259, 1966
15. Charny CW: Spermatogenesis potential of descended and non descended testis before and after treatment. J Urol 83:697, 1960
16. Comhaire F, Derom F, Vermeulen L: Recovery of spermatogenesis in an azoospermic patient after operation for bilateral undescended testes at the age of 25 years. Int J Androl 1:117, 1978
17. Cotelli F, Ferraguti M, Gambacorta M, Donin CLL: Ultrastructure of the tubular wall of the prepuberal cryptorchid human testis. Arch Androl 3:281, 1979
18. Czeizel A, Erödi E, Tóth J: Genetics of undescended testis. J Urol 126:528, 1981a
19. Czeizel A, Erödi E, Tóth J: An epidemiological study on undescended testis. J Urol 126:524, 1981b
20. Danner Ch, Frick J: Cryptorchidism in adults. Urol Int 38:351, 1983
21. Debre B, Gauthier F, Steg A: Tumors of the cryptorchid or previously cryptorchid testis. In Job JC (ed): Cryptorchidism, Diagnosis and Treatment, vol. 6: Pediatric and Adolescent Endocrinology Basel: S. Karger, 1979, p. 224
22. Donohue RE, Utley WLF, Maling TM: Excretory urography in asyntomatic boys with cryptorchidism. J Urol 109:912, 1973
23. Ehrlich RM, Dougherty LJ, Tomashefsky P, Lattimer JK: Effect of gonadotropin in cryptorchidism. J Urol 102:793, 1969
24. Eldrup J, Steven K: Influence of orchidopexy. J Urol 127:508, 1982
25. Farrington GH: Histologic observations in cryptorchidism: The congenital germinal-cell deficiency of the undescended testis. J Pediat Surg 4:606, 1969
26. Felton, LM: Should intravenous pyelography be a routine procedure for children with cryptorchidism or hypospadias? J Urol 81:335, 1959
27. Fonkalsrud EW: Current concepts in the management of the undescended testis. Surg Clin North Am 50:847, 1970
28. Frick J, Danner C, Kunit G, Galvan G, Bernroider G: The effect of chronic administration of a synthetic LH-RH analogue intranasally in cryptorchid boys. Int J Androl 3:469, 1980
29. Gendrel D, Roger M, Chaussain J, Canlorbe P, Job JC: Correlation of pituitary and testicular responses to stimulation tests in cryptorchid children. Acta Endocrinol 86:641, 1977
30. Gilbert J, Hamilton J: Studies in malignant testes tumors. III Incidence and nature of tu-

mors in ectopic testes. Surg Gynecol Obst 71:731, 1940
31. Glickmann MG, Weiss RM, Ltzchak Y: Testicular venography for undescended testes. AJR 129:67, 1977
32. Gotoh M, Miyake K, Mitsuya H, Hoshino T, Yamada K: Cytoplasmic inclusion bodies in Leydig cells from the testes of postpubertal cryptorchid patients. Int J Androl 6:221, 1983
33. Grantzow R, Zimmermann FA: Mikrochirurgische Autotransplantations eines Bauchhodens. Z Kinderchir 38:262, 1983
34. Gross RE, Replogle RL: Treatment of the undescended testis. Postgrad Med 34:266, 1963
35. Hadziselimovic F, Herzog B, Seguchi M: Surgical correction of cryptorchidism at 2 years: Electron microscopic and morphometric investigations. J Pediatr Surg 10:19, 1975
36. Hadziselimovic F, Herzog B, Girard J: Impaired intrauterine gonadotropin secretion as an eiological component of cryptorchidism (Abstr). Pediatr Res 10:883, 1976
37. Hadziselimovic F, Girard J, Herzog B, Stalder G: Hormonal treatment of cryptorchidism. Horm Res 16:188, 1982
38. Hagber S, Westphal O: Treatment of undescended testes with intranasal application of synthetic LH-RH. Eur J Pediatr 139:285, 1982
39. Hedinger C: Ueber den Zeitpunkt frühest erkennbarer Hodenveränderungen beim Kryptorchismus des Kleinkindes. Verh Dtsch Ges Pathol 55:172, 1971
40. Illig R, Bucher H, Prader A: Success, relapse and failure after intranasal LHRH treatment of cryptorchidism in 55 prepubertal boys. Eur J Pediatr 133:147, 1980
41. Jiménez FJ, Marina S, Sedano C: Criptorquidia y tumor de testiculo. An Fund Puigvert 6:90, 1976
42. Job JC, Gendrel D, Safar A, Roger M, Chaussain JL: Pituitary LH and FSH and testosterone secretion in infants with undescended testes. Acta Endocrinol 85:644, 1977
43. Johnston JH: The undescended testis. Arch Dis Child 40:113, 1965
44. Jones IRG, Young ID: Familial incidence of cryptorchidism. J Urol 127:508, 1982
45. Khademi M, Seebode JJ, Falla A: Selective spermatic arteriography for localization of an impalpable undescended testis. Radiology 136:627, 1980
46. Kiesewetter WB, Shull WR, Fetterman GH: Histologic changes in the testis following anatomically successful ochidopexy. J Pediatr Surg 4:59, 1969
47. Krabbe S, Skakkebaek NE, Berthelsen JG, Eyben FV, Volsted P, Mauritzen K, Eldrup J, Nielsen AH: High incidence of undetected neoplasia in maldescended testes. Lancet 1:999, 1979
48. Kroovand RL, Al-Ansari RM, Perlmutter AD: Urethral and genital malformations in prune belly syndrome. J Urol 127:94, 1982
49. Krueger RP, Hardy BE, Churchill BM: Cryptorchidism in boys with urethral valves. J Urol 124:101, 1980
50. Laron Z, Zilka E: Compensatory hypertrophy of testicle in unilateral cryptorchidism. J Clin Endocrinol Metab 29:1409, 1969
51. Laron Z, Dickerman Z, Ritterman I, Kaufman H: Follow-up of boys with unilateral compensatory testicular hypertrophy. Fertil Steril 33:297, 1980
52. Leape L: Torsion of the testis. Invitation to error. JAMA 200:669, 1967
53. Lipshultz LI, Carminos-Torres R, Greenspan CS, Snyder PJ: Testicular function after unilateral orchidopexy. N Engl J Med 295:15, 1976
54. Lopatkin NA, Gleizer YY, Marinbach AE: Scintigraphy of the testes: A new method in the diagnosis of undescended testes. Int Urol Nephrol 10:305, 1978
55. Mack WS, Scott LS, Ferguson-Smith MA, Lennox B: Ectopic testis and true undescended testis: A histological comparison. J Pathol Bacteriol 82:439, 1961
56. Marks LJ, Bergeson PS: The Silver-Russell syndrome: A case with sexual ambiguity, and a review of literature. Am J Dis Child 131:447, 1977
57. Marshall FF, Shermeta DW: Epididymal abnormalities associated with undescended testis. J Urol 121:341, 1979
58. Martin D, Menck H: The undescended testis: Management after puberty. J Urol 114:77, 1975
59. Mouiel J, Amiel J, Bertrand JC, Tire J, Schneider M: Tumeur maligne sur testicule cryptorchide abdominal reveélée par la torsion du cordon et diagnostiquée par l'artériographie. J Chir 116:201, 1979
60. Nistal M, Paniagua R, Díez-Pardo JA: Testicular microlithiasis in two children with bilateral cryptorchidism. J Urol 121:535, 1979
61. Nistal M, Paniagua R, Díez-Pardo JA: Histologic classification of undescended testes. Hum Pathol 11:666, 1980
62. Nistal M, Paniagua R, Abaurrea MA: Multivacuolated Leydig cells in human adult cryptorchid testes. Andrologia 13:436, 1981
63. Nistal M, Paniagua R, Abaurrea MA, Santamaría L: Hyperplasia and the immature appearance of Sertoli cells in primary testicular disorders. Hum Pathol 13:3, 1982
64. Nistal M, Ríos MJ: Citomegalia adrenal: Es-

tudio postmortem de 11 casos. Patología 6:171, 1973
65. Noe HN, Patterson TH: Screening urography in asymptomatic cryptorchid patients. J Urol 119:669, 1978
66. Noordhuizen-Stassen EN, Wensing CJG: The effect of transection of the main vascular and nervous supply of the testis on the development of spermatogenic epithelium in the pig. J Pediatr Surg 18:601, 1983
67. Numanoglu I, Kokturk I, Mutaf O: Light and electron microscopic examinations of undescended testicles. J Pediatr Surg 4:614, 1969
68. Pardo-Mindán FJ, Vargas-Torcal F, García-Julián G, Virto-Ruiz MT: Familial cryptorchidism. Pediatrics 56:616, 1975
69. Parra G, Seery W, Buchbinder M, Cole AT: Congenital total hemihypertrophy and carcinoma of undescended testicle: A case report. J Urol 118:343, 1977
70. Pirazolli P, Zappulla F, Bernardi F, Villia MP, Aleksandrowicz D, Scandola A, Stancari P, Cicogniani A, Cacciari E: LHRH nasal spray as therapy for undescended testicle. Arch Dis Child 53:235, 1978
71. Priebe CJ, Garret R: Testicular calcification in a 4-year-old boy. Pediatrics 46:785, 1970
72. Rajfer J, Tauber A, Zinner N, Naftulin E, Worthen N: The use of computerized tomography scanning to localize the impalpable testis. J Urol 129:972, 1983
73. Robinson JU, Engle ET: Some observations on the cryptorchid testis. J Urol 71:726, 1954
74. Saha SK: Cordopexy: A new approach to the undescended testis. Br J Urol 50:39, 1978
75. Saha SK: Cordopexy: A new approach to the undescended testis: A review of 2 to 5-year followup. J Urol 129:561, 1983
76. Salle B, Hedinger C, Nicole R: Significance of testicular biopsies in cryptorchidism in children. Acta Endocrinol 58:67, 1968
77. Schantz A, Milsten R: Testicular microlithiasis with sterility. Fertil Steril 27:801, 1976
78. Schindler AM. Díaz P, Cuendet A, Sizonenko PC: Follicle-stimulating hormone. IV. Study of the histology of pubertal cryptorchid and scrotal testes in relation to the secretion of gonadotropins. Fertil Steril 37:828, 1982
79. Schoorl M: Classification and diagnosis of undescended testis. Eur J Pediatr 139:253, 1982
80. Scorer CG, Farrington GH: Congenital deformities of the testis and epididymis. New York: Appleton-Century-Crofts, 1971, p. 19
81. Silber SJ: Recent advances in microsurgery of the male genitalia. Ann Chir Gynaecol 71:80, 1982
82. Smith DW: Recognizable patterns of human malformation. In Schaffer AJ (ed): Philadelphia: WB Saunders, 1970
83. Smolko MJ, Kaplan GW, Brock WA: Location and fate of the nonpalpable testis in children. J Urol 129:1204, 1983
84. Sniffen RC: Histology of normal and abnormal testes at puberty. Ann NY Acad Sci 55:609, 1952
85. Sohval AR: Histopathology of cryptorchidism: Study based on the comparative histology of retained and scrotal testes from birth to maturity. Am J Med 16:346, 1954
86. Stephens FD: Discussion-orchiopexy using microvascular surgical technique. AM Assoc Genitourin Surg 71:142, 1979
87. Van Vliet G, Caufriez A, Robyn C, Wolter R: Plasma gonadotropin values in prepubertal cryptorchid boys: Similar increase of FSH secretion in uni- and bilateral cases. J Pediatr 97:253, 1980
88. Vegni-Talluri M, Bigliardi E, Soldani P: Unusual incidence of binucleate spermatids in human cryptorchidism: A quantitative light and electron microscope study. J Submicrosc Cytol 10:357, 1978
89. Vegni-Talluri M, Bigliardi E, Vanni MG, Tota G: Testicular microliths: Their origin and structure. J Urol 124:105, 1980
90. Vitale PJ, Khademi M, Seebode JJ: Selective gonadal angiography for testicular localization in patients with cryptorchism. Surg Forum 25:538, 1974
91. Williams DI: Prune belly syndrome. In Harrison JH, Gittes RF, Perlmutter AD, Stamey TA, Walsh PC (eds): Campbell's Urology, 4th ed. Vol 2 Philadelphia: WB Saunders, 1979, p. 1743
92. Wolverson MK, Jagannadharao B, Sundaram M, Riaz MA, Nalesnik WS, Houttuin E: CT in localization of impalpable cryptorchid testes. AJR 134:725, 1980
93. Yamada E: Some observation on the fine structure of the interstitial cell in the human testis as revealed by electron microscopy. Gunma Symp Endocrinol 2:1, 1965
94. Yturriaga R: Criptorchidia: Diagóstico, tratamiento médico y quirúrgico, evolución y pronóstico. Laboratorios Leo. Madrid 1982 pp. 1–53

10

RETRACTILE TESTES

The term "retractile testes" designates testes that, having correctly descended into the scrotal pouch, may temporarily occupy a higher location (Scorer and Farrington, 1971). The retraction of the testis is due to the cremasteric reflex, which withdraws the testis from the scrotum into the superificial inguinal area. The strength of the cremasteric reflex varies with the age of the infant. At birth, it is absent or feeble, but after approximately 3 months it increases. Between 12 and 18 months of age, the cremasteric reflex is so strong that the testes ascend rapidly to either the higher portion of the scrotum or a superficial inguinal pouch. The cremasteric reflex is strongest at about 5 to 6 years of age. One or 2 years after puberty, it attenuates and even disappears, permitting most testes to return definitively to the lower portion of the scrotum (Schoorl, 1982; Scorer and Farrington, 1971).

Retractile testis diagnosis may present some difficulties, since several cases can be misinterpreted as cryptorchidism. Only when the testes are palpable in the inguinal area and can be manipulated into the scrotum with a stroking movement can they definitively be considered to be retractile testes.

Until now, it has been emphasized that retractile testes are a different entity from the other types of undescended testes, inasmuch as this condition does not require therapy. Whereas cryptorchid testes usually bear congenital lesions that indicate surgical treatment (Hadziselimovic, 1982; Hedinger, 1982), retractile testes do not show lesions and do find a permanent scrotal location at puberty (Lipshultz, 1976; Petit and Hennen, 1976; Schoorl, 1982; Scorer and Farrington, 1971). Nevertheless, Alexandre (1977) has suggested that retractile testes may have abnormalities or may constitute a degraded form of cryptorchidism, and we have observed that retractile testes are the only detectable anomaly in 6 percent of the patients being evaluated for infertility (Nistal and Paniagua, 1984). The semen analysis of these patients show oligospermia, asthenospermia, and severe teratospermia. Immature, tapering, and amorphous forms predominate among the anomalous spermatozoa. Hormonal assays reveal that luteinizing hormone (LH) and testosterone values are usually within normal levels, whereas follicle-stimulating hormone (FSH) levels are normal or slightly increased.

The testes are usually small and show several focal histological lesions that are distributed in a mosaic pattern in such a way that lesions vary from one testicular lobule to another, but all the seminiferous tubules from the same lobule exhibit the same lesions (Figs. 10–1 and 10–2). These lesions affect both the seminiferous tubules and the testicular interstitium.

Seminiferous tubule lesions cover a wide spectrum, ranging from tubules with hypospermatogenesis, dilated lumen, and many abnormally configurated spermatids, to fully sclerosed tubules (Fig. 10–2). The most frequent tubular lesions are (Fig. 10–1): slight, marked, or severe germ cell hypoplasia, with or without maturational abnormalities of the spermatid head; maturation arrest at the level of the spermatids, primary spermatocytes or spermatogonia; seminiferous tubules with only atrophic (oncocytic) Sertoli cells; and tubular sclerosis with peritubular lymphocytic infiltrates.

Other minor tubular alterations are

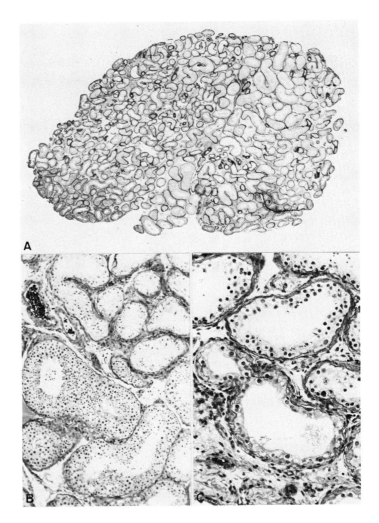

FIGURE 10–1. Retractile testis. A, Mosaic pattern of seminiferous tubule atrophy. Lobules showing seminiferous tubules with normal diameter are intermingled with lobules showing small, atrophic tubules (methenamine-silver, x10). B, Seminiferous tubules with only Sertoli cells beside tubules with complete, although reduced, spermatogenesis (H&E, x60). C, Dilation of the tubular lumen with severe hypospermatogenesis (top), and tubules with oncocytic transformation of Sertoli cells (bottom) (H&E, x125).

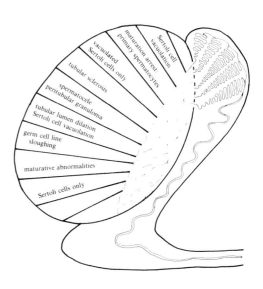

FIGURE 10–2. Characteristic lesions of retractile testes. Lobular affectation showing a progressive degree of tubular atrophy.

dilation of the tubule lumen, Sertoli cell athrocytosis (see chapter 7), cytoplasmic vacuolation of Sertoli cells, hypoplastic tubules and spermatocele-like lesions (tubules with atrophic seminiferous epithelium containing numerous spermatozoa in their lumen). Germ cell sloughing is a common finding, mainly in the seminiferous tubules with a higher degree of Sertoli cell vacuolation.

The interstitial lesions are primarily vascular lesions. In addition, perivascular lymphocytic infiltrates and apparently Leydig cell hyperplasia in the most atrophic lobules were seen. The most frequent vascular lesions are angiectasis, showing numerous dilated veins and venules, with or without thickening of the wall.

The semen analysis, the seminiferous tubule lesions, and the vascular lesions found in retractile testes recall those observed in varicocele (Cameron and Snydle, 1980; Hofman and others, 1982; Jecht and co-workers, 1982; MacLeod, 1965; Rodríquez-Rigau and co-authors, 1981). The causes of these lesions seem to be related to an obstructive mechanism that leads to progressive testicular atrophy. The less affected seminiferous tubules show a relatively well-preserved epithelium, an increased diameter with dilation of the lumen, which contains abundant spermatozoa, and athrocytosis at the apical Sertoli cell cytoplasm. This suggests an intermittent or partial occlusion, rather than a complete obstruction. It is not likely that the obstruction occurs at the level of the cauda epididymis or ductus deferens, since experimental studies as well as testicular biopsy in vasectomized patients have shown that the ligature at these distal levels has only a slight effect on the testicular parenchyma (Gupta and others, 1975). The complete atrophy of some tubules and the mosaic pattern of these lesions seem to indicate that the occlusion occurs in the intratesticular spermatic ducts. Venous ectasia, in the absence of varicocele, is due to venous obstruction.

The mechanism responsible for both venous and tubular obstruction is probably related to the positional changes experienced by the testis and epididymis during retraction. Contraction of the cremasteric muscle causes shortness of the spermatic cord, which becomes folded, causing a temporary partial occlusion of the spermatic veins and the subsequent venous ectasia (Fig. 10–3). The dilated large veins at the mediastinum testis would compress the tubuli recti causing their obstruction and the subsequent fluid ectasia. Such an ectasia is probably the cause of tubular lumen dilation, which leads to an increase of Sertoli cell phagocytosis, with accumulation of phagolysosomes in their cytoplasm (athrocytosis).

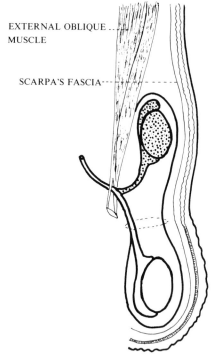

FIGURE 10–3. *Anatomical position of the retractile testis in comparison with that of the scrotal testis. (Modified from P.G. Jones.)*

This is followed by Sertoli cell vacuolation, which would facilitate germ cell sloughing, due to the disruption of the seminiferous tubule adluminal compartment, similar to that which occurs in varicocele (Cameron and Snydle, 1980).

If the Sertoli cell vacuolation progresses, germ cell sloughing will increase, giving rise to progressive maturation arrest, first at the level of primary spermatocytes, and afterward at the level of spermatogonia. Finally, the basal compartment is also affected and the most affected tubules only show atrophic Sertoli cells.

When this degree of Sertoli cell atrophy has been reached, the basement membrane becomes thickened, impeding the maintenance of Sertoli cells. The Sertoli cells become cuboidal or flattened and show an eosinophilic, granular cytoplasm. The final result is complete tubular sclerosis.

The different degrees of germ cell hypoplasia—slight, marked, and severe—observed in the retractile testes might be considered as either different degrees of germ cell affectation or a partial recovery of seminiferous tubules, probably due to an improvement in spermatic duct permeability. In relation to this, the seminiferous tubules with germ cell hypoplasia show sparse Sertoli cell vacuolation. On the other hand, the possibility that germ cell hypoplasia may be congenital, as has been suggested in cryptorchidism (see Chapter 9), should be taken into account.

Some retractile testes show only one type of tubular lesion instead of the several types of focal lesions distributed in a mosaic pattern. This might be attributed to several factors, including individual variations in the strength of the cremasteric reflex, the time of testicular retraction, the relative position of the testis with regard to the epididymis, and the reduced volume of the testicular biopsy.

The severe teratospermia, similar to that observed in varicocele, might also be secondary to venous ectasia and tubular obstruction. Although the causes of this relationship are not yet known, it is interesting to note that the retractile testes without venous angiectasis have sparse teratospermia.

Since retractile testes have severe lesions that lead to infertility, the fixation of these testes to the scrotum is recommended in order to prevent the progress of testicular lesions and further complications, such as torsion and infarct of the testes.

REFERENCES

1. Alexandre C: Les testicules oscillants. Forme dégradée de cryptorchidie? J Gynecol Obst Biol Reprod 6:71, 1977
2. Cameron DF, Snydle FE: The blood-testis barrier in men with varicocele: A lanthanum tracer study. Fertil Steril 34:255, 1980
3. Gupta AS, Kothati LK, Dhruva A, Bapna R: Surgical sterilization by vasectomy and its effect on the structure and function of the testis in man. Br J Surg 62:59, 1975
4. Hadziselimovic F: Pathogenesis and treatment of undescended testes. Eur J Pediatr 139:255, 1982
5. Hedinger CE: Histopathology of undescended testes. Eur J Pediatr 139:266, 1982
6. Hofman N, Hilscher B, Passia D, Hilscher W, Haider SG: Histological, morphometrical, and enzyme histochemical studies on varicocele orchiopathy. In Jecht EW, Zeitler E (eds): Varicocele and Male Infertility. Berlin: Springer Verlag, 1982, p. 27
7. Jecht EW, Müller R, Zieglwalner E: Varicocele and seminal cytology. In Jecht EW, Zeitler E (eds): Varicocele and Male Infertility. Berlin: Springer Verlag, 1982, p. 35
8. Lipshultz LI: Cryptorchidism in the subfertile male. Fertil Steril 27:609, 1976
9. MacLeod J: Seminal cytology in the presence of varicocele. Fertil Steril 16:735, 1965
10. Nistal M, Paniagua R: Infertility in adult males with retractile testes. Fertil Steril 41:395, 1984

11. Petit T, Hennen G: La cryptorchidie et son contexte endocrinien. Acta Urol Belg 44:101, 1976
12. Rodríguez-Rigau LJ, Smith KD, Steinberger E: Varicocele and the morphology of the spermatozoa. Fertil Steril 35:54, 1981
13. Schoorl M: Classification and diagnosis of undescended testes. Eur J Pediatr 139:253, 1982
14. Scorer CG, Farrington GH: Boyhood and adolescence: Retraction of the testis. In Congenital Deformities of the Testis and Epididymis. London: Butterworth and Co., 1971, p. 45.

11

HYPOGONADISM DUE TO PRIMARY TESTICULAR FAILURE

Classification of Hypogonadism

Classically, hypogonadism has been classified on a biochemical basis. Based on gonadotropin levels, three large groups have been distinguished: hypogonadotropic hypogonadism, hypergonadotropic hypogonadism, and normogonadotropic hypogonadism.

The increasing tendency to perform testicular biopsies and the standardization of the study of testicular abnormalities have enabled the pathologist to establish a morphological classification of hypogonadism. Morphological and clinical classification offer various viewpoints of a specific case, although generally they overlap.

The semen analysis, which actually constitutes the starting point in the evaluation of a patient for infertility, must be considered in the interpretation of hypogonadism. In order to differentiate between the types of hypogonadism, karyotype and sex chromatin studies are absolutely necessary. The functional study of other endocrine glands or that of certain organs is imperative in hypogonadism of obscure origin.

Following Wong and co-workers (1973) hypogonadism can be classified on an anatomical basis into three groups:

1. Hypogonadism due to primary testicular failure
2. Pretesticular hypogonadism
3. Post-testicular hypogonadism

Hypogonadism due to primary testicular failure is generally the most frequent. This group includes the different types of hypergonadotropic hypogonadism, hypospermatogenesis, maturation arrest, Del Castillo's syndrome, Klinefelter's syndrome, cryptorchidism, postradiation atrophy, postmumps orchitis atrophy, among others.

Pretesticular hypogonadism is generally hypogonadotropic hypogonadism and includes entities in which an accompanying endocrinological disorder exists. These include hypopituitarism that starts either at pre- or postpubertal ages and situations in which there is an excess of androgen and estrogen production of either exogenous or endogenous origin. An excess of endogenous estrogens is seen, for example, in functional adrenal tumors or in cirrhosis of the liver. An excess of androgens can be seen in the adrenogenital syndrome, or in adrenal-producing or testicular androgen-producing tumors. In these cases the testicular lesions are not only due to the direct action of the tumor on the testis, but also to the suppression of gonadotropin release by the pituitary. Hypogonadotropic hypogonadism can also be found in cases in which plasma glucocorticoids are increased, as in Cushing's syndrome, or in which they are administered in high doses, as in the treatment of ulcerative colitis, rheumatoid arthritis, bronchial asthma, in thyroid dysfunctions, such as hypo- or hyperthyroidism, in diabetes mellitus, and others.

Post-testicular hypogonadism is generally normogonadotropic and includes two types of patients: those who present with azoospermia due to spermatic obstruction, and a few who present with serious asthenospermia. Obstruction of the spermatic ducts includes congenital and acquired lesions, either postinflammatory or iatrogenic (due to surgery). Patients with asthenospermia have normal sperm counts and a normal testicular biopsy. The cause of the immobility of the spermatozoa can be found outside the testes, either in relation to inappropriate maturation during their course through the epididymis or to anomalies in the secretions of the seminal vesicles and prostate.

HYPOGONADISM LINKED TO SEX CHROMOSOME ABERRATIONS

Klinefelter's syndrome

Klinefelter's syndrome was described by Klinefelter and co-authors, (1942) as a hypogonadism characterized by the following: gynecomastia, azoospermia, testicular atrophy, and increase in gonadotropin production. As new cases were discovered, it was found that sometimes some of these symptoms were absent, and in 1945 by Heller and Nelson described syndromes without gynecomastia and with varying degrees of androgenic deficiency.

The clinical entity was completed when a systematic study of the presence of sex chromatin was performed on these patients. Two kinds of patients with the same phenotype were observed: chromatin positive and chromatin negative. This difference was the basis for the distinction between true Klinefelter's syndrome (chromatin positive) and false Klinefelter's syndrome (chromatin negative). However, there are cases in which both chromatin negative and chromatin positive patients have similar clinical features and testicular pattern (Paulsen and others, 1968).

Presently, the term "Klinefelter's syndrome" is usually used to designate only the chromatin positive patients. The chromatin negative patients must be accurately evaluated by such studies as hormonal assays and testicular biopsy for an exact diagnosis (Grabski and co-workers, 1979; Rimoin and others, 1968).

True Klinefelter's Syndrome

The frequency of Klinefelter's syndrome varies, depending on the population sample that is investigated. In the general population, the incidence is 1 per 1000 to 1400 of all male live births. In institutions for mentally retarded patients, it is 1 percent, and among males evaluated for infertility, 3 percent.

The karyotype shows a basic chromosomal constitution in all patients, 47,XXY, but there are numerous cases in which there are more than two X or Y chromosomes, or two or more cell lines, as in the mosaics: XY/XXY, XY/XXXY, XX/XXY, XY/XO/XXY, XX/XXY/XXXY, and XXXY/XXXXY.

The chromosomal constitution XXY originates from a nondysjunction or a failure in the separation of the sex chromosomes during the first or second meiotic division, in either parent, or in a mitotic nondysjunction in the zygote. Because of the study of X chromosome linked factors, such as color vision, or X_g blood group, 73 percent of extra X chromosomes were found to come from the mother, whereas only 27 percent were of paternal origin. Advanced maternal age has been implicated as a cause of a large number of XXY patients.

The most frequent clinical symptoms in 47,XXY Klinefelter's syndrome (Fig. 11–1) are the following:

1. A wide spectrum of traits corresponding to a variable degree of virilization: from patients with total absence of secondary sex characteristics to patients with almost normal development (Grabski and co-workers, 1979).
2. An eunuchoid phenotype, with tall stature and notably elongated length of the lower extremities. The relation

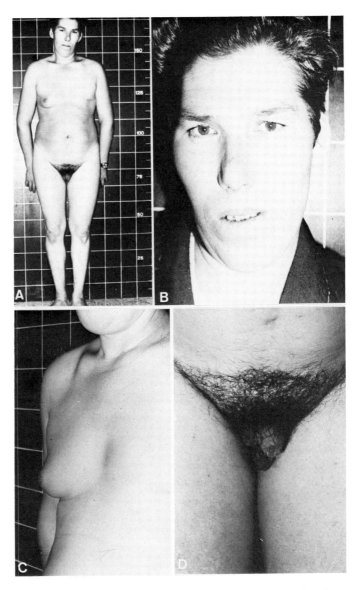

FIGURE 11-1. *47,XXY Klinefelter's syndrome. A 32-year-old patient with eunuchoid habitus, mental retardation, gynecomastia, and hypoplastic external genitalia.*

between span and height is less than one.

3. Gynecomastia is present in 55 percent of the cases and is usually bilateral. Histologically, severe periductal fibrosis replacing the adipose tissue with a slight proliferation of ductal epithelium can be observed. The pathophysiological mechanism is not entirely understood, although it is possible that an estrogen/androgen imbalance could be implicated. No correlation between gynecomastia and the degree of androgenization has been established.

4. Mental disorders are frequent in this syndrome and, although 80 percent of the patients have an IQ that enables them to play an active role in society, personality and behavioral disorders are frequently observed.

5. Other clinical entities frequently linked to Klinefelter's syndrome are: chronic bronchitis, varicose veins, cervical rib, kyphosis, scoliosis or pectus excavatum. A high incidence of

hypothalamic, hypophyseal, thyroid, and pancreatic dysfunctions have been found in Klinefelter's syndrome.

In most patients the external genitalia are normal. In 47,XXY patients, testicular size is generally less than 2.5 cm (Boisen, 1979), whereas in those patients with chromosomal mosaicism, testicular size can be almost normal. In 50 percent of the cases, the consistency of the testes is soft, and in 20 percent it is firm. In the XXY patients, cryptorchidism is rare, whereas it is frequent in patients with mosaicism of more than two X chromosomes (Becker, 1972).

The testes in the postpubertal patients present a pathognomonic pattern: most of the seminiferous tubules are completely sclerosed or hyalinized, the Leydig cells show an adenomatous hyperplasia, and the elastic fibers of the tunica propria are absent, indicating that the sclerosis was probably established early during puberty, before tunica propria maturation could occur (Fig. 11–2A).

In most biopsies, a few tubules with only Sertoli cells can also be seen (Fig. 11–2B). In some patients, these cells are sex chromatin negative, whereas a high percentage of others have positive sex chromatin. A small number of patients

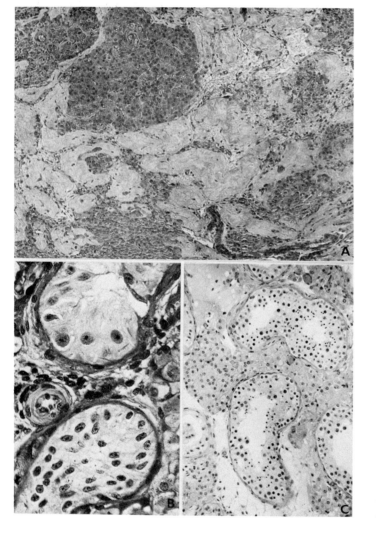

FIGURE 11–2. *47,XXY postpubertal Klinefelter's syndrome. A, Diffuse tubular sclerosis and adenomatous hyperplasia of the Leydig cells (Masson trichrome, x60). B, Seminiferous tubules with only Sertoli cells presenting various degrees of maturation. The Sertoli cells of the upper tubule contain Charcot-Böttcher crystals (Masson trichrome, x250). C, Focal spermatogenesis in 47,XXY Klinefelter's syndrome. Marked hyperplasia of the Leydig cells is seen (H&E, x125).*

show tubules with positive and negative sex chromatin Sertoli cells in the same biopsy. This leads to the distinction between two different types of seminiferous tubules containing only Sertoli cells (Frohland and Skakkebaek, 1971). Type A tubules present a central lumen lined with adult Sertoli cells with an ovoid nucleus characterized by a typical nucleolus, sparse, evenly distributed chromatin, and negative sex chromatin. Type B tubules are smaller and lack a central lumen. Their Sertoli cells adopt a pseudostratified disposition. The nucleus is round or ovoid, hyperchromatic, and has one or two small nucleoli. In some of the tubules the cells have positive sex chromatin in similar proportion to that of the Leydig cells or oral mucosal cells. In other type B tubules the cells have a low percentage of positive sex chromatin, and in still others the cells are sex chromatin negative.

Several hypotheses have been suggested to explain why patients with the 47,XXY karyotype, who do not have mosaicism in either blood, skin, or bone marrow cells, have negative sex chromatin in the Sertoli cells. Among these hypotheses are that both X chromosomes are isopyknotic, that Barr body is located beyond the nuclear limits, or that only one X chromosome is present in the cells of these tubules. The most probable explanation is the existence of testicular mosaics that may only be demonstrated after a testicular cell culture is done.

The Leydig cells form large clumps between the sclerosed tubules (Figs. 11-2A and 11-3). They present great variations in nuclear size, and some are multinucleated with multiple and prominent nucleoli. Many present telescoped cytoplasmic inclusions within the nucleus. In 40 to 70 percent of the cells the sex chromatin is positive. The cytoplasm is abundant and eosinophilic, with sparse lipids and lipofuscins. Reinke's crystals are difficult to observe, being either small or absent. Paracrystalline inclusions are abundant (Rubin and Mattei, 1971). In a small number of patients, Leydig cell hyperplasia is more moderate. Areas with spermatogenesis have been observed in some patients with the 47,XXY karyotype. Since testicular damage has been related to the presence of an extra X chromosome, it has been suggested that in these cases a mosaic would exist in the testicular cells. In patients with mosaicism, spermatogenesis is generally better preserved, and cases of paternity have been reported (Steinberger and co-authors, 1965) (Fig. 11-2C).

Ohno's cytological studies (1977) on meiosis in rat testes with an XXY chromosome complement demonstrated that germ cells with an extra X chromosome did not progress beyond spermatogonia formation, even if one of the two X chromosomes seemed to be heteropyknotic. Two types of germ cells were found resulting from nondysjunction of the X chromosome in the mitotic divisions in these rats: cells with a XXY complement that were eliminated; and cells with an XY complement that could differentiate into spermatogonia and complete the whole spermatogenetic process, giving rise to spermatozoa with an X or Y complement.

Leydig cell function, in spite of marked hypertrophy or hyperplasia, is inadequate, and the production of androgens generally does not exceed 50 percent of normal values. The reserve function, measured with human chorionic gonadotropin (HCG) stimulation, is also less than in the controls. Initially, testosterone levels are increased, although less than the controls, but later both basal testosterone levels and the reserve function decrease (Fukutani and others, 1983), although in some patients testosterone values remain higher than those found before performing the test. Although testosterone values may be normal in some patients, the free testosterone fraction is usually low. This may explain the failure of the feedback mech-

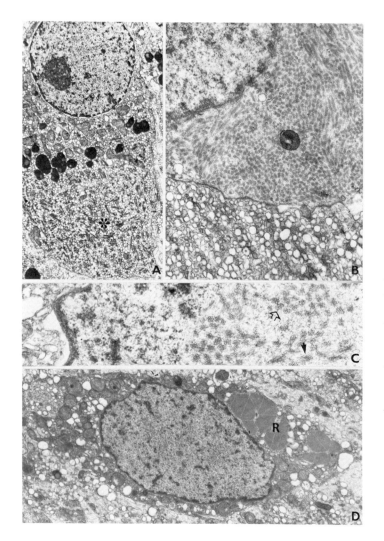

FIGURE 11-3. *Postpubertal Klinefelter's syndrome. Leydig cells. A, Leydig cells with sparse lipids and lipofuscins and abundant paracrystalline inclusions (asterisk) (×7500). B, Part of the cytoplasm of two adjacent Leydig cells showing a considerable disproportion in the number of paracrystalline inclusions (×20,000). C, Intranuclear paracrystalline inclusions. Those cut transversely present the image of a lamina folded four times (open arrow). Those cut longitudinally show a periodic structure formed by five parallel laminas (arrow) (×35,000). D, Leydig cells with minimal development of the smooth endoplasmic reticulum, abundant mitochondria containing dense granules, and numerous Reinke's crystals of reduced size (×6,500).*

anism of hormone control inhibiting the hypothalamus-pituitary axis. Total and free serum estrogen levels are normal or elevated. The conversion of testosterone into estradiol is increased (Gabrilove and co-workers, 1980).

The remaining hormonal determinations reveal a hypergonadotropic hypogonadism, with an increase in both follicle-stimulating hormone (FSH) and luteinizing hormone (LH) values. Examination of the hypothalamic-hypophyseal-gonadal axis shows proper functioning, in spite of great rigidity (Hsueh and co-workers, 1978). Exceptionally, low FSH and LH levels have been reported in patients with chromatin positive Klinefelter's syndrome (Nistal and others, 1980; Rabinowitz and co-authors, 1975). This suggests a hypogonadotropic hypogonadism associated with the primary hypogonadism in these cases.

The most frequent variants of true Klinefelter's syndrome are as follows:

1. XX/XXY. This constitutes, after the 47,XXY karyotype, the most frequent variant of Klinefelter's syndrome. Its most striking characteristics are the following: gynecomastia in only 33 percent of cases (compared with 55 percent in the XXY), azoo-

spermia in 50 percent (compared with 93 percent in the XXY), larger testes, and comparatively maintained spermatogenesis (Schreiber and others, 1976).
2. XXYY. Characteristics of this variety are the aggressive character and antisocial behavior of the patients. Their height is greater than that in XXY karyotype. Peripheral vein disorders are frequent. They can also present a characteristic dermatoglyphic pattern (Nistal and co-authors, 1978) (Figs. 11–4 and 11–5).
3. XXXY and XXXYY. Most salient characteristics are the mental retardation and skeletal malformations, such as radioulnar synostosis. It is in these variants of Klinefelter's syndrome that the highest incidence of cryptorchidism has been described (Ferguson-Smith and others, 1960).
4. XXXXY. A variant described by Fraccaro and co-workers (1960) refers to a group of patients presenting, in addition to the clinical symptoms of Klinefelter's syndrome, with severe mental retardation, hypoplasia of external genitalia, and, frequently, cryptorchidism and other anomalies, such

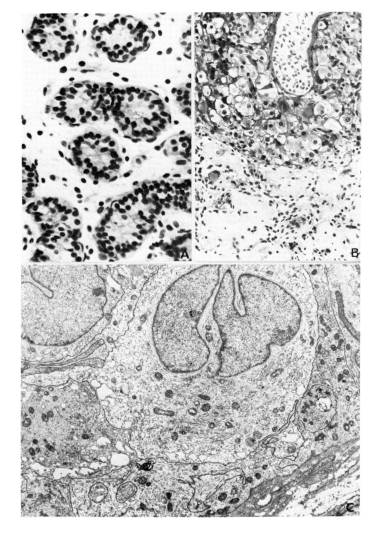

FIGURE 11–4. *48,XXYY Klinefelter's syndrome. A, Seminiferous tubules with slight reduction in mean tubular diameter and intense reduction in tubular fertility index in an 8-year-old boy (H&E, x250). B, Diffuse tubular sclerosis associated with Leydig cell adenomatous hyperplasia in a 17-year-old male. The seminiferous tubule located between the Leydig cells has a marked pseudostratification of the Sertoli cells and absence of apparent central lumen (Masson trichrome, x250). C, Sertoli cells corresponding to the seminiferous tubule mentioned in B, having intermediate characteristics between immature and mature Sertoli cells (x10,000).*

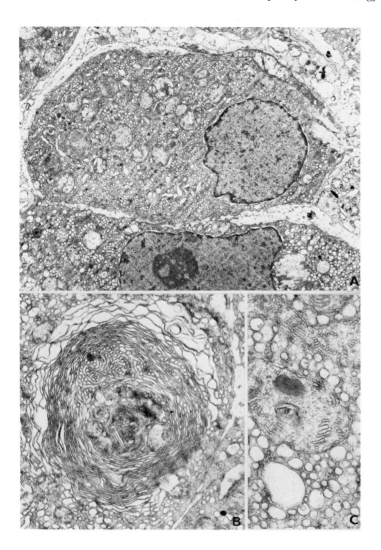

FIGURE 11–5. *48,XXYY Klinefelter's syndrome. Leydig cells. A, Leydig cells with abundant spherical and ovoid megamitochondria and absence of lipids and lipofuscins. Moderate development of the smooth endoplasmic reticulum is seen (x8500). B, Concentric laminar cisternae of the smooth endoplasmic reticulum enclosing cytoplasmic waste (x23,000). C, Megamitochondrion with an electron dense inclusion and a laminar inclusion (x52,000).*

as cardiac malformations, radioulnar synostosis, microcephaly, and high arched palate.

False Klinefelter's Syndrome

Negative sex chromatin Klinefelter's syndrome patients represent approximately 20 to 60 percent of all patients with Klinefelter's syndrome. In 40 percent of Klinefelter's syndrome patients with negative sex chromatin in buccal smears, a testicular mosaic has been observed. This fact, along with the presence of a phenotype similar to that of true Klinefelter's syndrome and some variable histological findings, makes it difficult to define the concepts that separate true and false Klinefelter's syndromes.

Ferguson-Smith (1966), on a histopathological basis, distinguished between two groups of patients with negative sex chromatin: those without germ cells and those with postpubertal testicular atrophy.

Negative sex chromatin Klinefelter's syndrome with an absence of germ cells rarely presents either tubular hyalinization or peritubular fibrosis. The tubules are lined with only Sertoli cells and a few isolated spermatogonia. The interstitium shows a diffuse Leydig cell hyperplasia.

The syndrome could be due to a defect in embryogenesis.

Negative sex chromatin Klinefelter's syndrome with postpubertal testicular atrophy is characterized by the presence of hyalinized seminiferous tubules. The tunica propria contains a great amount of elastic fibers, suggesting that the atrophy develops after puberty. Other tubules contain only Sertoli cells. Leydig cell number is increased. On the whole, the histological picture is similar to that observed in testicular atrophy secondary to mumps virus orchitis or testicular atrophy due to radiation.

Another group, constituted by negative sex chromatin Klinefelter's syndrome patients in which the histological findings reveal practically normal spermatogenesis, must be added to these two groups (Nasr and co-workers, 1971).

Prepubertal Klinefelter's Syndrome

Identification of a clinicopathological entity of Klinefelter's syndrome during childhood has been made possible by two factors: First, the systematic karyotype study of all newborns with positive sex chromatin; and second, the study of sex chromatin in all mentally retarded children (Ferguson-Smith, 1959).

Children with Klinefelter's syndrome present some interesting clinical symptoms that can be suggestive of the disorder: mental retardation or psychiatric problems, a taller stature than is normal for their age, with disproportionately long arms and small testes.

In most of the cases, testis development is abnormal. The mean tubular diameter is markedly decreased and the tubular fertility index is low. It is even possible to observe the absence of germ cells in some biopsies. The Sertoli cell index is decreased. Megatubules and ring-shaped tubules are frequent. The interstitium is ample and shows sparse Leydig cell precursors. On the whole, the histological pattern can be interpreted as that of a diffuse tubular hypoplasia. In those testes presenting spermatogonia, these progressively disappear during childhood (Gracia and co-authors, 1974) (Figs. 11-6A and B).

In the biopsies performed during puberty, a rapidly developing tubular sclerosis, in addition to a progressive increase in Leydig cell number, has been observed.

Hormonal assays carried out in infants with Klinefelter's syndrome reveal normal FSH and LH levels. This suggests that the pituitary hyperfunction begins at puberty, compared with the precocious manifestation of testicular lesions.

Klinefelter's Syndrome and Malignant Tumors

It has been shown that patients with Klinefelter's syndrome have a higher incidence of malignant tumors than normal males (Coley and others, 1971). Male breast cancer, first described in a patient with Klinefelter's syndrome by Jackson and co-authors (1965), is about 20 times more frequent than in normal males (Mies and others, 1982). Extragonadal germ cell tumors also have a higher incidence. The most frequent are: choriocarcinoma, teratoma, yolk-sac tumor, and embryonal carcinoma—all of which are located in the mediastinum—teratocarcinoma in the pineal region, and seminoma in both retroperitoneum and testis. Other tumor types, such as lymphoma, leukemia, transitional cell carcinoma of the bladder, prostate adenocarcinoma, and testicular interstitial cell tumor found in Klinefelter's syndrome do not seem to occur more frequently than in normal males (Curri and co-workers, 1981).

46,XX Males (La Chapelle Syndrome or 46,XX Klinefelter's Syndrome)

46,XX males have a male phenotype and male psychosexual behavior, but have hypogonadism of testicular origin.

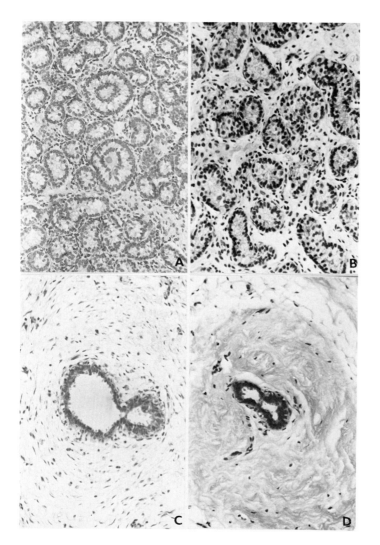

FIGURE 11-6. *A and B: 47,XXY prepubertal Klinefelter's syndrome. A, A 6-year-old boy. The seminiferous tubules have a reduced mean tubular diameter and lack germ cells. Two ring-shaped tubules can be observed (H&E, x125). B, A 9-year-old boy. Testicular parenchyma showing seminiferous tubules with or without germ cells displaying a mosaic distribution (H&E, x125). C and D, Two different patterns of mammary development in gynecomastia. C, Marked ductal proliferation, surrounded by loose connective tissue (H&E, x60). D, Lactiferous duct surrounded by an intensely collagenized stroma. This morphological variant can be seen in gynecomastia of long evolution (H&E, x60).*

This syndrome was described by La Chapelle and others (1964), and its incidence, both among patients evaluated for infertility and the general population, is very low. Statistics concerning male children reveal two XX males per 61,742 male births. La Chapelle confirmed the incidence of one case per 9000 births (1972).

XX males form a group of patients that has many common traits. Height, with some exceptions, is less than in males with normal karyotype, but greater than that of females. Body proportions are harmonious. Among the secondary sex characteristics, the most striking are the sparse beard and body hair, which in some cases has a feminine distribution. Nearly one-third of the patients have gynecomastia. Intelligence is usually normal (Fig. 11–6C and D).

The testicular histological pattern is that of tubular dysgenesis, the expression of which varies little from one case to the next, depending on whether the patients are pre- or postpubertal. In the infantile testes, the histological pattern varies from normal to absence of germ cells. In adult testes, three different patterns can be seen: (1) tubular sclerosis with adenomatous hyperplasia of the Leydig cells, which is the characteristic pattern of 47,XXY Klinefelter's syndrome (Nistal and others,

1975); (2) absence of germ cells with normality of the remaining tubular and interstitial components, compatible with the pattern seen in the Del Castillo's syndrome (Nistal and Paniagua, 1979; Romani and co-authors, 1977); (3) an intermediate pattern, with seminiferous tubules lined only with Sertoli cells, variable degrees of thickening of the tunica propria up to total sclerosis, and a marked diffuse nonadenomatous Leydig cell hyperplasia. This is the most frequent pattern. In isolated cases, some spermatogonia can be observed (Figs. 11–7 and 11–8).

In order to differentiate between XX males and Klinefelter's syndrome, the following criteria should be taken into account:

The general aspect of the XX male is typical male, as opposed to what occurs in Klinefelter's syndrome. However, while this is the general rule, one must not forget that a small group of XX males presents eunuchoid proportions and that XXY patients cover a clinical spectrum from the classical form to the completely viril.

A high incidence of Klinefelter's syndrome in population samples with mental retardation (four time greater than in the normal population) is not reflected in the XX males.

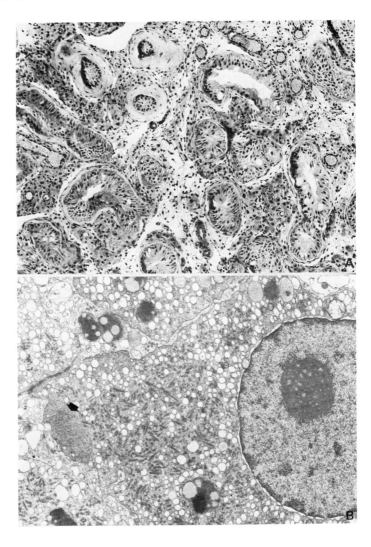

FIGURE 11–7. *46,XX male. A, Most of the seminiferous tubules show only Sertoli cells. In some of the tubules total or partial sclerosis can be seen. The Leydig cells present diffuse hyperplasia (Masson trichrome, x60). B, Leydig cells with paracrystalline inclusions and groups of microfilaments (arrow) (x17.000).*

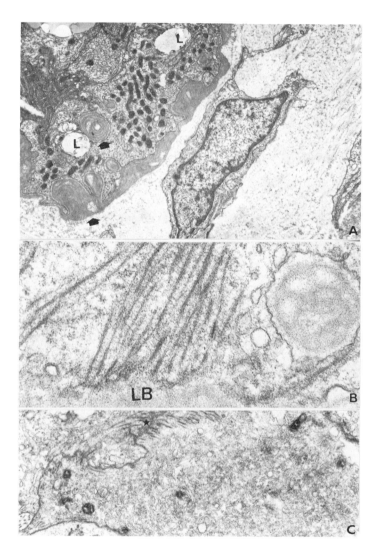

FIGURE 11-8. *46,XX male. Seminiferous tubules. A, Reduplication of the basal lamina with the formation of protrusions toward the inside of the Sertoli cells (arrows). The basal part of the Sertoli cells shows voluminous lipid inclusions (L), and abundant mitochondria (x12,000). B, Groups of thick, parallel microfilaments, perpendicular to the basal lamina (LB) in the lower portion of the Sertoli cell (x40,000). C, Abundant microfilaments irregularly distributed throughout the cytoplasm of the Sertoli cells. Thick filaments, similar to those in B, joining in the union zone of two Sertoli cells (star) (x20,000).*

In Klinefelter's syndrome, hormone assays reveal high gonadotropin levels, but in more than half of XX males those values are absolutely normal.

The testicular histological pattern presents two conditions in XX males that are not as marked as in the Klinefelter's syndrome: tendency to show tubular sclerosis and Leydig cell hyperplasia. Another interesting feature is the presence of elastic fibers in the majority of the seminiferous tubules of the XX males, whereas they are absent in true Klinefelter's syndrome.

The origin of the genetic anomaly that determines the occurrence of this syndrome still remains hypothetical, and the following tentative explanations have been offered:

1. The autosomal mutation gene theory. This hypothesis suggests a zygote that, after undergoing a mutation that would convert an autosomal gene into a masculinizing gene, would develop a male phenotype. This would avoid the necessity of the presence of a Y chromosome in order to assure male differentiation, as occurs in Drosophyla. Were this hypothesis true, consanguinity between XX male parents, a high familial incidence, and a higher proportion of boys over girls would

be frequently found in these patients.
2. Mosaic theory or Y chromosome line elimination. The zygote would have the same chromosomal constitution as XXY Klinefelter's syndrome. In later divisions, two cell lines would be formed: one with two X chromosomes, and one with XY chromosomes. The latter would cause gonadal differentiation and, ultimately, be lost or reduced to a minimal expression.
3. Translocation theory. The gene responsible for male differentiation would be translocated either onto an autosomal chromosome (which would have to be detectable) or onto the X chromosome or would remain in a small Y chromosome fragment (Ferguson-Smith, 1966).

This theory enjoys the widest acceptance. During the first meiotic division of primary spermatocytes, the X and Y chromosomes form the sex pair or sex vesicle, and establish synaptonemal complexes in several regions, allowing a reciprocal gene interchange. In this fashion, male gametes with normal X chromosomes or with X chromosomes with an incorporated Y chromosome fragment are formed. The latter, when fertilizing the ova, would form zygotes in which the sex would depend on whether or not the active X chromosome was female or male, leaving open the possibility of mosaicism. In this way, depending on the predominance or balance of the cell lines, either normal phenotypes with ovaries or testes or true hermaphrodites with ovotestes could arise (Butler and others, 1983).

Until now, no cases of XX males with spermatogenesis have been described; however, in rats with an XX complement, mosaics with tubules lacking germ cells and tubules with complete spermatogenesis have been observed. As in Klinefelter's syndrome with spermatogenesis, Ohno's interpretation of the mosaic resides in the formation of two germ cell types: one with an XXX karyotype that degenerates, and another with an XO karyotype that differentiates and produces spermatozoa with an X or O chromosome. However, these spermatozoa are infertile, suggesting that, in addition to the gene that determines the sex, the Y chromosome carries another, minor gene that is responsible for perfect spermatogenesis development.

H-Y antigen has been found in all XX males examined for this antigen, which suggests that the Y chromosome gene responsible for H-Y antigen is involved in gonadal differentiation (Wachtel, 1979).

XYY Syndrome

The existence of the karyotype 47,XYY was first described by Sanberg and others (1961) in a normal male (father of a mongoloid girl) whose only striking feature was his tall stature. Later, the frequency of this karyotype was studied in mental institutions and penitentiaries and found to be 3.6 percent (Jacobs and coworkers, 1965), so that it was linked to tall individuals, genetically predisposed toward a psychopathic personality and an antisocial behavior. More recent studies have shown that the frequency of this karyotype is 3 percent in institutions for subjects with antisocial behavior, compared with 1.8 percent in the general population. Most of the people belonging to this latter group are totally normal, well adapted individuals.

On the other hand, the sexual characteristics of these subjects have been studied during the past few years, and it has been found that the development of the external genitalia and secondary sex characteristics are normal, but that their fertility is slightly diminished.

Study of the testicular biopsy in carriers of the XYY karyotype shows that the seminiferous epithelium is affected in most cases. The changes observed are in the same testis and affect the tubules to varying degrees, forming a mosaic in which one can observe various patterns: tubules with only Sertoli cells, tubules with normal spermatogenesis, and tubules with maturation arrest at the primary spermatocyte level. The proportion in which these types of tubules combine is variable. In a large number of patients examined it was found that, in all, 50 percent of the seminiferous tubules in the XYY males have maturation arrest, and 30 percent have only Sertoli cells, with the remaining tubules being normal (Skakkebaek and co-authors, 1973a).

These numbers are in agreement with the low sperm levels found in most of the semen analyses. Although cases of paternity have been reported, in general, males with XYY karyotype have a diminished fertility (Kjessler and Berg, 1978).

Both the morphological pattern and the proportion of Leydig cells in the testicular interstitium are normal, which is in accordance with the normal androgren and gonadotropin levels observed.

The cause of this seminiferous tubule affect is as yet unknown. Although it has been suggested that spermatogenesis is reduced due to a decreased viability of the germ cells with decompensated genetic material. Studies in XYY males seem to indicate that the second Y chromosome is absent in most primary spermatocytes (Tettenborn and others, 1970).

Males with more than two Y chromosomes are very infrequent. Only a few men with three Y chromosomes (Hunter and Quaife, 1973) and recently one man with a 49,XYYYY karyotype have been reported (Sirota and co-workers, 1981).

Noonan's Syndrome

Noonan's syndrome (Noonan and Ehmke, 1963) refers to subjects with a male phenotype presenting various somatic anomalies similar to those observed in Turner's syndrome, but with a normal chromosomal pattern. In the past, these patients were considered to present a form of Turner's syndrome, which was termed "male Turner's syndrome." Lately, it has been found that Noonan's syndrome can also affect females with a normal female karyotype. In both cases, the gonads differentiate following the chromosomal sex. The syndrome is probably inherited as an autosomal dominant trait; however, no chromosomal anomalies have been found to be responsible.

In the male, Noonan's syndrome has the following characteristics in common with Turner's syndrome: short stature, webbing of the neck, and cubitus valgus. In addition, the affected subjects usually present other anomalous traits with greater frequency than do patients with Turner's syndrome: wide forehead, hypertelorism, micrognathia, inner epicanthal folds, flattened nose bridge, low set of posteriorly rotated ears, pectus excavatum, high arched palate, shield-shape chest, dental malocclusion, palpebral ptosis, abnormal dermatoglyphics, cryptorchidism, and congenital cardiovascular diseases (Figs. 11–9**A** and **B**). Whereas in Turner's syndrome the most characteristic cardiac abnormalities are aortic coarctation and stenosis, in Noonan's syndrome they are pulmonary stenosis, persistence of the ductus arteriosus, and defects of the interventricular septum (Hirsch and others, 1975). In these patients, marked mental retardation, Hashimoto's thyroiditis, and radiologically detectable urinary tract abnormalities, such as anomalous kidney rotation, duplication and hydronephrosis are also relatively frequent (Riggs, 1965). The hypogonadism present in Noonan's syndrome may be either hypergonadotropic or hypogonadotropic. Pubertal delay is also frequent (Schirren and Funey, 1982). Seventy percent of males with Noonan's syndrome have cryptorchidism, which is generally bilateral (Redman, 1973). In scrotal testes, prepubertal biopsies show a low tubular fertility index or absence of germ cells, and a minimal or marked decrease in tubular diameter.

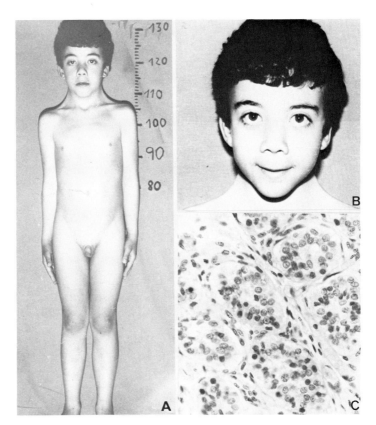

FIGURE 11-9. *Noonan's syndrome.* A and B, A 9-year-old boy presenting, in addition to other clinical features, pterygium colli, broad chest, cubitus valgus, and characteristic facies. C, Testis in the same patient with decreased tubular fertility index (H&E, x250).

Postpubertal biopsies have been found to be normal in some cases, but the most frequent changes are seminiferous tubules with immature Sertoli cells, marked germ cell hypoplasia, and progressive hyalinization of the basement membrane. In the interstitium, Leydig cells are sparse, accounting for the androgen deficiency found in most of these patients (Nistal and others, 1983). (Fig. 11-9C).

HYPOGONADISM LINKED TO AUTOSOMAL CHROMOSOME ABERRATIONS

With the growing practice of studying the karyotype of patients evaluated for infertility, it has been demonstrated that some autosomal anomalies can be responsible for failure in spermatogenesis, although, obviously, the presence of a chromosomal anomaly does not necessarily imply testicular alteration.

Among the autosomal anomalies most frequently found associatied with testicular defects are the following: Down's syndrome (trisomy 21) with or without linkage to other chromosomal defects; various translocations, such as those between D chromosomes, between chromosomes 14 and 21, and between chromosomes 10 and 15; patients with a small, central, extra chromosomal fragment; and t-balanced autosomal translocations (8-15).

The mechanisms by which these chromosomal alterations cause testicular deficiencies are unknown.

Down's Syndrome

The syndrome described by Langdon Down includes mental retardation, congenital malformations, such as short and thick fingers with clinodactyly, characteristic facies, flat facial traits, brachycephaly, articular laxity, Brushfield spots, and characteristic dermatoglyphics. Sixty percent of these patients die before the age of 10 years. The karyotype shows a triple chromosome 21 and, very often, translocations associated with this chromosome, such as those between chromosomes 13 and 21 or 2 and 21 (Miller and others, 1970).

The testes in these patients are either small or normal and can vary in the same individual. The secondary sex characteristics are normal. The semen analysis reveals oligospermia or azoospermia, and low quality semen (László, 1978). Histological study of these testes shows germ cell line alterations in most cases. The most frequent finding is that of a minimum reduction in germ cells with maturation arrest at the level of the primary spermatocyte. In some cases, the seminiferous tubules can have Sertoli cells only or Sertoli cells with some germ cells. These patterns often overlap, and, on occasion, the mosaic is even more heterogeneous, ranging from completely sclerosed tubules to normal ones. The interstitium has a normal aspect and Leydig cell alterations are not observed (Skakkebaek, and co-authors, 1973b).

Other Autosomal Aberrations

Although the number of testicular biopsies is not yet sufficiently large to allow generalizations, the data obtained permit us to maintain that a correlation between some chromosomal aberrations and testicular anomalies exists.

Patients with translocations between group D chromosomes show a normal phenotype, with testicular size and secondary sex characteristics being normal. However, histological study of the testis reveals maturation arrest at the level of the primary spermatocyte.

The carriers of translocations between chromosomes 14 and 21 on occasion have normal testes and spermatogenesis, but in other cases show maturation arrest at the level of the primary spermatocyte.

Testicular biopsies in a male with translocation between chromosomes 10 and 15, in whom the semen analysis revealed oligospermia and from 2 to 3 percent motile spermatozoa, show an incomplete maturation arrest of spermatogenesis in most of the seminiferous tubules.

Males with an extra small and central chromosomal fragment have normal-sized testes with germ cell hypoplasia or maturation arrest of the primary spermatocytes (Khurd and others, 1973; Skakkebaek and co-authors, 1973b).

DEL CASTILLO-TRABUCCO-DE LA BALZE SYNDROME (SERTOLI-CELL-ONLY SYNDROME)

In 1947 Del Castillo and others described a syndrome characterized by the complete absence of germ cells in the seminiferous tubule epithelium called Sertoli-cell-only syndrome. These patients have normal external genitalia and secondary sex characteristics, their only alteration being the reduced size of the testes and azoospermia. Del Castillo et al found low 17-ketosteroid levels in the urine and normal FSH levels. In order to explain the absence of germ cells, they suggested that no primordial germ cells were present during the embryonic differentiation of the gonads.

Later, the study of a greater number of these patients and the development of new hormonal determination techniques demonstrated that in general FSH levels were considerable increased. In many cases, it has been possible to verify that LH levels are also high, although not so high as FSH, and that on occasion testosterone levels are slightly lower than normal (Ishida and co-authors, 1976).

The testicular biopsies performed demonstrate seminiferous tubules with a slightly decreased diameter and with an enlarged basement membrane. The tubular epithelium contains only either immature (Nistal and others, 1982) or adult Sertoli cells (Chemes and others, 1977) with abundant microfilaments, extensive junctional complexes and deep interdigitations, and is completely devoid of germ cells. In the interstitium, the Leydig cells have a normal morphological pattern and may be slightly increased in number (Guay and co-workers, 1977). In some cases, multivacuolated Leydig cells and Leydig cells containing paracrystalline inclusions have also been found (Paniagua and co-authors, 1984), (Fig 11–10).

The Del Castillo's syndrome is considered to be a primary testicular disorder due to different causes, principally of congenital origin, although in some cases the possibility of acquired lesions cannot be discarded. Among the congenital lesions, failure in the migration of the primordial germ cells from the yolk sac to the genital ridge must be included. Among the acquired lesions are those caused by radiation, although testicular radiation almost never leads to the loss of germ cells exclusively, but rather to the progressive hyalinization of the basement membrane and from there to the sclerosis of the seminiferous tubules. The Leydig cells should also be somewhat damaged, since high LH

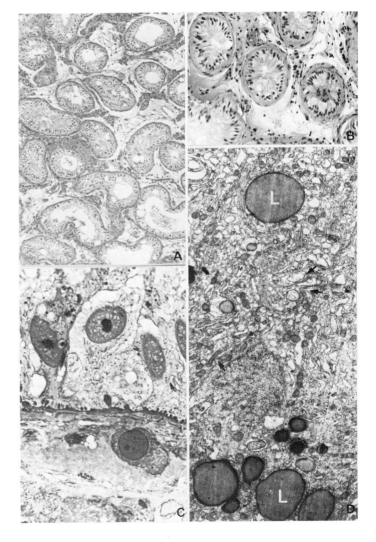

FIGURE 11–10. *Del Castillo's syndrome. A, Seminiferous tubules with decreased diameter and only Sertoli cells. Slight increase in Leydig cell number (H&E, x60). B, Thickening of the basement membrane and pseudostratification of Sertoli cells in the seminiferous tubules. Absence of germ cells (H&E, x125). C, Intense vacuolation of the Sertoli cell cytoplasm, 1 μm thick section (toluidine blue, x1250). D, Sertoli cells with increase in lipid content (L), complex interdigitations, and extensive junctional complexes between the Sertoli cells (arrows) (x7000).*

and low testosterone levels are observed. However, the reserve capacity of these cells is preserved, as shown by their stimulation with HCG.

Patients with 47,XXY Klinefelter's syndrome whose seminiferous tubules contain only Sertoli cells show much higher FSH and LH levels and a very deficient response to HCG stimulation in comparison with males with Del Castillo's syndrome (Ishida and co-authors, 1976).

WERNER'S SYNDROME (PROGERIA)

Werner's syndrome is inherited as an autosomal recessive disorder characterized by short stature, premature graying hair and baldness, cataracts, muscular and subcutaneous atrophy in which the adipose tissue is substituted by fibrous connective tissue that can become calcified, wrinkling of the skin, keratosis, osteoporosis, telangiectasia, atheroma, diabetes mellitus, gynecomastia, and hypogonadism. The testes have tubular atrophy, thickening of the basement membrane, and increase in Leydig cell number.

It has been suggested that the cause lies with an alteration in connective tissue metabolism, consisting in a shortening of fibroblast life span (Zucker-Franklin and others, 1968).

MYOTONIC DYSTROPHY

The myotonic dystrophy that is found in 30 percent of adult patients presenting with muscular disorders is generally associated with hypogonadism, cataracts, and frontal baldness in males (Fig. 11–11A and B). In most patients with myotonic dystrophy, the hypogonadism is of the hypergonadotropic type. It goes unnoticed until adulthood. The secondary sex characteristics are well-developed and the external genitalia are normal, although the testes are usually somewhat small. These patients are infertile and the testicular biopsy shows atrophy of the seminiferous tubules, with reduced diameter and fibrosis. The Sertoli cells appear vacuolated and degenerated. The germ cells are sparse. The Leydig cells are normal or hyperplastic. Hormonal determinations reveal high FSH levels and mormal, or at times high, LH levels. Testosterone levels are normal, or at times low. Generally, patients with normal testosterone levels are those who have Leydig cell hyperplasia. Morphological and histochemical findings suggest that the primary testicular lesion is a Sertoli cell insufficiency.

In another group of patients with myotonic dystrophy eunuchoid traits with infantile genitalia and failure in development of secondary sex characteristics have been described. Testosterone, LH, and FSH levels are very low. In this group of patients, the hypogonadism is of the hypogonadotropic type (Febres and co-authors, 1975).

PROGRESSIVE MUSCULAR DYSTROPHY

Hypogonadism is a frequent finding in progressive juvenile muscular dystrophy, which it inherited as an X-linked trait (Fig. 11–11C). The patients rarely reach the age of 20 years, and their last years are spent bedridden. The testicular histological pattern is similar to the one found in Klinefelter's syndrome (Fig. 11–11D).

ALSTRÖM-EDWARDS SYNDROME

In this syndrome, described by Alström and others (1959), hypogonadism associated with pigmentary retinopathy, neurogenous deafness, and anomalous glucose metabolism is present.

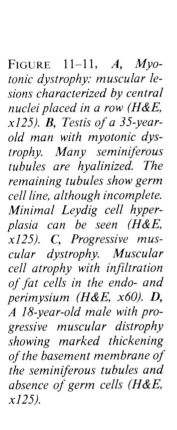
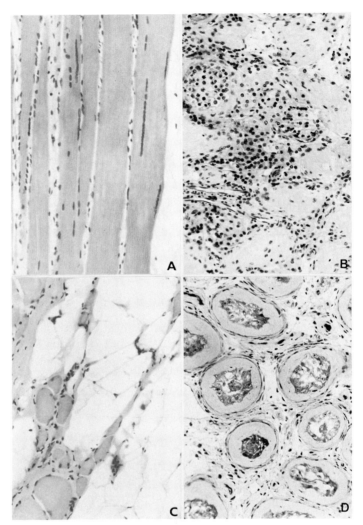

FIGURE 11-11, *A*, Myotonic dystrophy: muscular lesions characterized by central nuclei placed in a row (H&E, x125). *B*, Testis of a 35-year-old man with myotonic dystrophy. Many seminiferous tubules are hyalinized. The remaining tubules show germ cell line, although incomplete. Minimal Leydig cell hyperplasia can be seen (H&E, x125). *C*, Progressive muscular dystrophy. Muscular cell atrophy with infiltration of fat cells in the endo- and perimysium (H&E, x60). *D*, A 18-year-old male with progressive muscular distrophy showing marked thickening of the basement membrane of the seminiferous tubules and absence of germ cells (H&E, x125).

Obesity and diabetes mellitus are frequent.

The secondary sex characteristics are generally well-developed. In males, the penis is normal sized, but the testes are considerably smaller than normal. Patients having subvirilization, gynecomastia, and mental retardation, in addition to the described characteristics, have been reported as a variant of this syndrome (Edwards and co-workers, 1976).

Hormonal determinations reveal high FSH and LH levels, and testosterone levels within normal or below normal limits. The hypothalamic-hypophyseal-testicular axis is shown to function properly. Response to the administration of HCG is very limited. The hypogonadism is therefore of the hypergonadotropic type. Its familial presentation suggests that it is inherited as an autosomal recessive trait.

The testicular biopsy shows thickening and hyalinization of the basement membrane in the seminiferous tubules and absence of peritubular elastic fibers. An epithelium consisting of Sertoli cells and a few spermatogonia can be seen in the tubules not yet completely hyalinized. The interstitium shows hyperplasia of Leydig cells, which are arranged in clumps and contain Reinke's crystals. This histological pattern is similar to that of Klinefelter's syndrome, from which it can be differentiated by the absence of sex chromatin.

Androgen synthesis by the Leydig cells in patients with Alström's syndrome is considered to be sufficient for the development and maintenance of the secondary sex characteristics, but it is insufficient for producing normal testosterone levels, in spite of the high Leydig cell number and the high pituitary LH secretion.

Rudimentary Testes Syndrome

The term "rudimentary testes syndrome" was introduced by Bergada and others (1962) with reference to a clinical condition characterized by the presence of a hypoplastic penis and very small testes in male children with a male phenotype and negative sex chromatin. The testes measure less than 0.7 cm in length. Microscopically, they are formed by fibrous connective tissue with sparse nests of testicular parenchyma. During infancy, the seminiferous tubules can have both Sertoli cells and spermatogonia (Najjar and co-workers, 1974). After puberty, they only have Sertoli cells, although the testicular interstitium has some mature Leydig cells.

Hormonal assays performed in these males are like those characteristic of hypergonadotropic hypogonadism. The male phenotype, including absence of ambiguous genitalia, may be attributed to the normal testicular differentiation during the first 3 months of gestation, giving rise to complete male differentiation. The causes of the posterior testicular atrophy are unknown. There is no evidence of genetic anomaly in most cases studied (Glass, 1982).

Other Types of Hypergonadotropic Hypogonadism

Weinstein's Syndrome

This syndrome is characterized by a tubular dysgenesis similar to that found in Klinefelter's syndrome, from which it can only be differentiated by the absence of sex chromatin in the Leydig cells. The syndrome is completed by deafness, blindness, and metabolic anomalies (hyperuricemia, hypertriglyceridemia, and hyperprebetalipoproteinemia) (Weinstein and others, 1969).

Sohval-Soffer Syndrome

This syndrome was described in 1953 by Sohval and Soffer (1953) in two brothers and was characterized by mental retardation, multiple skeletal anomalies, and hypogonadism. The hypogonadism included small and soft testes, small penis, underdevelopment of the secondary sex characteristics, azoospermia, and gynecomastia. Histological study shows two types of seminiferous tubules: one formed by tubules containing only Sertoli cells and lacking a lumen and another with hyalinization. Leydig cells were sparse in one of the brothers and distributed in clumps in the other. The gonadotropin determinations gave high values.

REFERENCES

1. Alström CH, Hallgren B, Nilssen LB, Asander H: Retinal degeneration combined with obesity, diabetes mellitus and neurogenous deafness. Acta Psychiatr Neurol Scand [Suppl] 129:34, 1959
2. Becker KL: Clinical and therapeutic experi-

ences with Klinefelter's syndrome. Fertil Steril 23:568, 1972
3. Bergada C, Cleveland WW, Jones HW, Wilkins L: Variants of embryonic testicular dysgenesis, bilateral anorchia and the syndrome of rudimentary testes. Acta Endocrinol 40:521, 1962
4. Boisen E: Testicular size and shape of 47,XYY and 47, XXY men in a double-blind, double-matched population survey. Am J Hum Genet 31:697, 1979
5. Butler MG, Walzak MP, Sanger WG, Todd CT: A possible etiology of the infertile 46XX male subject. J Urol 130:154, 1983
6. Chapelle A de la, Hortling H, Niemi M, Wennstrom J: XX sex chromosomes in a human male. First case. Acta Med Scand [Suppl] 412:25, 1964
7. Chapelle A de la: Analytic review: Nature and origin of males with XX sex chromosomes. Am J Hum Genet 24:71, 1972
8. Chemes HE, Dym M, Fawcett DW, Javadpour N, Sherins RJ: Patho-physiological observations of Sertoli cells in patients with germinal aplasia or severe germ cell depletion. Ultrastructural findings and hormone levels. Biol Reprod 17:108, 1977
9. Coley GM, Otis RD, Clark WE: Multiple primary tumors including bilateral breast cancer in a man with Klinefelter's syndrome. Cancer 27:1476, 1971
10. Curri WA, McKay CE, Richardson RL, Greco A: Klinefelter's syndrome and mediastinal germ cell neoplasms. J Urol 125:127, 1981
11. Del Castillo EB, Trabucco A, de la Balze FA: Syndrome produced by absence of the germinal epithelium without impairment of the Sertoli or Leydig cells. J Clin Endocrinol Metab 7:493, 1947
12. Edwards JA, Sethi PK, Scoma AJ, Bannerman RM, Frohman LA: A new familial syndrome characterized by pigmentary retinopathy, hypogonadism, mental retardation, nerve deafness and glucose intolerance. Am J Med 60:23, 1976
13. Febres F, Scaglia H, Lisker R, Espinosa J, Morato T, Shkurovich M, Pérez-Palacios G: Hypothalamic-pituitary-gonadal function in patients with myotonic dystrophy. J Clin Endocrinol Metab 41:833, 1975
14. Ferguson-Smith MA: The prepubertal testicular lesion in chromatin positive Klinefelter's syndrome as seen in mentally handicapped children. Lancet 1:219, 1959
15. Ferguson-Smith MA, Johnston AW, Handmaker S: Primary amentia and microorchidism associated with an XXXY sex-chromosome constitution. Lancet 2:184, 1960
16. Ferguson-Smith MA: X-Y chromosomal interchange in the etiology of true hermaphroditism and of XX Klinefelter's syndrome. Lancet 1:475, 1966
17. Fraccaro M, Kaijser K, Lindsten J: A child with 49 chromosomes. Lancet 2:899, 1960
18. Frohland A, Skakkebaek NE: Dimorphism in sex chromatin pattern of Sertoli cells in adults with Klinefelter's syndrome: Correlation with two types of "Sertoli-cell-only" tubes. J Clin Endocrinol Metab 33:683, 1971
19. Fukutani K, Ishida H, Shinohara M, Minowada S, Niijima T, Isurugi K: Responses of serum testosterone levels to human chorionic gonadotrophin stimulation in patients with Klinefelter's syndrome after long-term androgen replacement therapy. Int J Androl 6:5, 1983
20. Gabrilove JL, Freiberg EK, Nicolis GL: Testicular function in Klinefelter's syndrome. J Urol 124:825, 1980
21. Glass AR: Identical twins discordant for the "rudimentary testes" syndrome. J Urol 127:140, 1982
22. Grabski J, Pusch H, Schirren C, Passarge E, Held K, Bartsch W, Wernicke I: Klinische hormonale, histologische und chromosomale Untersuchungen beim Klinefelter-Syndrom. Andrologia 11:182, 1979
23. Gracia R, Martín-Alvarez L, Figols J, Lledó G, Nistal M, Barreiro E: Síndrome XXY (Klinefelter) en el periodo prepuberal. Estudio de ocho observaciones. Ann Esp Pediatr 7:510, 1974
24. Guay AT, Tuthill RJ, Woolf PD: Germinal cell aplasia: Response of luteinizing hormone (LH), follicle-stimulating hormone (FSH), and testosterone to LH/FSH-releasing hormone with histopathologic correlation. Fertil Steril 28:642, 1977
25. Heller CG, Nelson WC: Hyalinization of the seminiferous tubules associated with normal or failing Leydig cell function. Discussion of relationship to eunuchoidism, gynecomastia, elevated gonadotropins, depressed 17-ketosteroids and estrogens. J Clin Endocrinol Metabol 5:1, 1945
26. Hirsch H, Gelband H, Garcia O, Gottlieb S, Tamer D: Rapidly progressive obstructive cardiomyopathy in infants with Noonan's syndrome. Report of two cases. Circulation 52:1161, 1975
27. Hsueh WA, Hsu TS, Federman DD: Endocrine features of Klinefelter's syndrome. Medicine 57:447, 1978
28. Hunter H, Quaife A: 48 XYYY male: A somatic and psychiatric description. J Med Genet 10:80, 1973
29. Ishida H, Isurugi K, Aso Y, Takayasu H, Ta-

makoi B: Endocrine studies in Sertoli-cell-only syndrome. J Urol 116:56, 1976
30. Jackson AW, Muldal S, Ockey CH, O'Connor PJ: Carcinoma of male breast in association with the Klinefelter's syndrome. Br Med J 1:223, 1965
31. Jacobs PA, Brunton M, Melville NM, Brittain RP, McClemont WF: Aggressive behavior, mental subnormality and the XYY male. Nature 208:1351, 1965
32. Khurd G, Naftolin F, Benirschke K, Zárate A, Guzmán-Toledano R: Unusual translocations and reproductive failure. Obst Gynecol 41:542, 1973
33. Kjessler B, Berg AA: Testicular steroid metabolism in vitro and spermatogenesis in male with an XYY-karyotype. Int J Androl 1:122, 1978
34. Klinefelter HF, Reifenstein EC, Albright F: Syndrome characterized by gynecomastia, aspermatogenesis with aleydigism and increased excretion of follicle-stimulating hormone. J Clin Endocrinol Metab 2:615, 1942
35. László H: Down Férfiak spermatogramjai. Anthrop Közl 22:117, 1978
36. Mies R, Fischer H, Pfeiff B, Winkelmann W, Würz H: Klinefelter's syndrome and breast cancer. Andrologia 14:317, 1982
37. Miller JR, Dill FJ, Corey MJ, Rigg JM: A rare translocation (47,XY, t(2p−; 21q+), 21+) associated with Down's syndrome. J Med Genet 7:389, 1970
38. Najjar SS, Takla RJ, Nassar VH: The syndrome of rudimentary testes: Occurrence in five siblings. J Pediatr 84:119, 1974
39. Nasr H, Chen JC, Pearson OH, Wieland RG: Chromatin-negative Klinefelter's syndrome with normal testes and serum gonadotropins and testosterone. Fertil Steril 22:761, 1971
40. Nistal M, Barreiro E, Herruzo A, López-Pajares I, Figols J: Varón con cariotipo 46,XX. Arch Esp Urol 28:263, 1975
41. Nistal M, Paniagua R, López-Pajares I: Ultrastructure of Leydig cells in Klinefelter's syndrome with 48,XXYY karyotype. Virchows Arch [Cell Pathol] 28:39, 1978
42. Nistal M, Paniagua R: Ultrastructure of testicular biopsy from an XX male. Virchows Arch [Cell Pathol] 31:45, 1979
43. Nistal M, Paniagua R, Abaurrea MA, Pallardo LF: 47,XXY Klinefelter's syndrome with low FSH and LH levels and absence of Leydig cells. Andrologia 12:426, 1980
44. Nistal M, Paniagua R, Abaurrea MA, Santamaría L: Hyperplasia and the immature appearance of Sertoli cells in primary testicular disorders. Hum Pathol 13:3, 1982
45. Nistal M, Paniagua R, Pallardo LF: Testicular biopsy and hormonal study in a male with Noonan's syndrome. Andrologia 15:415, 1983
46. Noonan JA, Ehmke DA: Associated noncardiac malformations in children with congenital heart disease. J Pediatr 63:468, 1963
47. Ohno S: Control of meiotic process. In Troen P, Nankin HR, (eds): The Testis in Normal and Infertile Men. New York: Raven Press, 1977, p.1
48. Paniagua R, Nistal M, Bravo MP: Leydig cell types in primary testicular disorders. Hum Pathol. 15:181, 1984
49. Paulsen CA, Gordon DL, Carpenter RW, Gandy HM, Drucker WD: Klinefelter's syndrome and its variants: A hormonal and chromosomal study. Recent Prog Horm Res 24:321, 1968
50. Rabinowitz D, Cohen MM, Rosenmann E, Rosenmann A, Segal S, Bell J, Rosler A, Spitz I: Chromatin-positive Klinefelter's syndrome with undetectable peripheral FSH levels. Am J Med 59:584, 1975
51. Redman J: Noonan's syndrome and cryptorchidism. J Urol 109:909, 1973
52. Riggs W: Roentgen findings in Noonan's syndrome. Radiology 96:48, 1965
53. Rimoin DL, Borganonkar DS, Asper SF: Chromatin-negative hypogonadism in phenotypic men. Am J Med 44:225, 1968
54. Romani F, Terquem A, Dadoune JP: Le testicule chez l'homme 46,XX. A propos d'une observation ultrastructurale. J Gynecol Obst Biol Rep 6:1049, 1977
55. Rubin P, Mattei A: Les lesions de la cellule de Leydig dans la maladie de Klinefelter, apport de la microscopie electronique. Rev Fr Endocrinol Clin Nutr Metabol 5:397, 1971
56. Sanberg AA, Koepf GF, Ishihara T, Hauschka TS: XYY human male. Lancet 2:488, 1961
57. Schirren C, Funey S: Andrologische Befunde bei Turner-Noonan-Syndrom. Andrologia 14:68, 1982
58. Schreiber D, Palutke W, Cohen MP: Hypothalamic hypothyroidism and XXY/XY sex chromosome mosaicism. Am J Clin Pathol 65:675, 1976
59. Sirota L, Zlotogora Y, Shabtai F, Halbrecht I, Elian E: 49,XYYYY. A case report. Clin Genet 19:87, 1981
60. Skakkebaek NE, Hulten M, Jacobsen P, Mikkelsen M: Quantification of human seminiferous epithelium. II. Histological studies in eight 47,XYY men. J Reprod Fertil 32:391, 1973a
61. Skakkebaek NE, Hulten M, Philip J: Quantification of human seminiferous epithelium. IV. Histological studies in 17 men with numerical and structural autosomal aberrations. Acta Pathol Microbiol Scand 81:112, 1973b
62. Sohval AR, Soffer LJ: Congenital testicular

deficiency. Defective Sertoli cell differentiation in hypogonadism of so-called "obscure origin." J Clin Endocrinol Metab 13:408, 1953
63. Steinberger E, Smith KD, Perloff WH: Spermatogenesis in Klinefelter's syndrome. J Clin Endocrinol Metab 25:1325, 1965
64. Tettenborn V, Gropp A, Murken ID, Tinnefeld W, Fuhrmann W, Schwinger E: Meiosis and testicular histology in XYY males. Lancet 2:267, 1970
65. Wachtel SS: Primary sex determination. Arthritis Rheum 22:1200, 1979
66. Weinstein RL, Kliman B, Scully RE: Familial syndrome of primary testicular insufficiency with normal virilization, blindness, deafness and metabolic abnormalities. N Engl J Med 281:979, 1969
67. Wong TW, Straus FH, Warner NE: Testicular biopsy in the study of male infertility. I Testicular causes of infertility. Arch Pathol 95:151, 1973
68. Zucker-Franklin D, Rifkin H, Jacobson HG: Werner's syndrome: An analysis of ten cases. Geriatrics 23:123, 1968

12

HYPOGONADISMS DUE TO SECONDARY TESTICULAR FAILURE

There are a group of clinical syndromes, characterized by gonadal hypofunction, that appear at a prepubertal age and are related to gonadotropin deficiency. These disorders are due to a hypothalamic-hypophyseal lesion and are referred to as "secondary or hypogonadotropic hypogonadisms (hypogonadotropic eunuchoidisms)." These patients present eunuchoid habitus and underdevelopment and incomplete genital maturation (Nistal and others, 1973).

On an etiopathological basis the following disorders can be included within this group: constitutional delay of puberty; idiopathic hypogonadotropic hypogonadism; hypogonadism with anosmia (Maestre de San Juan-Kallmann syndrome); the fertile eunuch syndrome (Pasqualini syndrome); hypogonadotropic hypogonadism associated with cerebelar ataxia; the Laurence-Moon-Rozabal-Bardet Biedl syndrome; hypogonadism associated with congenital ichthyosis; diabetes mellitus with hyperlipemia; mental retardation with microcephaly; and Moebius syndrome. Excluded from this group are: prepubertal hypogonadotropic hypogonadisms due to global pituitary deficiency (pituitary dwarfism), and hypogonadisms appearing at a postpubertal age.

CONSTITUTIONAL DELAY OF PUBERTY

This disorder is characterized by a delay in sexual maturation. It is often associated with genital or generalized adiposity and does not require hormonal treatment. It is generally accepted that this syndrome is due to a delay in the maturation of the hypothalamus.

The limits between normal and delayed puberty on one hand, and between delayed puberty and hypogonadotropic hypogonadism on the other, are not easy to establish. The most apparent physical change at puberty is the increase in testicular size (at approximately 13.5 years of age in 99 percent of boys), followed by an increase in stature and the appearance of secondary sex characteristics one or two years later. If there is not testicular size increase at 14 years of age, this suggests a delayed puberty. The familial presentation of delayed puberty is a frequent finding. Familial histories of pubertal development at ages between 14 and 18 years facilitate the diagnosis.

The limits between delayed puberty and hypogonadotropic hypogonadism are more difficult to define since there are histories of males who reached puberty at 18 years or even 20 years of age. When a delayed puberty is suspected, a prolonged observation of the patient is advisable. During this time, the gonadotropin tests are useful for diagnosis. If the gonadotropin levels are similar to those of prepubertal boys, or the repeated gonadotropin determinations reveal progressive increased values, the diagnosis of delayed puberty is strongly supported. The LH-RH test may have similar results.

IDIOPATHIC HYPOGONADOTROPIC HYPOGONADISM (ISOLATED GONADOTROPIN DEFICIT)

This disorder is characterized by a deficient synthesis or release of FSH and LH, with otherwise normal pituitary function. Patients with this syndrome never reach normal puberty; their proportions are eunuchoid, their body hair and beard are scarce, and their genitalia underdeveloped. Furthermore, they have a high-pitched voice, a slight muscular build, and are not able to ejaculate. Although this form of hypogonadism is not very frequent, it can occasionally affect various families belonging to the same generation. This defect has been shown to be inherited as an autosomal dominant (Ewer, 1968) or X-linked (Paulsen, 1968) recessive trait.

Hormone determinations for patients with this syndrome reveal very low gonadotropin, testosterone, and estrogen levels. The HCG stimulation test is frequently positive, but stimulation with clomiphene fails to produce an increase in either FSH, LH, or testosterone levels (Boyar and others, 1973). Stimulation with LH-RH can induce an increase in FSH and LH levels in some cases (Pallardo and others, 1972), but it has no effect in others. The lack of gonadotrophin response to LH-RH can be overcome by frequent administration of low doses of natural LH-RH in a pulsatile fashion (Varela DaCosta and co-workers, 1982; Donald and associates, 1983). Adequate androgenization and spermatogenesis has been reached in some patients after a prolonged treatment with either clomiphene, LH-RH, or a combination of HMG and HCG (Spitz and others, 1978) (Fig. 12-1). In patients undergoing treatment with HCG, one must realize that additional injections of HCG within a period of 48 hours does not cause an increase in the amount of testosterone produced by the Leydig cells (Smals and others, 1979). When fertility is not desired, secondary sex development can be induced with the administration of testosterone.

Maestre de San Juan-Kallmann-De Morsier Syndrome

In 1856, Maestre de San Juan described for the first time a syndrome characterized by the association of hypogon-

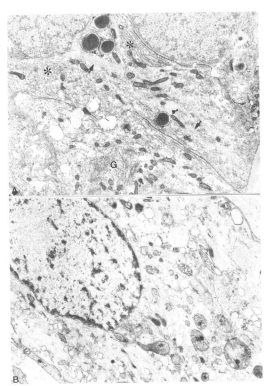

FIGURE 12-1. *Idiopathic hypogonadotropichypogonadism after 6 months treatment with HCG and HMG. A, Sertoli cells in which persist some of the characteristics of differentiating immature Sertoli cells, such as prominent Golgi complex (G), numerous rough reticular endoplasmic cisternae (asterisks) and numerous microfilaments (arrows) (x20,000).* ***B,*** *Differentiating Leydig cells with marked signs of hormonal stimulation: mitochondrial pleomorphism, absence of lipids, and moderate development of smooth endoplasmic reticulum (x20,000).*

adism and anosmia. Eighty-eight years later, Kallmann and others (1944) studied the same syndrome in three families, suggesting that a genetic factor was involved in its transmission. In 1954 De Morsier reviewed 31 cases in the literature of olfactory bulb agenesis and found that in 14 of the cases there was evidence of testicular atrophy as well. He designated the syndrome "olfacto-hypothalamo-genital dysplasia." The syndrome retains this name as well as that of the three mentioned authors and can be characterized as the congenital association of hypogonadotropic hypogonadism and anosmia or hyposmia, with or without the presence of additional cerebral or systemic malformations and anomalies. The syndrome represents almost 13 percent of all male hypogonadisms (Agulhon, 1971). Its presentation is familial or sporadic and affects, with preference, the male sex (De Morsier and Gauthier, 1963; Santen and Paulsen, 1973).

The anosmia can be either partial or selective for determinate smells (hyposmia), and can be confirmed on an anatomical basis by determining whether there is partial or complete agenesis of the olfactory bulbs and whether it is either uni- or bilateral (Fig. 12-2A). A hypoplastic hypothalamus and cryptorchidism can be associated with hypogonadism in these patients.

Other disorders associated with this syndrome include: mental retardation; color blindness; eunuchoid skeletal structure; facial asymetry; neurogenic deafness; epilepsy; shortening of the fourth metacarpals; tarsal navicular fibrous dysplasia; familial cerebelar ataxia; diabetes mellitus; hyperlipemia; Laurence-Moon-Rozabal-Bardet Biedl syndrome, gynecomastia; and cleft lip, maxilar, or palate.

Hormone determinations generally reveal low gonadotropin values in urine and serum, as well as low total testosterone and estrogen levels. Levels of 17-ketosteroid and 17-OH-ketosteroid remain

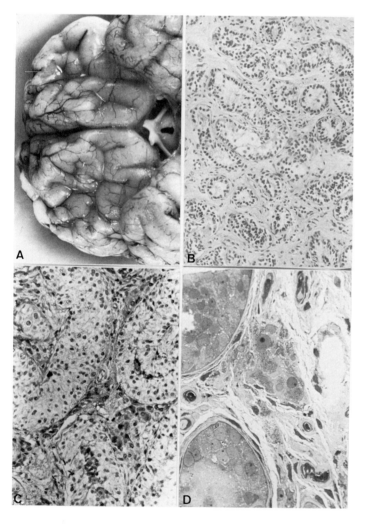

FIGURE 12-2. Maestre de San Juan-Kallmann-De Morsier syndrome. A, Absence of olfactory bulbs and tracts. B, Testis in a male of 20 years with prepubertal development (Mean tubular diameter 60µ; tubular fertility index 30 percent. H&E (x80). C, After treatment with HCG and HMG the testis in the same patient shows proper Leydig cell development and a certain development of the germinal line up to primary spermatocyte stage in some of the tubules. Masson trichrome (x125). D, Detail of the Leydig cells in the same patient after treatment showing normal characteristics with the exception of Reinke chrystals. 1 micron-thick section of epon-embedded material. Toludine blue (x450).

either low or within the lower limits of normality. All other hormone determinations, including those of the anterior lobe of the pituitary, are normal (Rodríguez and Woodhead, 1972). The karyotype also is normal in this syndrome. Many of the described cases show a familial incidence, and it has been supposed that the inheritance of the disorder is an X-linked dominant trait, but with incomplete penetrance, which would in turn justify the appearance of numerous sporadic cases (Sebaoun and associates, 1975).

The penis and testes have a prepubertal appearance in patients with this defect and the secondary sex characteristics are either lacking or scarce. The histologic pattern of the testes is characteristically prepubertal showing seminiferous tubules with a decreased diameter—in some cases devoid of central lumen—containing immature Sertoli cells and scarce spermatogonia (Pervaiz and co-authors, 1979). The remaining germinal line cells are absent. The testicular interstitium is formed by a loose connective tissue that generally lacks mature adult Leydig cells, although some precursor cells can be recognized. On the whole, the histologic pattern can be defined as a diffuse tubulo-interstitial hypoplasia (Enríquez and others, 1973) (Fig. 12-2**B**). The pituitary gland, although small in size, is histologically normal and the hypothalamus can be either hypoplastic or normal.

With regards to the etiopathogenesis of the hypogonadism, the possibility of an organic or functional hypothalamic lesion has been suggested. On the developmental basis this syndrome represents the least severe form of holoprosencephaly-hypopituitarism complex, a spectrum of developmental anomalies associated with impaired midline cleavage of the embryonic forebrain, aplasia of the olfactory bulbs and tracts, and midline dysplasia of the face (Rimion and Schimke, 1971). The consequence would be either a deficient integration between hypothalamus and olfactory tracts—the latter having connections with the lateral hypothalamus—or a failure in gonadotropin release secondary to a defect in the activation of the hypothalamic releasing factors. The anatomical deficiencies are in agreement with clinical data on the lack of response to clomiphene tests. The experimental removal of the olfactory bulbs has been shown to inhibit gonadotropin release (Signoret, 1962). Since the evagination of the prosencephalon to form the olfactory bulbs occurs at sixth week of embryonic life, the lesion would probably appear at this time.

The treatment with low-dose pulsatile LH-RH causes an increase of both FSH and LH plasma levels to normal values. After treatment with HCG and HMG there is a notable Leydig cell maturation as well as a certain development of the germinal cell line up to primary spermatocyte stage. The latter occurs only in some tubules (Enríquez and others, 1973) (Fig. 12-2**C** and **D**; 12-1).

Due to unresponsiveness to gonadotropin treatment observed in many patients, it has been suggested that the testicular structures could be refractory to gonadotropins. The alteration might affect either the Leydig cells, the seminiferous tubules, or both (Check and others, 1979).

The development of a seminoma has been reported in a patient with hypogonadotropic hypogonadism, who had not previously received gonadotropin treatment (Albers and Males, 1981).

Pasqualini-Bur-McCullagh Syndrome (Syndrome of the Fertile Eunuch; Isolated Deficiency in LH)

In 1950, Pasqualini and Bur (Pasqualini and Bur, 1950 and 1955) first described a syndrome characterized by hypogonadism and conserved spermatogenesis. In 1953, McCullagh and associates found in patients with this syndrome: an LH deficiency; the presence of spermatozoa; and Leydig cell absence. This defect was then termed the "syndrome of the fertile eunuch."

Clinically, these patients display the following characteristics: eunuchoid habitus; small or markedly reduced testicular size; a hypoplastic penis; feminine hair distribution; an infantile voice; and a marked diminution of the libido. Additional features, such as gynecomastia; anosmia; ocular lesions; malformations; or pituitary tumors have been reported (Kjessler and Lundberg, 1973). Characteristic features of these patients are the low LH and testosterone levels. FSH levels, however, are normal (Faiman and others, 1968). An increased response of LH levels and a less increased response of FSH levels are obtained after LH-RH stimulation. The clomiphene test is negative in most patients (Del Pozo and associates, 1975).

Testicular biopsy studies reveal seminiferous tubules that are normal, or slightly below normal, in diameter and that have complete, although scarce, spermatogenesis. Leydig cells are scarce or absent (Fig. 12–3A).

The etiopathogenetic mechanism of this syndrome might consist in a hypo-

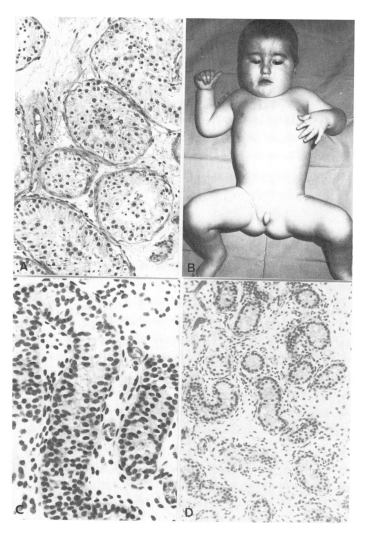

FIGURE 12–3. *A*, Pasqualini syndrome. Male consulting for sterility showing oligospermia and very low testosterone levels. The seminiferous tubules show hypospermatogenesis and the interstice absence of mature Leydig cells. H&E (x125). *B*, Child of 4 months with Prader-Willi syndrome. Note the external genitalia hypoplasia. *C*, Prader-Willi syndrome (8 months old) with seminiferous tubules showing Sertoli cells with a pseudostratified distribution and reduction in germinal cell number. H&E (x250). *D*, Testicular biopsy in a male of 19 years with Prader-Willi syndrome. The tubular and intersticial development are prepubertal (x125).

thalamic lesion, with the subsequent alteration of the feedback mechanism of hormone control, and in Leydig cell alteration. The nature of these lesions is unknown.

The maintenance of the spermatogenesis has been explained as follows (Makler and others, 1977). Under FSH stimulation Sertoli cells would secrete normal amounts of androgen-binding-protein (ABP); this would aid in the maintenance of sufficient intratesticular testosterone levels to conserve spermatogenesis, in spite of the reduced levels of plasma testosterone.

During the treatment of these patients it must be noted that, with advancing age, the Leydig cells become less sensitive to LH or human chorionic gonadotropin (HCG) stimulation than younger Leydig cells, and that the effects of testosterone administration are also decreased (Vague and Sardo, 1982).

Prader-Labhart-Willi Syndrome (HHHO Syndrome)

Prader-Labhart-Willi syndrome (1956) is a clinical entity characterized by: obesity; muscular hypotonia; psychophysical retardation; acromicria; and hypogonadism. The hormonal determinations are usually within normal range, except for the gonadotropin and testosterone values, which are low in the adult. The syndrome is often associated to hypersensitivity to exogenous insulin and, at a later date, these patients can develop clinical diabetes. The karyotype is normal in these patients, and the manifestation of the syndrome is usually sporadic, although a few isolated cases of familial occurence have been reported. The disorder is 2.5 times more frequent in males than it is in females (Fig. 12-3B).

In male patients, the hypogenitalism is apparent since early childhood. Seventy percent of patients present with cryptorchidism, which is bilateral 45 percent of the time. The scrotum is hypoplastic and has a smooth surface and the penis is small or curved. When the testes are palpable in the scrotum, they are found to be small and soft. The histologic study of the infantile testes shows a marked decrease of both mean tubular diameter and tubular fertility index. The seminiferous tubules contain immature Sertoli cells and low spermatogonium number (Martín-Zurro and others, 1972) (Fig. 12-3C) or Sertoli cells only (Uehling, 1980). When these patients reach adulthood the infantile testicular pattern persists (Fig. 12-3D). Clomiphene administration at this time causes an adequate gonadotropin response—with increases almost reaching normal levels—although after a few days the hormone levels return to their previous values. A positive response to the administration of hypothalamic gonadotropin releasing factors can also be observed.

The response to clomiphene seems to exclude that the hypothalamus is directly responsible for the lesion because its structure, at least partially, is conserved. The nature of this syndrome remains unknown.

Laurence-Moon-Rozabal-Bardet Biedl (LMB Syndrome)

LMB syndrome is a congenital disorder which, in its complete form, is characterized by: obesity; sexual infantilism; short stature; insipid diabetes; mental deficiency; retinitis pigmentosa; polydactyly; and syndactyly. Hypogenitalism is present in 74.4 percent of the males (Bell, 1958). Males are affected more often than females, and no male patient has been reported to have been fertile.

The aspect of the external genitalia tends to reflect the degree of testicular development. Bell's statistics (1958) show that cryptorchidism is present in 42 percent of patients affected with this syndrome. In 28 percent of the cases the cryptorchidism is bilateral, and in 14 percent it is unilateral. Severe alteration can be observed in the testicular structure and the testes have been described as atrophic and hypoplastic. Among 78 male patients, 23 were found to have bilateral testicular atrophy. The scrotum has been described as either hypoplastic, or bifid and hypoplastic, coinciding on the same side as the cryptorchid atrophic testis. The penis can be small, even when the size of the testes is normal. A hypoplastic penis can be associated with bilateral cryptorchidism and to a hypoplastic scrotum as well.

Gonadotropin and 17-ketosteroids determinations have made it possible to confirm that the hypogonadism is hypogonadotropic (Reinfrank and Nichols, 1964). Cases described as hypergonadotropic hypoganodisms seem to correspond to the Almstrom syndrome (see Chapter 11). The testicular histologic pattern shows a diffuse tubulo-interstitial hypoplasia with an infantile or pubertal maturation pattern.

Hypogonadism and Ichthyosis

Ichthyosis, isolated or coinciding with neurological disorders, can be associated to hypogonadism. In these cases, cryptorchidism is very frequent, and can show a familial presentation. Gonadotropin determinations reveal low or undetectable values (Lynch and others, 1960). The testicular biopsy shows small seminiferous tubules with immature Sertoli cells and a decreased number of spermatogonia (Fig. 12-4). Ichthyosis, associated with hypogonadism, mental retardation, and epilepsy, constitutes the Rud syndrome (McGillivray, 1954). Other skin disorders in which hypogonadism is frequently observed are poikiloderma congenitale (Rothmund-Thomson syndrome) and dyskeratosis congenita (Zinsser-Cole-Engman syndrome). Both ichthyosis and dyskeratosis congenita are inherited as a sex-linked trait (Falk and others, 1967), whereas poikiloderma congenitale is inherited as an autosomal recessive trait.

Hypogonadism with Hypomentia and Microcephaly (Kraus-Ruppert Syndrome)

In 1956 Kraus-Ruppert described a syndrome characterized by microcephaly; severe mental retardation; syndactyly; and hypogonadism, in three brothers from a consanguineous marriage. The syndrome was found to be inherited as an autosomal recessive trait.

The testicular biopsy study revealed absence of spermatogenesis and Leydig cells. The postmortem examination of the brain showed a marked hypoplasia of the hypothalamic nuclei.

Hypogonadism and Ataxia

Hypogonadism is frequent in Louis-Bar syndrome, characterized by cerebelar ataxia; mucocutaneous telangiectasia; growth delay; and frequent respiratory infections, presumably secondary to a deficit in IgA and IgE immunoglobulins and to an alteration in delayed hypersensitivity (Dunn and others, 1964). The disease is inherited as an autosomal recessive trait (Ryan, 1961). Among the lesions that have been observed in the pituitary, the presence of cytomegalic cells with telescoped nuclear inclusions is characteristic. In most patients, the hypogenitalism is hypogonadotropic (Amman and associates, 1970). In Friedreich's ataxia, there is hypogonadism, sometimes of the hypergonadotropic type and sometimes of the hypogonadotropic variety. In Marie's ataxia the hypogonadism is hypogonadotropic.

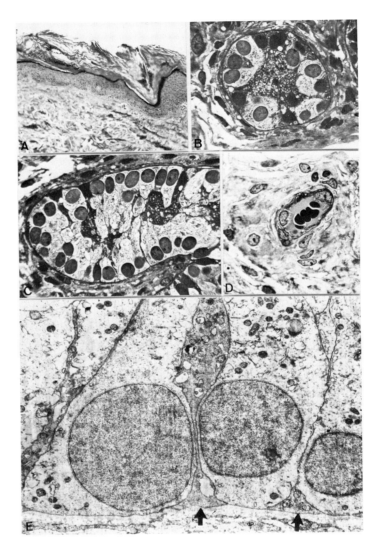

FIGURE 12–4. *Hypogonadism associated with ichthyosis in an 18-year-old patient. A, Skin with marked hyperkeratosis with orthokeratosis. H&E (x60). B and C, Transverse section of seminiferous tubules (B) and longitudinal section (C) showing a tubular diameter of about 60 μm and Sertoli cells with a spherical or oval nucleus and small nucleolus. 1 micron-thick section of epon-embedding material. Toluidine blue (x450). D, Interstitium with numerous fibroblasts and probably undifferentiated Leydig cells around a venule. 1μm section. Toluidine blue (x450). E, Pseudostratified and immature aspect of Sertoli cells with the electron microscope. The arrows point to the basal portion of the cells, in which the nucleus appears closer to the lumen than do those seen in the picture (x9000).*

HYPOGONADISM AND DWARFISM

A defect in the secretion of gonadotropins can appear to be associated with other deficiencies relating to the secretion of a determinate pituitary hormone. In order to confirm the association between a gonadotropin deficiency and dwarfism, the remaining tropic hormones must be found to be normal. If puberty can seem to be delayed in dwarfs, a variable degree of infantilism can be seen in adult patients with dwarfism and hypogonadism (Laron and Sarel, 1970).

OTHER HYPOGONADOTROPIC HYPOGONADISMS

In addition to the aforementioned, other syndromes that often present hypogonadism are the following:

1. Carpenter syndrome: acrocephaly; peculiar facies; braquisyndactyly of the fingers; preaxial polydactyly; syndactyly; obesity; mental retardation; and hypogonadism.
2. Biedmond syndrome: coloboma iris;

obesity; postaxial polydactyly; and hypogonadism.
3. Borjeson syndrome: mental retardation; obesity; grotesque facies; dwarfism; hypometabolism; and hypogonadism.
4. Richards-Rundle syndrome: ketoaciduria; mental retardation; deafness; ataxia; peripheral muscle wasting; and lack of secondary sexual development.

REFERENCES

1. Albers DD, Males JL: Seminoma in hypogonadotropic hypogonadism associated with anosmia (Kallmann's syndrome). J Urol 126:57, 1981
2. Agulhon G, Philbert M, Moreau L: A propos d'un cas de dysplasia olfactogénitale: étude des 34 cas publiés. Ann Endocrinol 32:777, 1971
3. Ammann AJ, Duquesnoy RJ, Good RA: Endocrinological studies in ataxia-telangiectasia and other immunological deficiency diseases. Clin Exp Immun 6:587, 1970
4. Bell J: Unhereditary digital anomalies. In the Treasury of Human Inheritance. London: Cambridge University Press, 1958, vol. 3
5. Boyar RM, Finklestein JW, Wilkins M, Kaper S, Weitzmann E, Hellman L: Studies of endocrine function in isolated gonadatropin deficiency. J Clin Endocrinol Metabol 36:64, 1973
6. Check J, Caro JF, Criden L, Meltz R, Brownstein K: Leydig cell responsiveness with germinal cell resistance to gonadotropin therapy in Kallmann's syndrome. Am J Med 67:495, 1979
7. Del Pozo E, Bolte E, Very M: Suprasellar disturbance in the syndrome of fertile eunuchoidism: case report. Acta Endocr 80:165, 1975
8. De Morsier G: Études sur les dysraphies cranio-encephaliques. Agenesis des lobes olfactifs (telencephaloschizis lateral) et des commisures calleuse et anterieure (telencephaloschizis median) la dysplasie olfacto-genitale. Arch Neurol Psychiat 74:351, 1954
9. De Morsier G, Gauthier G: La dysplasie olfato-génital. Rapport aus II^c Journées Internationales d'Endocrinologie de Marseille 6:6, 1963
10. Donald RA, Wheeler M, Sönksen PH, Lowy C: Hypogonadatrophic hypogonadism resistant to HCG and responsive to LH-RH: report of a case. Clin Endocrinol 18:385, 1983
11. Dunn HG, Meuwissen H, Livingstone CS, Pump KK: Ataxia telangiectasia. Canad Med Ass J 91:1106, 1964
12. Enríquez L, Díaz-Rubio M, Zamarron A, González-Páramo P, Nistal M: Hypogonadismo hypogonadotrópico con anosmia. Rev Clin Esp 131:383, 1973
13. Ewer RW: Familial monotropie pituitary gonadotropin insufficiency. J Clin Endocrinol Metab 28:783, 1968
14. Faiman C, Hoffman DL, Ryan RJ, Albert A: The "fertile eunuch" syndrome, demonstration of isolated luteinizing hormone deficiency by radio-immunoassay technique. Mayo Clin Proc 43:661, 1968
15. Falk AB, Traisman HS, Ahern GJ: Ichtyosis congenita. J Dis Child 93:259, 1967
16. Kallmann F, Schönfeld WA, Barrera SE: The genetic aspects of primary eunuchoidism. Am J Med 28:203, 1944
17. Kjessler B, Lundberg PD: Dysfunction of the neuroendocrine system in nine males with aspermia. Fertil Steril 23:1007, 1973
18. Kraus-Ruppert R: Zur Frage vererbter diencephaler Storungen: infantiler Eunuchoidismus sowie Mikrocephalie bei recesivem Erbgang. Z Menschl Vererb 34:643, 1956
19. Laron Z, Sarel R: Penis and testicular size in patients with growth hormone insufficiency. Acta Endocrinol 63:625, 1970
20. Lynch HT, Ozer FL, McNutt W, Johnson JE, Jampolsky NA: Secondary male hypogonadism and congenital ichtyosis. Association of two rare genetic defects. Am J Hum Genet 12:440, 1960
21. Maestre de San Juan A: Falta total de los nervios olfatorios con anosmia en un individuo en quien existía una atrofia congénita de los testículos y del miembro viril. Siglo med 131:211, 1856
22. Makler A, Glezerman M, Lunenfeld B: The fertile eunuch syndrome. An isolated Leydig-cell failure. Andrologia 9:163, 1977
23. Martín-Zurro A, Sánchez-Franco F, Cerdán-Vallejo A, Nistal M: Síndrome de Prader-Willi. Rev Clin Esp 125:450, 1972
24. McCullagh EP, Beck JC, Schaffenburg CA: A syndrome of eunuchoidism with spermatogenesis, normal urinary FSH, and low-normal ICSH ("Fertile eunuchs"). J Clin Endocrinol Metab 13:489, 1953

25. McGillivray RC: The syndrome of Rud. Am J Mental Defic 59:62, 1954
26. Nistal M: Testículo humano. Hipoplasia túbulo-intersticial difusa (hipogonadismo hipogonadotrópico). Arch Esp Urol 26:253, 1973
27. Pallardo LF, Santiago-Corchado M, Cerdán-Vallejo A, Nistal M: Algunos aspectos del eunucoidismo hipogonadotrópico. Med Clin 59:390, 1972
28. Pasqualini RQ, Bur GE: Síndrome hipoandrogénico con gametogénesis conservada: clasificación de la insuficiencia testicular. Rev Asoc Méd Argent 64:6, 1950
29. Pasqualini RQ, Bur G: Hypoandrogenico syndrome with spermatogenesis. Fertil Steril 6:144, 1955
30. Paulsen AA: The testes. In Williams RH (ed) Textbook of Endocrinology Philadelphia: WB Saunders Co., 1968, p. 405
31. Pervaiz N, Hagedoorn J, Miniberg DT: Electron microsopic studies of testes in Kallman syndrome. Urology 14:267, 1979
32. Prader A, Labhart A, Willi H: Ein Syndrom von Adipositas, Kleinwuchs, Kryptorchidismus und Oligospermia nach Myotonie-Artigem Zunstand im Neugeborenalter. Schweiz Med Wschr 86:1260, 1956
33. Reinfrank RF, Nichols FL: Hypogonadotrophic hypogonadism in the Laurence-Moon syndrome. J Clin Endocr 24:48, 1964
34. Rimoin DL, Schimke NR: Disorders of anterior pituitary. In Genetic Disorders of the Endocrine Glands. C.V. Mosby and Co., St. Louis 1971, pp. 26–28
35. Rodríguez FR, Woodhead DM: Olfactory genital dysplasia (Kallmann's syndrome): An unsuspected urological endocrinopathy. J Urol 107:78, 1972
36. Ryan RJ: Male hypogonadism. Disease-a-month. Chicago, Ill: Year Book Publ, 1961
37. Santen RJ, Paulsen CA: Hypogonadotropic hypogonadism. I. Clinical study of inheritance. J Clin Endocrinol Metabol 36:47, 1973
38. Sebaoun J, Delzant G, Weisselberg C, Attali JR, Tamboise A: Syndrome de De Morsier chez 2 fréres dont l'un porteur d'une gonosomie XXY. Ann Endocr 36:345, 1975
39. Signoret JP, Mauleon P: Action de l'ablation des bulbes olfactifs sur les mécanismes de la reproduction chez la truie. Ann Biol Anim 167:101, 1962
40. Smals AG, Pieters GF, Drayer JI, Bernraad, TJ, Kloppenborg PW: Leydig cell responsiveness to single and repeated human chorionic gonadotropin administration. J Clin Endocrinol Metab 49:12, 1979
41. Spitz IM, Schumert Z, Steiner J, Rosen E, Segal S, Slonim A, Rabinowitz D: Induction of spermatogenesis in hypogonadotrophic hypogonadism. Postgraduate Medical Journal 54:694, 1978
42. Uehling D: Cryptorchidism in the Prader-Villi syndrome. J Urol 124:103, 1980
43. Vague J, Sardo J: L'hypoandrogénisme avec spermatogénèse. Sem Höp. Paris 58:767, 1982
44. Varela da Costa C, Tovar Ruiz J. Alvarez Santirso R, Zurita Sepulveda P: Deficit aislads de gonadatropinas. Respuesta al tratamiento con hormona hipotalamica liberadora de gonadatropinas (LH-RH). Rev Clin Esp 164:233, 1982

13

TESTICULAR LESIONS SECONDARY TO DISORDERS OF DIFFERENT ENDOCRINE GLANDS

The maintenance of normal spermatogenesis and proper androgenic functioning requires functional harmony among all endocrine glands. The failure of any one of these often results in an alteration of the hypothalamic-hypophyseal-gonadal axis and indirect damage to the testis.

PITUITARY

The role played by the pituitary as an intermediate link between the hypothalamus and the testis has been commented on in Chapter 5 and in the section on hypogonadotropic eunuchoidism in Chapter 12. We shall now study those hypogonadisms in which there is a demonstrable lesion in the pituitary. It is important to separate hypopituitarisms that commence postpubertally from those that commence prepubertally. The difference in the clinical symptoms is related to whether or not there has been normal sexual development during puberty.

Prepubertal Hypopituitarism

There are various causes for this syndrome; cysts or tumors in the sella turcica or suprasellar area and in clinical cases of "empty sella" (Thomas and associates, 1973). In many cases panhypopituitarism with failure of somatic development and thyroid and adrenal functions is associated to this condition (Fig 13-1**A**).

Histologically, the testes maintain prepubertal characteristic at adulthood. They contain only spermatogonia and immature Sertoli cells. The tunica propria is thin, lacking elastic fibers, and Leydig cells are in a stage of nondifferentiation (Wong and others, 1974) (Fig. 13-1**B**).

In some patients a thickening in the basement membrane may appear in the seminiferous tubules. The conservation of the tubular fertility index (TFI), associated with such a hyalinization, permits the differentiation of this histological picture from that of tubular dysgenesis. In other cases, tubular maturation with mitosis in the spermatogonia and meiosis in some primary spermatocytes begins during puberty.

Postpubertal Hypopituitarism

The most frequent causes of gonadal failure secondary to postpubertal hypopituitarism are: lesions located in the pituitary gland or nearby; pituitary adenomas; craneopharyngiomas; or lesions secondary to trauma affecting the sella turcica, such as fractures of the cranial base (Fig. 13-1**C** and **D**).

The testes progressively shrink due to advancing tubular atrophy. The seminiferous tubules show successively: maturation arrest; germinal hypoplasia; reduction of the tubular diameter; and thickening and hyalinization of the tunica propria. Elastic fibers are present in the wall of the atrophied tubules; this directly proves that there was normal pubertal hormonal stimulation (Fig. 13-2**A** and **B**). In postpubertal hypopituitarism the Leydig cells decrease in size, their nuclei become pyknotic and their cytoplasms show abundant lipofuchsin pigment bodies (Wong and others, 1974). These patients usually recuperate normal spermatogenesis with a treatment based on HMG and

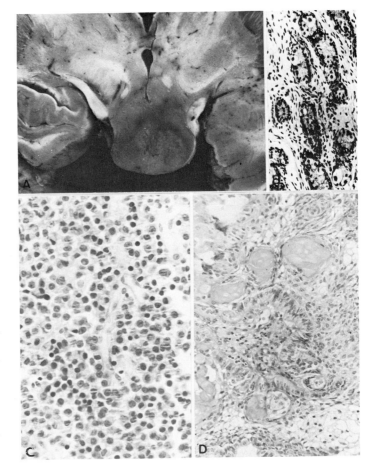

FIGURE 13-1. *A*, Frontal section of the hypothalamus showing a voluminous tumor which has destroyed an ample area of the hypothalamus in a 18-year-old patient. *B*, Testis from the same patient in which seminiferous tubules with prepubertal development and an absence of Leydig cells can be observed. H&E (x125). *C* and *D*, Hypogonadism secondary to destructive pituitary lesions. *C*, Characteristic solid pattern of pituitary acidophil cell adenoma. H&E (x250). *D*, Epithelial tumor in which the peripheral pallisade position of the cells, keratin nodular formations and vacuolization of the remaining epithelial cells are notable. The picture corresponds to a surgically resected pituitary tumor in a 19-year-old patient. H&E (x125).

HCG administration. Spermatogenesis is then maintained only with HCG (Johnsen, 1978).

Hyperprolactinemia and Hypoprolactinemia

Hyperprolactinemia is not uncommon as the cause of infertility in women. An increase of prolactin is observed in between 15 percent and 20 percent of patients with amenorrhea. Various cases of azoospermia or oligospermia associated with high levels of prolactin have been observed in men. One percent of male sterility has been estimated to be related to hyperprolactinemia (Hargreave and associates, 1977).

The causes of hyperprolactinemia are multiple: lesions in the hypothalamus, the pituitary stalk, and in the pituitary; treatment with drugs like phenothyazines, antidepressives tricycles, alpha-methyldopa, reserpine, TSH, or "ectopic" secretion of prolactin by tumors in other organs (Peillon and others, 1975).

Although the relation between hyperprolactinemia and hypogonadism is not completely understood, three possibilities have been considered:

1. A lesion in the pituitary stalk capable of producing a drop in gonadotropin secretion can also cause an increase in prolactin secretion through a drop in the inhibitory factor.
2. A second hypothesis attributes the gonadotropin secretion interference to prolactin.
3. The third possibility is that prolactin

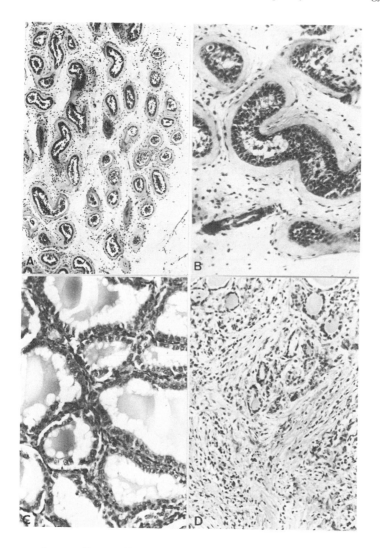

FIGURE 13–2. *A and B,* Testicular biopsy in a 17-year-old patient with pituitary adenoma. The seminiferous tubules show diffuse hyalinosis of the basement membrane. Some spermatogonia and primary spermatocytes can be seen. The interstitium shows an involution of the Leydig cells. H&E (A: x60; B: x125). *C,* Characteristic follicular pattern in thyroid adenomatous hyperplasia. The follicular cells are tall and the colloid shows signs of reabsorption. H&E (x125). *D,* Diffuse thyroid atrophy in a patient with mixedema secondary to chronic lymphocytic thyroiditis. The picture corresponds to autopsy material from a 45-year-old male whose testes displayed marked hypospermatogenesis. H&E (x60).

has a direct effect on testicular function.

Today we have ergot alkaloids (bromocriptine) that inhibit prolactin secretion and reinstates gonadal function (Roulier and associates, 1976; Hargreave and others, 1977).

There are two syndromes secondary to abnormal prolactin secretion in boys:

1. Hyperprolactinemia, testicular enlargement and primary hypothyroidism (Roitman and others, 1978).
2. Prolactin deficiency, obesity and enlarged testes (Roitman and associates, 1980).

THYROID GLAND

Thyroid malfunction is a rare cause of male infertility (0.6 percent in Dubin and Amelar 1971 statistics), but it has the peculiarity of being reversible if the correct treatment is established (Fig. 13–2C and D).

Hyperthyroidism

Testicular biopsies on patients with hyperthyroidism show varying degrees of germinal hypoplasia or incomplete maturation arrest. The causes are not well understood and have been related to stress or to the increase of temperature. Hormonal studies shows that the alteration may be more complicated.

An increase of testosterone and gonadotropins have repeatedly been observed. These findings have been interpreted as an increase in the binding capacity of testosterone-estradiol binding globulin (TeBG). Upon increasing the binding of testosterone by TeBG the clearance of testosterone drops while testosterone plasma levels rise; but as the formation of free testosterone drops, the levels of gonadotropins consequently rise (Clyde and associates, 1976).

Hypothyroidism

Generally patients with hypothyroidism have reduced fertility. Testicular biopsy shows a slight or markedly reduced hypospermatogenesis. Many times, fertility is improved with substitutive therapy.

On the other hand, a small group of children with hypothyroidism shows precocious testicular maturation. This condition is treated in more detail in Chapter 8 on precocious testicular maturation. Primary hypothyroidism; the increase of testicular size; and hyperprolactinemia are a frequent association (Roitman and others, 1978).

ADRENAL GLAND

Congenital Adrenal Hyperplasia

There are congenital disorders, characterized by failure of steroidogenesis, which is secondary to enzyme defects in cortisol synthesis. They are inherited and linked to a recessive autosomic gene. Both sexes are affected, but the proportion is higher in women than in men. The frequency of the disorder is 1 in every 5000 to 7000 births (Pato-Castel, 1977).

A consequence of the drop in cortisol synthesis is the appearance of adrenal hyperplasia. Since the true regulator of adrenocorticotrophic hormone (ACTH) secretion is cortisol, an excessive hypothalamic CRF secretion is produced in these patients, which consequently increases ACTH secretion. Under this stimulus the adrenal cortex undergoes hyperplasia and their cells produce large quantities of cortisol precursors. The resulting clinical syndrome is as much due to the effects of these precursors as to the lack of the hormones that should have been produced.

The following types of congenital adrenal hyperplasia, defined by their characteristic enzyme deficiency, are known: a 21-hydroxylase deficiency; an 11-β-hydroxylase deficiency; a 20-α-hydroxylase deficiency; an 18-hydroxylase deficiency; and an 18-hydroxysteroid-dehydrogenase deficiency. Ninety-five percent of the patients have a 21-hydroxylase deficiency and the remaining five percent are distributed among the other deficiencies.

These varieties of congenital adrenal hyperplasia can be grouped according to their effects on the male genital tract as follows: virilizing adrenal hyperplasia; feminizing adrenal hyperplasia; and adrenal hyperplasia that does not affect the genital sphere (non genital affecting adrenal hyperplasia).

Virilizing Adrenal Hyperplasias

21-Hydroxylase Deficiency. 21-hydroxylase controls the change of 17-OH-progesterone to form 11-desoxycortisol and of progesterone into desoxycorticosterone. The resulting clinical condition is one of androgenic hyperproduction that may or may not be associated with a salt-loss syndrome.

Females are born with a pseudohermaphroditic condition whereas males, whose genitals may be normal at the moment of birth, soon begin to experience increased growth in the penis, which continues throughout infancy until it becomes disproportionately large. These patients grow rapidly with great muscular development and experience an early onset of puberty. The testes maintain a small size throughout infancy, or begin to atrophy due to the constant supression of LH secretion caused by excess androgen secretion.

The adrenal glands' weight is several times greater than normal, demonstrating a correlation between the degree of virilization and the hyperplasia. The hyperplasia is initially diffuse and regular and may later become nodular. Patients without salt loss have light brown adrenals during childhood and brown adrenals in adulthood. The adrenal cortex is composed of: the zona glomerulosa that is wider than normal, a narrow zona fasciculata, and the zona reticularis that constitutes the main part of the cortex. The cells in this layer contain large quantities of lipofuchsin. When salt loss occurs the adrenal cortex demonstrates numerous foldings, which because of their resemblance to the cerebral cortex have given this condition the name of cerebriform hyperplasia. In these cases the adrenal glands are grey. Histologically we can appreciate that the cortex is almost entirely constituted by the zona fasciculata. The cytoplasm in these cells has hardly any lipids or lipofuchsin, and if vacuolization is present, it is due to hydropic degeneration (Fig. 13–3 **A**, **B**, **C**, and **D**).

During infancy the testes either show no development or, in the more serious cases, are clearly atrophied. During puberty the Leydig cells do not differentiate and the seminiferous tubules show incomplete or no spermatogenesis. Some testis development during puberty and spermatogenesis in adult testes can occur in the less serious forms. The number of spermatozoa formed is low, which causes these patients to consult a physician about sterility (Herrera-Pombo and others, 1971; Molitor and associates, 1972).

Small nests of adrenal cortical cells, even in tumoral form, develop in the testis as well as in the epididymis in some patients. The adrenal intratesticular ectopia can clinically and histologically simulate a Leydig cell tumor (Chrousos and others, 1981). The differential diagnosis can only be definitively established when an involution of testicular size is observed after proper treatment of the congenital adrenal hyperplasia.

In patients with the salt-loss syndrome, hyperplasia in the basophil cells has been observed at the level of the pituitary glands, as well as in the juxtaglomerular cells of the kidney.

11-β-hydroxylase Deficiency. 11-β-hydroxylase acts on 12-hydroxy-progesterone or 11-desoxycortisone to form corticosterone. The patients present varying states of virilization and hypertension occurs in half of the cases. The adrenal glands suffer hyperplasia in the zona fasciculata and the zona reticularis (Bongiovanni and associates, 1967) (Fig. 13–3E).

Feminizing Adrenal Hyperplasias

In certain forms of adrenal hyperplasia the enzymatic block on steroidogenesis can affect the synthesis of androgens. The lack of an androgenic stimulus determines the slight or abnormal development of the urogenital sinus during the male fetal stage that results in undifferentiated or incompletely masculinized genitals. The following enzymatic deficiencies are responsible for these conditions.

20-α-hydroxylase Deficiency. Lipoid congenital adrenal hyperplasia or Prader's syndrome. This enzymatic deficiency blocks steroidogenesis during the change from cholesterol to 20-α-cholesterol. It primarily affects the adrenals as well as the testes. The boys display external female genitals. The adrenal glands are voluminous and intensely yellow due to the large quantities of stored lipids. Histolog-

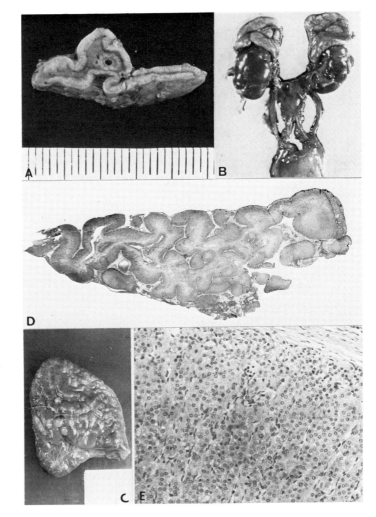

FIGURE 13-3. Congenital adrenal hyperplasia. A, Sagittal section of a normal adrenal gland displaying a smooth surface and a uniform cortex thickness. B, Congenital adrenal hyperplasia in a newborn. Compare the size of the adrenals with that of the kidneys. C, Histological section of an adrenal gland in a patient with 21-hydroxylase deficiency. Note the cerebriform appearance of the cortex. H&E (x10). D, Adrenal gland cerebriform appearance in a patient with 11-β-hydroxylase deficiency. E, Hyperplasia of the zona fasciculata is recognizable in a patient with 11-β-hydroxylase deficiency. H&E (x125).

ically they may demonstrate dystrophic calcifications, cholesterol crystals, and giant multinucleated cell reactions.

These patients' testes are macroscopically normal throughout infancy. Histologically they show an excess of lipids, as do the adrenal cells (Pato-Castell, 1977). **3-β-hydroxysteroid-dehydrogenase Deficiency.** This enzyme is necessary for the change from pregnenolone into progesterone and for the change of 17-OH-pregnenolone into 17-OH-progesterone. The boys have incompletely masculinized external genitals and a salt-loss syndrome. **17-α-hydroxylase Deficiency.** This enzyme defect blocks the change of pregnenolone into progesterone. The low level of androgens produced is responsible for the ambiguous external genitals. With the arrival of puberty, secondary sexual development fails and gynecomasty appears. The clinical symptoms may notably present a hypermineralocorticoidism.

Nongenital Affecting Adrenal Hyperplasias

These hyperplasias are caused by either an 18-hydroxylase or 18-hydroxysteroid-dehydrogenase deficiency. Both enzymatic defects provoke salt-loss syndromes due to a breakdown in aldosterone synthesis.

Adrenal Cortical Carcinoma

Adrenal carcinomas are frequently associated with an excessive production of: glucocorticoids; mineralocorticoids; androgens; and estrogens, which can cause Cushing syndrome; hyperaldosteronism; virilism; or feminization (Cahill and others, 1942). The clinical symptoms are related to the moment of development in which the tumor appears and the hormones are produced. If the tumors develop during infancy or childhood, precocious pseudopuberty along with breakdown in testicular maturation occurs, which, after the neoformation's removal, may retrogress.

In the adult, virilizing tumors produce large quantities of dehydroepiandrosterone (DHEA) and testosterone. The peripheric aromatization of these adrenal steroids causes a rise in estradiol. This should be responsible for the suppression of the hypothalamic-pituitary-gonadal axis. The testes show a drop in spermatogenesis and Leydig cell function.

The symmetric increase in size in both testes has been observed in isolated cases with a tubular hypertrophy secondary to the tumoral androgenic action (Drago and associates, 1979).

In the feminizing tumors, elevated estrogen production can alter secondary sex characteristics and give rise to irreversible lesions in organs. The clinical symptoms first include gynecomastia, which is always bilateral, sometimes associated with galactorrhea and pigmentation of the areola. Then a loss of masculine hair distribution, a drop in libido and feminine adiposity occur. The tumors are usually voluminous, cystic, or solid with areas of hemorrhage. The differential diagnosis between a malignant or a benign growth is habitually difficult to make.

An excess of estrogens suppress gonadotropic secretion and lead to a testicular deficiency. The testes show a breakdown in the development of germinal cells and thinning of the seminiferous epithelium along with thickening and hyalinization of the tunica propria. The Leydig cells progressively atrophy. The lesions are identical to those in postpubertal hypopituitarism. A similar condition of testicular atrophy can be observed in other alterations in which there is an increase in the levels of circulating estrogens, as in hepatic cirrhosis, Sertoli cell tumors, in estrogen secreting Leydig cell tumors, or when estrogens are administered to patients with prostatic carcinoma.

Cushing's Syndrome

Patients with Cushing's syndrome or those in whom corticosteroids are administered as prolonged treatment (as in treatments for ulcerative colitis, rheumatoid arthritis, or bronchial asthma) have diminished fertility. Their ejaculates show severe oligospermia and the testicular biopsies show a maturation arrest or hypospermatogenesis that are compatible with the patients' hypogonadotropic hypogonadism. A marked improvement has been observed when the excess of glucocorticoids is corrected (Luton and others, 1977).

Adrenoleukodystrophy

This is a sex-linked disease that primarily affects the central nervous system and adrenal cortex and develops in boys between 5 and 15 years of age. This disease is usually fatal. The white matter of the central nervous system shows inflammatory, demyelinative lesions. The adrenal cortex displays noninflammatory cytotoxic atrophy. Adrenoleukodystrophy is considered to be a hereditary metabolic disease in which the cholesterol esters contain long-chain fatty acids.

In those cases when adrenoleukodystrophy or its adrenomyeloneuropathic variant begin in an adult, impotence, diminished libido, and infertility are observed (Powers and Schaumburg, 1980).

In adrenoleukodystrophy characteristically needle-shaped cytoplasmic inclusions are found in the Leydig cells.

PANCREAS

Diabetes Mellitus

A large number of diabetic patients manifest alterations in sexual function — impotence and diminished fertility are most common. Diabetic patients have a hypothalamic-hypophyseal malfunction with a low LH response to LH-RH stimulation. Testosterone is normal in those patients treated with oral antidiabetics (Shahwan and associates, 1978).

Testicular biopsy study shows changes principally in the seminiferous tubules, with the most frequent being a more or less marked hypospermatogenesis. The Leydig cells are normal. The arterioles display subendothelial hyalinosis (Fig. 13-4A). The spermiograms manifest variable affectations of the different parameters, with a diminishing sperm mobility, followed in order by morphological spermatozoon alterations, a decrease in ejaculate volume and spermatozoon number

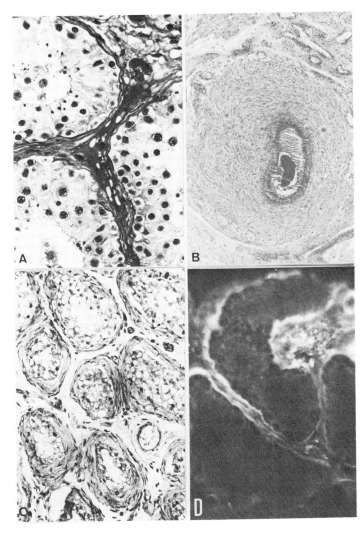

FIGURE 13–4. *A, 48-year-old patient, whose diabetes had been diagnosed 5 years earlier, showing marked hypospermatogenesis. Masson trichrome. (x450). B, Markedly hypoplastic ductus deferens that shows a dark plug in its lumen. From a 3-year-old patient with cystic fibrosis, whose death resulted from pulmonary complications. P.A.S. (x10). C, Peritubular fibrosis and marked diminishment of tubular diameter and germinal line in a 52-year-old patient with a history of alcoholic cirrhosis. H&E (x125). D, Seminiferous tubules with IgG at the level of the basement membrane in a patient with multiple (adrenal, thyroid, and testicular) endocrine gland insufficiency. H&E (x250).*

(Barták, 1979). There may be a double cause for this lesion—diabetic neuropathy or arteriosclerosis.

Diabetic neuropathy of the pelvic nerves appears to be responsible for the impotency, lack or breakdown of ejaculate or retrogressive ejaculates, and germinal line lesions. The mechanism (ischemic or thermic) by which the nervous lesion affects spermatogenesis is unknown (Faerman and associates, 1974).

Arteriosclerosis in the testicular arteries or their branches, which is frequent in these patients, causes hypospermatogenesis and tubular atrophy, which overlap the earlier lesions in patients with long standing diabetes. The main cause of impotence in diabetic patients is arteriosclerosis of the pudendal arteries or their branches (Lehman and Jacobs, 1983)

Cystic Fibrosis

With improved medical care the number of adults diagnosed as having cystic fibrosis has increased considerably and it is not infrequent for them to seek evaluation for sterility. Obstructive azoospermia is discovered in the majority of patients. In Landin and associates' (1969) series of 32 cases of cystic fibrosis, 28 patients displayed absence, atrophy, or fibrosis in the epididymis and ductus deferens; 2 patients displayed atresia of the ductus deferens and atrophy of the epididymis; in 1 case the spermatic cords were normal. The epididymis manifested a prominent caput, caused by dilatation of the ductuli efferens, with atrophied or absent corpus and cauda.

Histological studies performed on children show, even in the early years, that the epididymis and ductus deferens may be lacking or extremely thin; in this case their lumen can show a mucous plug (Fig. 13–4B).

Testicular studies performed during infancy are said to be normal. Postpubertal testes show slight or marked hypospermatogenesis, and a large number of small and round-headed spermatozoa that were binucleated or had abundant cytoplasm.

The cause of these lesions in the spermatic cord is probably genetic, and their insufficient development or atrophy manifests itself precociously (Feigelson and others, 1969). The cause of the hypospermatogenesis and the maturation abnormalities in the spermatozoa could be secondary to obstruction of the spermatic cord (Holschaw and associates, 1971; Gordon and Schwachman, 1979) or to malabsorption (see discussion concerning lack of vitamins A and E in Chapter 14).

LIVER

Chronic Liver Diseases

The affectation of testicular function in patients with chronic liver illnesses is a well-known fact. The patients complain of a loss of libido, and frequently display a loss of facial and body hair, small testes, and gynecomastia (Silvestrini-Corda syndrome).

The hypogonadism observed in cirrhosis does not appear to have a single cause. In those patients with advanced cirrhosis, the hypogonadism is hypergonadotropic. The majority of these patients have high levels of estradiol. This is due to the transformation of estrone into diol in the liver as well as the peripherical conversion of testosterone. However, since the clearance of the estrogens is normal, there is some disagreement as to whether the signs classically attributed to an excess of estrogens, such as gynecomastia, vascular spiders, or palmar erythema, have any direct relation to these hormones (Baker and others; Mowat and associates, 1976; Geisthövel and Mühlen, 1978).

Testicular lesions observed in patients with hemocromatosis support the existence of hypogonadotropic hypogonadism. Histologically, an abundant iron deposit in the pituitary and fibrotic areas are found (Bergeron and Kovacs, 1978). The testes display a secondary atrophy. Iron deposits are selectively detected in the wall of small blood vessels (Sheldon, 1935).The hypothesis that the hypogonadism may be secondary to a diabetic neuropathy can not be discarded in some cases.

Ethanol, by itself, is capable of producing the symptoms just described, in either a normal or cirrhotic liver. Acute alcohol ingestion supresses plasma testosterone levels in non-alcoholic volunteers. Chronic and excessive use of alcohol leads to morphological and functional defects in the testis. These include: changes in the concentration of testosterone binding globulins; impaired synthesis of testosterone in the testis; altered metabolism of testosterone in the liver; defects in the hypothalamic-pituitary functions through possible changes in the mechanisms associated with release of luteinizing hormone; and defects related to zinc deficiency and impaired metabolism of vitamin A (Morgan, 1982; Bhalla and others, 1983). The testes display small calibre seminiferous tubules, intense hypospermatogenesis, an increase of the tunica propria with abundant myofibroblasts, and a drop in the number of Leydig cells (Fig. 13–4C) (Galvão-Teles and others, 1983).

Intrahepatic Bile Duct Hypoplasia

Hypogonadism has been observed in patients who have manifested cholestasis during their first months of life that is secondary to bile duct hypoplasia. These patients sometimes display vertebral, cardiac, and facial malformations as well as mental retardation.

The hypogonadism is reflected by a decrease in testicular size, delay of puberty, and, in adulthood, lack of germinal cell line maturation. The endocrine assays reveal a slight increase of FSH levels. The cause is unknown (Alagille and others, 1975).

KIDNEY (CHRONIC RENAL INSUFFICIENCY)

Uremia is frequently accompanied by serious alterations in gonadal function. Many patients present with infertility, impotence, and loss of libido. Plasma testosterone levels are low and FSH levels are elevated, while LH levels are normal. Spermiograms show oligospermia or azoospermia. Testicular biopsy studies show atrophy of the seminiferous epithelium, which spreads from hypospermatogenesis to germinal cell aplasia. The following are different attempts at the explanation of these disorders: (1) low levels of plasma testosterone; (2) lesions that may be secondary to uremic neuropathy; and (3) a breakdown in the conversion of testosterone into its active metabolite dihydrotestosterone; and (4) zinc deficiency.

These lesions may originate from both the testis and the hypothalamus. Since the clomiphene test is positive, there is an alteration, not in the storage or the liberation of gonadotropins, but in the reception and integration of the peripheric messages (Lim and Fang, 1975).

In spite of treatment with immunosuppressors, kidney transplantation improves testicular function (Baumgarten and others, 1977; Rodrigues-Netto and associates, 1980). Patients with chronic nephropathy who undergo periodic hemodialysis develop gynecomastia in more than a third of the cases. The gynecomastia may be due to the different drugs employed, their undernourished condition, or an increase in the plasma prolactin levels.

PLURIGLANDULAR INSUFFICIENCY

The frequency of, and association between, insufficiencies in various glands is well known. Among these can be mentioned: adrenal and thyroid hypofunction; the association between Addison's disease and gonadal insufficiency; the association between primary adrenal, thyroid, and gonadal insufficiencies; the relationship between diabetes mellitus and Addison's disease; and the link between hypoadrenalism, hypothyroidism, diabetes, and primary hypogonadism.

The condition in which we are principally interested is the association between hypogonadism and Addison's disease. This association is so high that not less than 25 percent of the patients with primary adrenal insufficiency display gonadal dysfunction (Perlmutter and others, 1961). The hypogonadism is primary and therefore causes elevated levels of gonadotropins. The testes show atrophy, which irregularly affects the seminiferous tubules. Basement-membrane immunoglobulin deposits have been detected with immunofluorescence techniques in some patients.

Less frequently the association between primary adrenal, thyroid, and gonadal insufficiencies with diabetes mellitus is recognized. In these cases, if the proper hormonal assays are not done, a diagnosis of multiple endocrine gonadal insufficiency can be confused with pituitary lesions.

The cause of pluriglandular insufficiency is unknown. Histological findings of the same lesion (lymphocyte infiltration and fibrosis) in different organs support the hypothesis of a common cause. Observations of adrenal, thyroid, and gonadal tissue serum antibodies suggest an autoimmune response (Appel and Holub, 1976) (Fig. 13–4D).

REFERENCES

1. Alagille D, Odièvre M, Gautier M, Dommergues JP: Hepatic ductular hypoplasia associated with characteristic facies; vertebral malformations; retarded physical, mental, and sexual development; and cardiac murmur. J Pediatr 86:63, 1975
2. Appel GB, Holub DA: The syndrome of multiple endocrine gland insufficiency. Am J Med 61:129, 1976
3. Baker HWG, Burger HC, Kretser DM de, Dulmais A, Hudson B: A study of the endocrine manifestation of hepatic cirrhosis. Quant J Medic 117:145, 1976
4. Barták V: Sperm quality in adult diabetic men. Int J Fertil 24:226, 1979
5. Baumgarten SR, Lindsay GK, Wise GJ: Fertility problems in the renal transplant patient. J Urol 118:991, 1977
6. Bergeron C, Kovacs K: Pituitary siderosis: a histologic, immunocytologic, and ultrastructural study. Am J Pathol 93:295, 1978
7. Bhalla VK, Rajan VP, Newman ME: Alcohol-induced luteinizing hormone receptor deficiency at the testicular level. Alcoholism: Clin Exp Res 7:153, 1983
8. Bongiovanni AM, Eberlein WR, Goldman AS, New M: Disorders of adrenal steroid biogenesis. Rec Progr Horm Res 23:375, 1967
9. Cahill GF, Melicow AM, Darby MM: Adrenal cortical tumors: the types of nonhormonal and hormonal tumors. Surg Gynecol Obstet 74:281, 1942
10. Chrousos GP, Loriaux DL, Sherins RJ, Cutler GB: Unilateral testicular enlargement resulting from inapparent 21-hydroxylase deficiency. J Urol 126:127, 1981
11. Clyde HR, Walsh PC, English RW: Elevated plasma testosterone and gonadotropin levels in infertile males with hyperthyroidism. Fertil Steril 27:662, 1976
12. Drago JR, Olstein JS, Tesluk H, Sheikholislam B, Palmer JM, Link D: Virilizing adrenal cortical carcinoma with hypertrophy of spermatic tubules in childhood. Urology 14:70, 1979
13. Dubin L, Amelar RD: Etiologic factors in 1294 consecutive cases of male infertility. Fertil Steril 22:469, 1971
14. Faerman I, Glocer L, Fox D, Jadzinsky MN, Rappaport M: Histological studies of the autonomic nervous fibers of the corpora cavernosa in impotent diabetic males. Diabetes 23:971, 1974
15. Feigelson J, Pecau Y, Schwachman H: A propos d'une paternité chez un malade atteint de mucoviscidose. Etudes des fonctions genitales et de la filiation. Arch Franc Péd 26:937, 1969
16. Galvão-Teles A, Gonçalves L, Carvalho H, Monteiro E: Alterations of testicular morphology in alcoholic disease. Alcoholism: Clin Exp Res 7:144, 1983
17. Geisthövel W, Mühlen A von zur: Untersuchungen über die Hypophysen-Testes-Funktion bei Männern mit chronischen Lebererkrankungen. Klin Woschenschrift 56:929, 1978

18. Gordon F, Schwachman H: Cystic fibrosis in adults. Pathology Annual 2:377, 1979
19. Hargreave TB, Kyle KF, Kelly AM, England P: Prolactin and gonadotropins in 208 men presenting with infertility. Brit J Urol 49:747 1977.
20. Herrera-Pombo JL, Ramos F, Rodríguez-Miñón JL: El síndrome adrenogenital del varón adulto. Rev Clin Esp 122:413, 1971
21. Holschaw DS, Perlmutter AD, Jockin H, Schwachman H: Genital abnormalitities in male patients with cystic fibrosis. J Urol 106:568, 1971
22. Johnsen SG: Maintenance of spermatogenesis induced by HMG treatment by means of continuous HCG treatment in hypogonadotrophic men. Acta Endocrinol 89:763, 1978
23. Landing BH, Wells TR, Wang CI: Abnormality of the epididymis and vas deferens in cystic fibrosis. Arch Path 88:569, 1969
24. Lehman TP, Jacobs JA: Etiology of diabetic impotence. J Urol 129:291, 1983
25. Lim VS, Fang VS: Gonadal dysfunction in uremic men. A study of the hypothalamo-pituitary testicular axis before and after renal transplantation. Am J Med 58:655, 1975
26. Luton JP, Thieblot P, Valcke JC, Mahoudeau JA, Bricaire H: Reversible gonadotropin deficiency in male Cushing's disease. J Clin Endocrinol Metab 45:488, 1977
27. Molitor JT, Chertow BS, Fariss BL: Long-term follow-up of a patient with congenital adrenal hyperplasia and failure of testicular development. Fertil Steril 24:319, 1972
28. Morgan MY: Sex and alcohol. Brit Med Bull 38:43, 1982
29. Mowat NA, Edwards CRW, Fisher R, McNeilly AS, Green JRB, Dawson AM: Hypothalamic-pituitary-gonadal function in men with cirrhosis of the liver. Gut 17:345, 1976
30. Pato-Castel J: In Palacios-Mateos JM (ed) Endocrinología en la práctica médica Madrid: Paz Montalvo, 1977, p.406
31. Peillon F, Boyet F, André C, Dreyfus G: La fonction gonadotrope dans les adénomes à prolactine. Ann Endocr 36:331, 1975
32. Perlmutter M, Numeroff M, Manulklin T: Primary adrenocortical insufficiency and hypogonadotrophic eunuchoidism. Metabolism 10:647, 1961
33. Powers JM, Schaumburg HH: A fatal cause of sexual inadequancy in men: adrenoleukodystrophy. J Urol 124:583, 1980
34. Rodrigues-Netto N, Pecorano G, Sabbaga E, Menezes de Goes G: Spermatogenesis before and after renal transplant. Int J Fertil 25:131, 1980
35. Roitman A, Assa S, Laron Z: Hyperprolactinaemia in a boy with hypothyroidism due to an ectopic thyroid. Acta Paediatr Belg 31:155, 1978
36. Roitman A, Assa S, Kauli R, Laron Z: Prolactin deficiency, obesity, and enlarged testes—a new syndrome? Arch Dis Child 55:647, 1980
37. Roulier R, Mattei A, Reuter A, Franchimont P: Etude de la prolactine dans les stérilités et les hypogonadismes masculins. Ann. Endocr. 37:285, 1976
38. Shahwan MM, Spathis GS, Fry DE, Wood PJ, Marks V: Differences in pituitary and testicular function between diabetic patients on insulin and oral anti-diabetic agents. Diabetologia 15:13, 1978
39. Sheldon JH: Haemochromatosis. Oxford University Press. London, 1935
40. Thomas BM, Lufkin EG, Ellis GJ, Hartman CR, Hofeldt FD, Herman RH: Hypogonadotropism and "empty sella:" improvement in 2 cases with clomiphene citrate. Fertil Steril 23:252 1973
41. Wong TW, Strauss FH, Warner NE: Testicular biopsy in the study of male infertility. Pretesticular causes of infertility. Arch Pathol 98:1, 1974

14

TESTICULAR LESIONS SECONDARY TO PHYSICAL-CHEMICAL AGENTS, DIETARY DEFICIENCIES, AND PERIPHERAL NERVOUS SYSTEM LESIONS

The following etiologically diverse conditions (induced by either physical or chemical agents or occurring secondary to malnutrition) frequently produce seminiferous epithelium lesions. In relation to these conditions, references are made throughout this chapter to experimentally produced pathologies (models). By studying these models, a better understanding of human disorders can be achieved.

Testicular Lesions Caused by Physical-Chemical Agents

X-Rays

The testicular parenchyma is one of the most radiation sensitive tissues. Its extreme sensitivity converts it into a precise tissue dosimeter when accidental exposure to radiation occurs (Hacker and others, 1981).

Since Albers-Schönberg's (1903) first studies, the reduction of testicular size even after exposure to moderate irradiation has merited attention. This macroscopic finding translates into important germinal-line alterations conferring temporary sterility while conserving the libido. As a result, this was used as a male contraceptive method until it was discovered a few decades ago that genetic changes could be produced.

This type of testicular atrophy has been investigated in humans in the following situations: after accidental irradiation; after irradiation of the groin subsequent to orchiectomy due to a tumor; or in the testes of prisoners who had volunteered for the experiment.

The most serious lesions occur in the seminiferous tubules. The germinal cells are the most radiosensitive with great variations in relation to the stage of differentiation. Rugh (1960) graphically established that if we assign a value of 1 to the radiosensitivity of type B spermatogonia, type A would be 70 times less sensitive, spermatids 200 times, spermatocytes 400 times and spermatozoa 10,000 times less sensitive. The pale spermatogonia form is the most resistant of the spermatogonia to irradiation.

Sertoli cells are extremely resistant, even when they are in immature or fetal form. Doses of 5000 rads have barely produced ultrastructural changes in these cells and have only very discretely increased their phagocytic activity against tubular lumen cells or their wastes.

The distribution of the testicular atrophy varies in accordance with different species. Rats display a patchy appearance of the lesion with atrophied tubules surrounded by others that had been better respected. In humans, the lesion is more diffuse and uniform. This different behavior is related to the organization of the rat's germinal line into perfectly individualized spermatogenetic stages of their cycle, as compared to human's in which cellular association is less apparent and the characteristic associations occupy smaller areas.

The seminiferous tubules show a reduction of both their length and caliber, without lesions of the tunica propria. Even though there are no morphological repercussions, the genetic material alterations that the spermatogonia can suffer is notable.

Leydig cells are very radiation resistant and usually appear accumulated into groups covering larger-than-normal areas. This false appearance of hyperplasia is caused by the diminishing of tubular volume. Androgen secretion maintains lower, but close to normal, values. Biochemical methods have proved that there is a certain incapacity in steroid transformation, which induces a gonadotropin increase in an attempt to accelerate the enzymatic reactions of this secretion. This gonadotropin increase is parallel to germinal epithelium destruction (Ellis, 1970).

Little is known about the effects of irradiation on prepubertal testis. Leiper and others' (1983) studies in children with acute lymphoblastic leukemia suggest that the ability of the Leydig cells to produce testosterone—as detected by the HCG test—is appreciably reduced after irradiation, and that tubular dysfunction may sometimes be predicted by a raised FSH response to LH-RH administration.

Two factors that influence testicular reaction to irradiation are the subject's age and the doses received. The younger the subject, the more serious are the lesions produced. Repeated exposures are more pernicious than sporadic ones, even when the latter are of higher levels: doses of 300 rads lead to sterility, which, if the doses are repeated, can require two or three years to reach recuperation.

The number of spermatozoa in an irradiated testis do not represent a faithful index of fertility, since pregnancies have been produced with recount levels of no more than 50,000 spermatozoa, and even with only a few spermatozoa in the extensions.

Heat

In animal experiments it has been seen that rodent testes transplanted to the abdominal cavity rapidly lose their germinal line. The first lesions appear after 5 to 7 days and at 20 days the germinal epithelium disappears. Similar effects have been obtained by transplanting the testes to the anterior chamber of the eye as well as by applying heat directly to the scrotum, which leads to testicular atrophy. Very similar results have been observed in dogs. In humans, it has been demonstrated that an elevation of body temperature to 40.5°C (or 104.9°F) causes a reduction in spermatogenesis, which is accentuated between the 25th and 55th day. If the scrotum is heated directly, spermatogenesis significantly falls between the fifth and ninth weeks, to subsequently return with normal temperatures. Robinson and coworkers (1968) have observed that scrotal heating is followed by a spermatozoon number drop in normospermic men, but that the number of spermatozoa subsequently returns to normal. In oligospermic patients the drop in spermatogenesis is less marked.

Procope (1965) studied the effects of saunas on twelve normal men whom he exposed to heat during twelve days for a total of eight hours. He was able to observe that between the 30th and 39th day after the experiment was over, spermatogenesis was reduced to 50 per cent of normal. A decrease in mobility was found in a lower proportion, while the appearance of abnormal forms was in a higher proportion than in normal men.

The rise in temperature also appears to be responsible for the low spermatozoon counts obtained in individuals who work seated on hot machines; wear close-fitting underpants; or in Europeans who work in the tropics during the acclimatization period.

Not all germinal line cells are especially sensitive to heat. The most affected are the intermediate stages (spermatocytes and spermatids), followed by spermatozoa and last, by spermatogonia. Nuclear pyknosis and meiotic alterations are observed in the spermatocytes. Multinucleated forms are very frequent in the spermatids (Fig. 14–1A).

The action of heat on the testicular

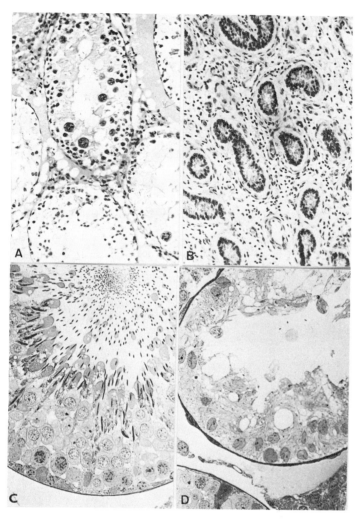

FIGURE 14–1. *A*, Thermic lesions. Seminiferous tubules displaying marked germinal cell loss and numerous multinucleated cells in a rat exposed to elevated temperatures. H&E (x125). *B*, Tubular atrophy in a nine-year-old boy with acute lymphoblastic leukemia. The atrophy was induced by the treatment of the leukemia with cyclophosphamide + vincristine + Adriamycin. H&E (x60). *C* and *D*, Experimentally produced lesions induced by cyclophosphamide in rat testis. *C*, Initial lesions consist of Sertoli cell vacuolation. 1-μm-thick section of epon-embedded material. Toluidine blue borax (x450). *D*, Highly developed lesions in which the absence of the germinal line and intense Sertoli cell vacuolation can be detected. 1-μm-thick section of epon-embedded material. Toluidine blue borax (x450).

endocrine function has also been investigated. Short-term exposures to elevated temperatures hardly produce alterations on the basal testosterone levels; however, the Leydig cell capacity under stimulation to produce androgens is affected. Since the temperature required to produce this functional change (41°C in the rat) is the same as the one that determines a spermatozoon production reduction, it has been suggested that the germinal line lesion may be secondary to the alteration in the Leydig cells (Dambert and others, 1978).

Testicular hormone regulation has been explored in burned male patients. A markedly decreased serum testosterone level and severe impairment of spermatogenesis have been found (Doleček and others, 1983).

Other physical agents capable of producing—by themselves or in conjunction with heat—low spermatozoon counts are vibrations. In a comparison between agricultural or industrial heavy machinery drivers and other drivers, it has been proved that the former display a higher incidence of pathologic seminograms (Sas and Szöllösi, 1979).

Chemical Agents

A great variety of chemical agents produce testicular atrophy, particularly in the seminiferous epithelium. In many cases the testicular atrophy is the lesser evil of a treatment for leukemia, lymphoma, or other tumors, and is therefore without important clinical repercussion. But there are other occasions when avoidable testicular lesions occur. Workers who use certain pesticides (dibromochloropropane); who make batteries; who mine lead; or who handle organic solvents such as xylol, benzol, or toluene, are at special risk.

There are enough data to think that the number of drugs capable of producing germinal line damage is much greater than would appear initially. From year to year the percentage of normal spermiograms drops in industrial populations. A 1950 U.S. study showed that 44 percent of 1000 healthy men had spermatozoon counts of over 100 million/ml; in another 1977 report only 22 percent of 2000 healthy men reached that figure. The percentage of men with spermiograms between 20 and 40 millions was 12 percent in 1950; by 1977 it had risen to 22 percent (Lee and Dixon, 1978).

The action on the testis of various drugs has been repeatedly studied (Delafontaine and others, 1979). Hodgkin disease patients with proven fertility prior to MOPP (prednisone + procarbazine + chlormetine + vincristine) treatment manifest severe oligospermia or azoospermia afterwards. FSH levels rise after the first months of treatment while the LH and testosterone levels remain unchanged. Procarbazine is probably the primary agent responsible for the germinal line lesion, without discarding the possibility that its effect is potentiated by the other drugs used in the treatment.

Patients with metastases of testicular cancer who have been treated with VACAM (vincristine + adriamycine + cyclophosphamide + medroxyprogestrone acetate) develop azoospermia (Fossa and associates, 1980).

Leydig cells can be affected during treatment with alkylating agents and low testosterone levels and the appearance of gynecomasty have been detected in some patients. These last symptoms are probably due to androgen-estrogen imbalances (Friedman and Plymate, 1980; Vermeulen, 1981). Conclusive data on fertility in these patients have not been provided, and there is evidence of spermatogenesis recovery in some patients (Lange and others, 1983).

1. *Cyclophosphamide* used to treat lymphomas as well as renal and hepatic diseases, and collagenosis, causes testicular atrophy when the dosage is over or at 3 mg/kg/day for over 3 months. The result is permanent azoospermia. The seminiferous tubules contain only Sertoli cells and isolated spermatogonia. Months after completing the treatment an incomplete spermatogenesis occurs only in isolated tubules. The administration of cyclophosphamide during puberty may quite probably be responsible for sterility (Miller, 1971) (Fig. 14–1B, C, and D; 14–2A).

2. *Clorambucil,* widely used as a treatment for lymphomas, gives rise to a loss of seminiferous epithelium and marked peritubular fibrosis. Total dosages of over 400 mg produce an azoospermic condition (Fig. 14–2B).

3. *Colchicine* has well known effects on spermatogenesis in experimental animals. Meiosis stops selectively during metaphase. Cases of azoospermia during this treatment are known (Merlin, 1972). Another effect that can be attributed to colchicine is the high frequency of patients with 47 chromosomes in their lymphocyte cultures, due to which the risk of producing trisomic offspring is emphasized.

4. The influence of *antibiotics* over spermatogenesis has been experimentally studied in rats. In humans the studies carried out on patients treated with gentamycine show the existence of some interference during meiosis and an increase in the amount of abnormal primary spermatocytes.

5. *Spironolactones* suppress adrenal as well as testicular androgen production by

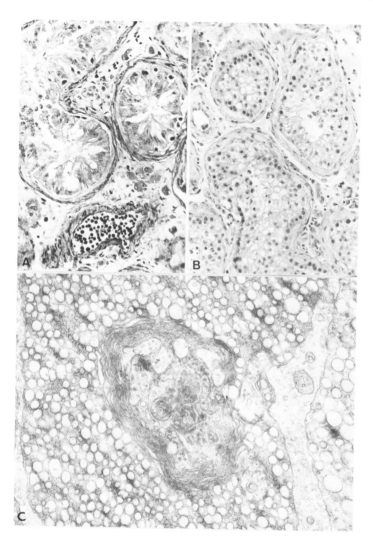

FIGURE 14–2. *A, Seminiferous tubules with marked fibrosis in the tunica propria and isolated spermatogonia persistance. The picture corresponds to a chronic myeloid leukemia in a patient treated with busulphan. Masson trichrome (x125). B, Seminiferous tubules with intense hypospermatogenesis, fibrosis, and basement membrane hyalinization, observed in a patient with chronic lymphoid leukemia treated with chlorambucil. H&E (x125). C, Smooth endoplasmic reticulum transformed into concentric cisternae in a Leydig cells after treatment with spironolactone (x23,500).*

inhibiting the progesterone's change into diverse androgens. Pseudomyelinic figures, like concentric cisternae of the smooth endoplasmic reticulum, have been observed in the cytoplasm of Leydig cells (Baba and others, 1978) (Fig. 14–2C).

6. *Diethylstilbestrol* is a synthetic hormone that has been tested on women with histories of repeated miscarriages to prevent the miscarriage as well as in large doses as an abortive to prevent the egg's implantation. It is responsible for the high incidence of vaginal adenosis and clear cell adenocarcinoma in women. Benign as well as malignant lesions have been reported in men. The sons of mothers treated with diethylstilbestrol show a high incidence of epididymal cysts; testicular hypoplasia; maldescended testes; varicocele; and thickening of the albuginea (Whitehead and Leiter, 1981). In adult patients exposed to diethylstilbestrol in utero a drop in spermatogenesis has been found (Gill and associates, 1977). Recently, the possibility of carcinogenesis has been suggested in diethylstilbestrol-exposed males (Conley and others, 1983). Since the exposure to this synthetic estrogen was most common in the 1950's, the group at greatest risk would be expected to be seen in the 1980's.

7. *Estrogens* have been widely used to

suppress testicular androgen function in prostate carcinoma patients. Its prolonged administration leads to a complete loss of germinal cells and causes a decrease in the number of Leydig cells (Jones and co-authors, 1978) (Fig. 14–3A). Antiandrogens are used in the same way (Fig. 14–3B).

8. *DBCP (Dibromo-chloro-propane)* is a nematocide of proven toxicity for the people who work with it. Males exposed to environments having 0.4 to 0.6 parts per million display azoospermia with high levels of FSH and LH after three years of exposure. Intermittant or seasonal exposure of field workers of over two months is accompanied by significant drops in spermatozoon numbers and in FSH elevation (Glass and associates, 1979).

9. *Testosterone* has long been known as an inhibitor of spermatogenesis. Continuous testosterone treatment produces a marked decrease in spermatozoon number and testicular size due to the suppression of gonadotropic hormones. This type of treatment, therefore, converts testosterone into a male contraceptive agent (Soufir and others, 1983). Testosterone treatment has been used in oligospermic males with relative success, attempting to provoke an increase in semen quality after finishing the treatment (testosterone rebound therapy).

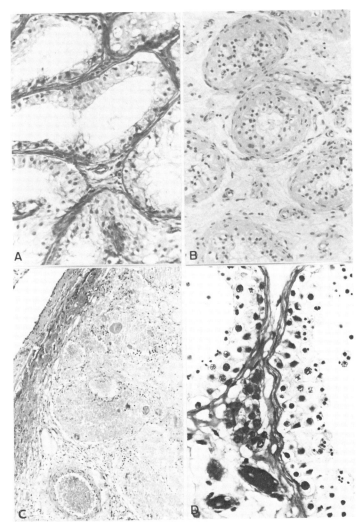

FIGURE 14–3. *A*, Seminiferous tubules lacking germinal cells in an estrogen-treated patient. P.A.S. (x125). *B*, Absence of germinal cells and peritubular fibrosis observed in antiandrogen treatment. H&E (x125). *C*, Hemorrhagic necrosis of the testicular parenchyma produced in a rat after cadmium administration. H&E (x60). *D*, Marked hypospermatogenesis observed in the testicular biopsy of a paraplegic patient. The Leydig cells exhibit Reinke's crystals. H&E (x250).

Testicular Abnormalities Secondary to Dietary Deficiencies

Malnutrition

The perfect functioning of the endocrine system requires adequate, healthy nutrition. This is the only way to guarantee the synthesis and liberation of the hormones that maintain the equilibrium of testicular function and the proper trophic state.

Hyponourishment situations in prepubescence are responsible for genital infantilism and frequently for cryptorchidism along with often irreversible lesions in the testicular parenchyma. Hypogonadotropic hypogonadism is frequent in malnourished adults. The testicular pattern shows small seminiferous tubule diameter, thickening of the tunica propria, and a drop in Leydig cell size. Histochemically there is a lessening of β-hydroxysteroid dehydrogenase (Leathem, 1970).

The pathogenic mechanism is established through the hypothalamic-hypophyseal-testicular axis. This mechanism is known as a "pseudo-hypophysectomy" state and has low hypothalamic concentrations of releasing factors and obvious pituitary lesions, such as cytoplasmic vacuolation and nuclear pyknosis and, at times, cystic transformation in the gland.

An experimental reduction of *protein* intake affects spermatogenesis. These results are not only related to protein quantity, but also to the amino acid composition of the proteins. Nine days after beginning a diet lacking in arginine there is a great drop in spermatozoon counts in men. Lysine and tryptophane deficiencies, contrary to what occurs with experimental animals, do not appear to diminish spermatogenesis in humans. A drop in spermatogenesis is considered to be caused by a lessening of pituitary hormone synthesis.

The most studied *carbohydrate*-metabolism alterations in human pathology are those associated with diabetes mellitus. A marked hypospermatogenesis with frequent morphological anomalies is known to exist in diabetic patients (Faerman and others, 1972). In rats, tolbutamide and insulin produce germinal line lesions that can be prevented by simultaneous glucose administration.

Diets poor in essential *fatty acids* can produce seminiferous epithelium degeneration in experimental animals (rats). This is believed to occur through the pituitary, which shows alterations in the adenohypophysis.

Avitaminosis

Liposoluble vitamin absorption is greatly disturbed, especially in the absorption of the tocopherols, in the severe fat-metabolism disorders (for example, congenital biliary atresia; cystic fibrosis; chronic pancreatitis; idiopathic steatorrhea; sprue; coeliac disease; Whipple's disease; and lymphatic vessel blocks of differing etiology) observed in biliary system, pancreas, or in intestine illness.

Vitamin E deficiency is very frequent in tropical populations as their diets are rich in carbohydrates and low in fats. Tullock and Sood (1967) found that approximately 30 percent of their subjects in an extensive population in Uganda displayed an extremely low tocopherol serum index.

Although it is difficult to establish the way in which one specific vitamin deficiency contributes to the production of a particular lesion in human pathology, a chronic vitamin deficiency must exist before the lesion can manifest itself. The information concerning the development of the deficiency can be more important than the intensity of the steatorrhea itself. Binder and Spiro (1967) feel that unless the steatorrhea has lasted at least a year, there has not necessarily been any development of vitamin E deficiency.

Experimentally, the deficiency of vitamin E produces lesions in guinea pigs, hamsters, and bird testes. These lesions are particularly intense in the rat, where vitamin E deficiency can even lead to testicular atrophy. If three-week-old rats are subjected to a diet entirely lacking in vitamin E, lesions are produced in the following stages. *First stage*: After one to two months, pyknosis and spermatozoon head atrophy are observed while the germinal epithelium is still preserved. *Second stage*: After two or three months there is an intense drop in spermatozoon number and degeneration signs in the spermatids and secondary spermatocytes. *Third stage*: Intratubular sloughing of spermatocytes and spermatids and the appearance of giant cells in the seminiferous epithelium or in the tubular lumen are the most characteristic features. These giant cells are spermatids without cytoplasmic segmentation. *Fourth stage*: Secondary spermatocytes and spermatogonia degeneration and fatty degeneration and lysis in the giant cells are observed. *Fifth stage*: Three to six months after the imposition of the avitaminosis the germinal epithelium has disappeared and Leydig cells may appear retracted, normal, or even slightly augmented. Biochemically there is a proven drop in glucogen, aspartic transaminase, esterase, and β-glucuronidase (Shina and co-authors, 1964).

Vitamin A deficiency can be present in human pathology as part of a generalized state of malnutrition, especially when a lack of protein predominates. In gestating females, vitamin A deficiency manifests in complex malformations in the fetus that affect virtually all the structures of the organism. Cryptorchidism and testicular hypoplasia are the most notable effects in the genital area. In numerous adult experimental animals (mice, rats, guinea pigs, cats, bulls) vitamin A has been proven to take part in the maintenance of testicular function and structure. Deficiencies that are not very severe determine effects that spread from rapid drops in spermatogenesis to testicular atrophy in which the seminiferous tubules only display Sertoli cells and spermatogonia (Huang and Hembree, 1979; Sobhon and others, 1979). Spermatogenesis can be restored after three months of an appropriate diet. Leydig cells do not usually display alterations (Huang and co-authors, 1983).

Among other biochemical determinations a drop in phospholipids, (although not as intense as in vitamin E deficiency) and an absence of liposomic enzyme liberation are manifested (Reddy and Khanna, 1983).

It is now believed, despite some disagreement, that the active mechanism of vitamin A deficiency acts directly, either upon the germinal cells or through the Sertoli cells, but in either case without significant hypothalamic-hypophyseal axis intervention. These findings are based on Palludan's (1966) studies. The injection of vitamin A into boar testes displaying testicular atrophy caused by dietary deficiency, is followed by maturation of the seminiferous epithelium in the tubules in the vicinity of the injected material, but not in the more distantly located tubules nor in the contralateral testis.

Prolonged *vitamin C* deficiency in rodents can cause atrophy in the Leydig cells as well as in the seminiferous tubules. Acute deprivation causes important changes in DNA and RNA.

Biotin deficiency during fetal life produces cryptorchidism and, later, testicular development delay with selective damage to germinal cells.

Pantothenic acid and *pyridoxine* deficiencies produce sterility in rats, principally due to their effect on the seminiferous epithelium, which eventually leads to the disappearance of the germinal line (Delost and Terroine, 1966). *Thiamin, folic acid,* and *vitamin B_{12}* deficiencies produce less serious testicular lesions.

Minerals

Zinc is present in high concentrations in spermatogonia, spermatocytes, and spermatozoon heads and, to a lesser degree, in Leydig and Sertoli cells. The progressive incorporation of zinc into spermatids during the last stages of their maturation into spermatozoa is necessary for normal spermiogenesis (Björndahl and Kvist, 1982; Reyes and associates, 1983). An insufficient supply of zinc during adolescence results in an important delay in pubertal maturation. In adults, it may lead to severe oligospermia (Abbasi and associates, 1980).

Experimentally, (after imposing a zinc-poor diets on rats) it is found that there is a drop in lactic, malic, and alcoholic dehydrogenase activity as well as some diaforase activities. These experiments also showed a reduction of testicular lipids, which is not as intense as in vitamin E deficiency, as well as an increase in protein catabolism without an affect on protein synthesis. These alterations, in principle, are felt to be due to inanition and a pituitary trophic hormone deficit. This hypothesis is corroborated in clinical practice where hypogonadotropic hypogonadisms are frequently observed in adolescent's between 12 and 20 years of age whose diets are lacking in zinc.

In adults, the administration of gonadotropins does not prevent seminiferous tubule atrophy. Therefore it is assumed that zinc acts directly on the testis.

Patients with cretinism or those with *iodine* deficient diets display great testicular development delay and their seminiferous tubules contain few germinal cells, with some spermatocytes. Atrophy of Leydig cells is also observed. In hypothyroidism, vitamin A carotene conversion is reduced, vitamin B requirements are higher, and protein synthesis lower. Myxedematous men manifest androgen metabolism alterations and an exiguous androsterone production. Thyroid hormones can reverse these situations.

Iron is one of the metals found in semen and it is appears bound to the proteins in the spermatozoon tail. Experiments with guinea pigs have shown that prolonged iron administration leads to tubular atrophy. However, Prasad and coauthors (1961) tell us that inhabitants of some villages in Iran who suffer from malnutrition present a syndrome characterized by sideropenic anemia, hypogonadism, and dwarfism. The iron present in the diet of these patients, while in normal quantity, is poorly absorbed due to high phosphate consumption. This hypogonadism is related to malnutrition, and to a zinc or iron deficiency.

Lead's harmful effects have been known since the last century and it is admitted that the high frequency of sterile couples and miscarriages among lead workers is due to its harmful effect on the testes (Lancrajan and associates, 1975; Thomas and Brogan, 1983).

Cadmium is extremely toxic to the testis. Even when the dosage received does not produce lesions in other organs, hemorrhagic necrosis occurs in the testis, which continues with seminiferous tubule calcification and Leydig cell atrophy (Fig. 14–3C).

By experimentation, other mineral dietary deficiencies or excesses have been proven to affect the testis. For example, *calcium*-poor diets, if maintained, reduce Leydig cell number and *Phosphorus* and *manganese* deficiencies condition maturation arrest. Impotence is one of the most precocious symptoms of intoxication by these elements.

Testicular Abnormalities Secondary to Peripheral Nervous System Lesions

Thoraco-lumbar sympathectomy produces in most animals the loss of a great number of the vasomotor fibers in the testis, epididymis and ductus deferens. Partial extirpation of the sympathetic chain in man (Monro, 1959), as well as in animals, is followed by testicular lesions. At the tubular level, germinal cell degeneration with a lower mitotic index is established. Intense vasodilation is produced at the interstitial level. The explanation of the mechanism behind this atrophy has followed several hypothesis: loss of pampiniformis plexus tone (Baumgarten and associates, 1968); seminiferous epithelium anoxia, which is secondary to vascular stagnation; and functional obstruction caused by spermatozoa in an epididymal region close by the ductus deferens (Hodson, 1965).

Light testicular atrophy with hypospermatogenesis is observed in spinal cord transection. These lesions are difficult to explain with the former theories since vasomotor tone is regulated by lateral horn neurons and persists even when connections with superior centers are interrupted (Fig. 14–3D). Similar testicular atrophies have been found after rectal cancer surgery.

REFERENCES

1. Abbasi AA, Prasad A, Rabbani P, Du Mouchelle E: Experimental zinc deficiency in man. Effect on testicular function. J Lab Clin Med 96:544, 1980
2. Albers-Schönberg HE: Ueber eine bisher Unbekannte Wirkung der Röntgen-strahlen auf den Organismus der Tiere. Münch Med Wochschr 50:1859, 1903
3. Baba S, Murai M, Jitsukawa S, Hata M, Tazaki H.: Antiandrogenic effects of spironolactone: hormonal and ultrastructural studies in dogs and men. J Urol 119:375, 1978
4. Baumgarten HG, Falck B, Holstein AF, Owman C, Owman T: Adrenergic innervation of the human testis, epididymis, ductus deferens and prostate: A fluorescence, microscopic, and fluorometric study. Z Zellforsch 90:81, 1968
5. Binder HJ, Spiro HM: Tocopherol deficiency in man. Amer J Clin Nutr 20:594, 1967
6. Björndahl L, Kvist U. Importance of zinc for human sperm head-tail connection. Acta Physiol Scan 116:51, 1982
7. Conley GR, Sant GR, Ucci AA, Mitcheson HD: Seminoma and epididymal cysts in a young man with known diethylstilbestrol exposure in utero. JAMA 249:1325, 1983
8. Dambert JE, Janson PO: The effects of LH, adrenaline, and noradrenaline on testicular blood flow and plasma testosterone concentrations in anesthetized rats. Acta Endocrinol 88:390, 1978
9. Delafontaine D, Marmor D, Roux C: Influence sur la fertilité du traitement de la maladie de Hodgkin par MOPP. La Nouvelle Presse Médicale 34:2757, 1979
10. Delost P, Terroine T: Origin of sexual disturbations in the male on pyridoxine deficiency. Hormonal and vitamin treatment. Arch Sci Physiol 20:65, 1966
11. Doleček R, Dvořáček C, Ježek M, Kubis M, Sajnar J, Závada M: Very low serum testosterone levels and severe impairment of spermatogenesis in burned male patients. Correlations with basal levels and levels of FSH, LH and PRL after LHRH + TRH. Endocrinol Exp (Bratisl) 17:33, 1983
12. Ellis LC: In: The Testis III Johnson AD, Gomes WR, and Vandemark NL (eds) New York: Academic Press, 1970
13. Faerman J, Vilar O, Rivarola MA, Rosner JM, Jadzinsky MN, Fox D, Lloret AP, Bernstein-Hahn L, Saraceni D: Impotence and diabetes. Studies on androgenic function in diabetic impotent males. Diabetes 21:23, 1972
14. Fossa SD, Klepp O, Aakvaag A, Molne K: Testicular function after combined chemotherapy for metastatic testicular cancer. Int J Androl 3:59, 1980
15. Friedman NM, Plymate SR: Leydig cell dysfunction and gynecomastia in adult males treated with alkylating agents. Clin Endocr 12:553, 1980
16. Gill WB, Schumacher GF, Bibbo M: Pathological semen and anatomical abnormalities of the genital tract in human male subjects exposed to diethylstilbestrol in utero. J Urol 117:477, 1977
17. Glass RI, Lyness RN, Mengle DC, Powell KE, Kahn E: Sperm count depression in pesticide applicators exposed to dibromochloropropane. Am J Epidemiol 109:346, 1979
18. Hacker U, Schumann J, Göhde W, Müller K: Mammalian spermatogenesis as a biologic dosimeter for radiation. Acta Radiol Oncol Radiat Phys Biol 20:279, 1981
19. Hodson N: Sympathetic nerves and reproductive organs in the male rabbit. J Reprod Fertility 10:209, 1965
20. Huang HFS, Dyrenfurth I, Hembree WC: Endocrine changes associated with germ cell loss during vitamin A deficiency and vitamin A-induced recovery of spermatogenesis. Endocrinology 112:1163, 1983
21. Huang HF, Hembree WC: Spermatogenic re-

sponse to vitamin A in vitamin A deficient rats. Biol Reprod 21:891, 1979
22. Jones TM, Fang VS, Landau RL, Rosenfield R: Direct inhibition of Leydig cell function by estradiol. J Clin Endocrinol Metabol 47:1368, 1978
23. Lancrajan I, Popescu HI, Gavanescu O: Reproductive ability of workmen occupationally exposed to lead. Arch Environ Health 30:396, 1975
24. Lange PH, Narayan P, Vogelzang NJ, Shafer RB, Kennedy BJ, Fraley EE: Returns of fertility after treatment for nonseminomatous testicular cancer: changing concepts. J Urol 129:1131, 1983
25. Leathem JH: In The Testis III Johnson AD, Gomes WR, Vandemark NL (eds) New York: Academic Press, 1970
26. Lee IP, Dixon RL: Factors influencing reproductive and genetic toxic effect on male gonads. Environ Health Perspect 24:117, 1978
27. Leiper AD, Grant DB, Chessells JM: The effect of testicular irradiation on Leydig cell function in prepubertal boys with acute lymphoblastic leukemia. Arch Dis Child 58:906, 1983
28. Merlin HE: Azoospermia caused by colchicine. A case report. Fertil Steril 23:180, 1972
29. Miller DG: Alkylating agents and human spermatogenesis. JAMA 217:1662, 1971
30. Monro PA: In Sympathectomy. New York: Oxford University Press, 1959
31. Palludan B: Direct effect of vitamin A on boar testis. Nature 211:639, 1966
32. Prasad AS, Halsted JA, Nadimi M: Syndrome of iron deficiency anemia, hepatosplenomegaly, hypogonadism, dwarfism, and geophagia. Am J Med 31:532, 1961
33. Procope BJ: Effect of repeated increase of body temperature on human sperm cells. Int J Fertil 10:333, 1965
34. Reddy TS, Khanna A: Effect of undernutrition and vitamin A deficiency on the phospholipid composition of rat tissues at 21 days of age. II. Lung, Heat and Testes. Internat J Vit Nutr Res 53:9, 1983
35. Reyes R, Magdaleno VM, Hernández O, Rosado A, Delgado NM: Effect of zinc on decondensation of human spermatozoa nuclei by heparin. Arch Androl 10:155, 1983
36. Robinson D, Rock J, Menkin MF: Control of human spermatogenesis by induced changes of intrascrotal temperature. JAMA 204:290, 1968
37. Rugh R: In Errera M, Forsberg A (eds) Mechanism in radiobiology, Vol. II New York: Academic Press, 1960
38. Sas M, Szöllösi J: Impaired spermiogenesis as a common finding among professional drivers. Arch Androl 3:57, 1979
39. Shina KK, Roy S, Mukherjee AK: Vitamin E and carbohydrate metabolism. Indian J Physiol Allied Sci 18:134, 1964
40. Sobhon P, Mitranond V, Tosukhowong P, Chindaduan-Grat W: Cytological changes in the testes of vitamin A-deficient rats. Ultrastructural study of the seminiferous tubules. Acta anat. 103:169, 1979
41. Soufir JC, Jouannet P, Marson J, Soumah A: Reversible inhibition of sperm production and gonadotropin secretion in men following combined oral medroxiprogesterone acetate and percutaneous testosterone treatment. Acta Endocrinol (Copenh) 102:625, 1983
42. Thomas JA, Brogan WC.: Some actions of lead on the sperm and on the male reproductive system. Am J Industr Medic 4:127, 1983
43. Tullock JA, Sood NK: Vitamin E deficiency in Uganda. Amer J Clin Nutr 20:884, 1967
44. Vermeulen A: Effects of drugs on Leydig cell function. Int J Androl (Suppl) 5:163, 1982 Whitehead ED, Leiter E: Genital abnormalities and abnormal semen analyses in male patients exposed to diethylstilbestrol in utero. J Urol 125:47, 1981

15

VASCULAR DISORDERS OF THE TESTIS

Experimental Bases of Ischemic Lesions

Experimental studies on the effects of ischemia on the testis have been carried out in numerous laboratory animals. The findings on the human testis come for the most part from the observation of testicular lesions that involve ischemia as in spermatic cord torsion. Experimental studies show that the occlusion of the testicular artery leads, within a very short period of time, to necrosis of the parenchyma and a drop in androgen levels.

Testicular Artery Occlusion

Experiments done on rats show that three days after arterial clamping, numerous tubules develop necrosis: After six days the testis displays considerable weight loss and a lack of living cells in most of the testicular parenchyma except for the periphery, which is less affected (Fig. 15–1). The resulting degenerative changes can be outlined as follows:

Seminiferous tubules display alterations as soon as one hour after the suppression of arterial flow. Sertoli cells show an increase in lipids and lysosomes and many vesicles and vacuoles that originated from the smooth endoplasmic reticulum have appeared. The cytoplasm in the spermatogonia has become electron-dense and vacuolated while the chromatin has condensed into small clumps, forming a peripheral band, attached to the nuclear envelope.

Similar changes are observed in spermatocytes and spermatids. The latter are the first affected, so that only an hour after suppression of arterial flow, sloughed spermatids can be found in the tubular lumen. After three hours the changes in the seminiferous epithelium are accentuated and cellular degeneration is quite marked. After approximately six hours, spermatids and spermatogonia are detached from the seminiferous epithelium. Sertoli cells are the most resistant cell type. After 24 hours most cells in the seminiferous epithelium are completely necrosed. Leydig cells begin to degenerate approximately six hours after arterial occlusion. They display intense cytoplasmic vacuolation and abundant lipofuchsin granules.

With ischemia, connective testicular tissue also undergoes visible changes after 24 hours. The tunica albuginea as well as the intertubular spaces appear to be swollen and contain fibrin deposits. The mesothelium of the tunica albuginea sloughs and the albuginea thickens noticeably. After three days the epithelium sheds the basement membrane around the seminiferous tubules. Myofibroblasts begin to degenerate, their cytoplasm becomes denser and the lysosome content increases. Some myofibroblasts die, so that, after six days, the number of these cells have considerably decreased. The remaining connective cells acquire macrophagic properties that, after two weeks, are very obvious. Some weeks later the seminiferous tubules completely disappear and the entire testis is invaded by fibroblasts, collagen fibers, and neoformed blood vessels (Kaya and Harrison, 1975).

The possibilities for testicular recuperation after temporary ischemia are in proportion to the intensity of damage done and the duration of the ischemia. If the arterial occlusion lasts for less than one hour (producing light or moderate damage) the testis can completely recuperate after several weeks. However, if the ischemia lasts between two and six hours,

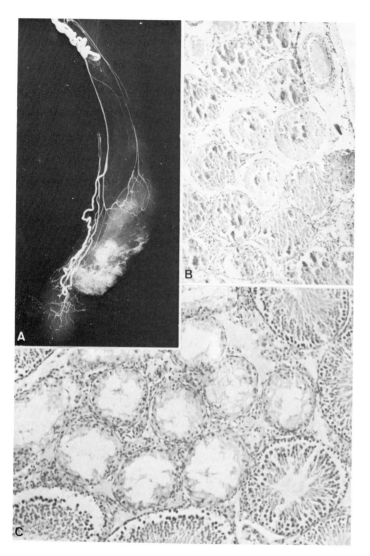

FIGURE 15–1. Experimental rat ischemia. A, Arteriography performed 15 days after testicular artery occlusion. A scarcity of blood vessels in the testicular parenchyma and numerous calcifications are observed. Vascularization is attained via anastomoses with other arteries of the spermatic cord. B, Total seminiferous epithelium necrosis with focal intratubular calcifications. Testis observed six days after testicular artery clamping. H&E (x60). C, A group of seminiferous tubules containing only Sertoli cells, surrounded by normal seminiferous tubules, in a zone close to the tunica albuginea. The picture was taken one month after testicular artery clamping. H&E (x60).

spermatogenesis will resume in only a few tubules and the remaining tubules will only contain Sertoli cells. Finally, if the ischemia should last over six hours, not even tubules containing only Sertoli cells will recuperate, even long after the return of arterial flow (Steinberger, 1970).

Contralateral Testis

The testis opposite to the one that suffered testicular artery occlusion will also manifest some transitory changes of unknown origin (Kaya and Harrison, 1975). Three days after the ischemia is produced the contralateral testis will show an increase in lysosomes and lipid droplets and cytoplasmic vacuolation can be observed in the Sertoli cells. After 18 days the cells are recuperated and present an almost normal appearance. Spermatogonia also show changes after the third day: the cytoplasm presents vacuolation and contains some increased lipid inclusions. Recuperation takes place some 14 days later.

Spermatocytes begin to degenerate 3 days after arterial occlusion. Many die and can be seen to slough within the tubular lumen. They are replaced by new spermatocytes that have developed from recuperated spermatogonia.

Spermatids are the most strongly affected cells. They begin to degenerate only a few hours after the onset of ischemia. Most of them die and are sloughed. New, immature spermatids can be seen replacing the sloughed ones (after 18 days). Many of these new spermatids display alterations such as the presence of two or more nuclei. This is caused by karyokinesis without cytokinesis occuring during their development. This defect does not arrest their maturation and eventually they form infertile binucleate spermatozoa.

Situations that recall these experimental models occur in human pathology. Testes affected by an acute ischemia also rapidly develop a testicular infarct. The infarct is hemorrhagic in spermatic cord torsions, vena cava thrombosis, and compression of the cord caused by a strangled hernia (Waldbaum and others, 1976). It is diffuse in the majority of the cases. Segmentary or focal infarcts are associated with stages of hypercoagulability and polycythemia for example. The infarct in ischemic is arterial obstructions secondary to emboli, thrombosis, or inflammations of the testicular artery or its branches. The lesions produced by chronic ischemia (for example, arteriosclerosis and hypertension) are focal and multiple.

Testicular Lesions in Arteriosclerosis

Small groups of sclerosed seminiferous tubules can be observed in 60 percent of normal adult testes. These findings become more and more frequent with advancing age. Other groups of seminiferous tubules, close by or not to the sclerosed tubules, show hypoplasia of germ cells. The arterioles show thickenings of their walls that vary with age. The small ones (12 microns in diameter) can reach diameter of 50 microns or more—the largest ones (50 microns in diameter) can reach diameters of 250 microns. The most sensible areas are located under the tunica albuginea and they are supplied by recurrent centrifugal arteries (Fig. 15–2A and B). The chronology of the most frequently observed testicular lesions is as follows:

1. *Early lesions*: a patchy distribution of light spermatogenesis; isolated sclerosis in the seminiferous tubules or lineal scars; and minimal fibrosis of the testicular artery, its branches and/or focal arteriolar hyalinosis.
2. *Evolved lesions*: a patchy distribution of severe hypospermatogenesis; seminiferous tubule sclerosis, forming perpendicular scars to the tunica albuginea; fibrosis in the tunica intima and tunica media of the great arteries and arterioles, and a normal or decreased Leydig cell number (Fig. 15–2C).
3. *Late lesions*: tubular sclerosis that is either total or respects some groups of tubules that lack germinal cell line and show variable basement membrane thickening; fibrosis primarily in the tunica intima with severe luminar stenosis in the testicular, centripetal, and centrifugal arteries. Angiography shows irregular or absent arterial bending and a marked decrease in the number of arterioles, capillaries, and veins is observed. Scarce and vacuolated Leydig cells are observed in the interstitium (Fig. 15–3A, B, and C).

With reference to the relation between testicular lesions and the systemic vascular lesions of arteriosclerosis, in general, it may be said that there is no direct correlation between the intensity of the testicular lesions and the degree of systemic arteriosclerosis. Nevertheless, if we consider the degree of arteriosclerosis in the coronary vessels, the aorta, and the arteries of the brain base, the following interesting observations can be made (Krus and associates, 1971). Patients with severe arteriosclerosis and who have had a myocardial infarct at an early age usually do not have testicular lesions and their testicular histology and spermatogenesis is normal. However, patients with advanced arteriosclerosis in the vessels of

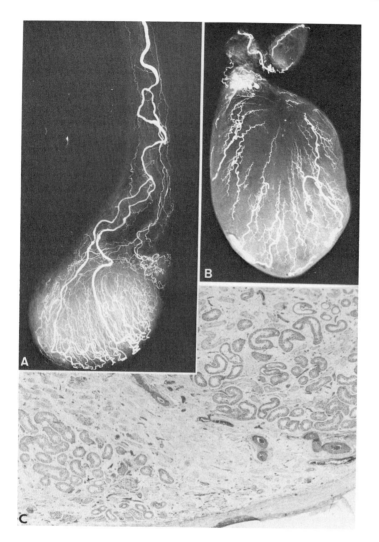

FIGURE 15–2. *Arteriosclerosis A, Arteriography showing multiple stenoses along the principal branches of the testicular artery. B, Reduction in parenchymatous arterial branch number. C, Wedge atrophy of seminiferous tubules following testicular blood vessel distribution. The base of the wedge is located at the periphery of the testicular parenchyma and the apex towards the center of the testis. H&E (x40).*

the brain base show characteristic testicular lesions with patchy seminiferous tubule sclerosis and decreased spermatogenesis. Advanced focal tubular sclerosis is observed in over a half of the patients with severe aortic arteriosclerosis.

TESTICULAR LESIONS IN HYPERTENSION

Testicular size appears slightly decreased, and there are diffuse arterial and parenchymatous lesions in patients with hypertension. The lesions are more related to the time elapsed since the hypertension began than to its intensity. Hypertrophy of the tunica media, and a proliferation of the inner elastic sheath and connective tissue cells and fibers is observed in the arterioles. These lesions are usually associated with arteriolar hyalinosis and/or arteriosclerotic lesions in the large blood vessels.

The testicular parenchyma lesions affect the seminiferous tubules as well as the intertubular spaces. The seminiferous tubules show a slight caliber reduction without a notable thickening of either the basal lamina or of the tunica propria. The spermatogenesis is very reduced; many tubules show maturation only to spermatocytes and there is a marked reduction of the numbers of type A and B spermatogonia.

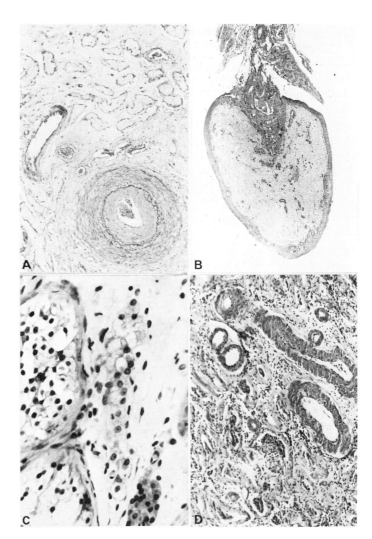

FIGURE 15-3. *Testicular arteriosclerosis. A, Concentric thickening of the tunica intima and diffuse tubular sclerosis in the testicular arteries. Van Gieson elastic fibers (x60). B, Diffuse testicular atrophy in severe testicular arteriosclerosis. H&E (x5). C, Leydig cells with pyknotic excentric nucleus and intense cytoplasmic vacuolation. H&E (x400). D, Testicular amyloidosis. Artery and arteriole walls show thickening of hyaline appearance. The testicular parenchyma shows diffuse tubular sclerosis. Congo red (x60).*

Some tubules are collapsed and no cells can be seen in their interiors. The interstitial connective tissue is found to be augmented, with intense collagenization and occasional lymphoplasmacyte cell infiltrations.

TESTICULAR ARTERIOLAR HYALINOSIS

Arteriolar hyalinosis is characterized by an accumulation of a PAS positive, eosinophilic, amorphous substance—which is unaccompanied by necrosis or other inflammatory processes—below the arteriole endothelium. These deposits adopt a segmented distribution and are eccentric, assymetric, and irregular; at times completely stenosing the arteriolar lumen. Arteriolar hyalinosis is frequently found in childrens' and adults' follicular arterioles of the spleen. In adults, it is a constant finding in the hepatic, choroidal, and retinal arterioles, where its presence is closely related to hypertension and/or diabetes. It is also very common in the hepatic, pancreatic, and adrenal arterioles, and in the arterioles of the limbs of elderly patients.

Testicular arteriolar hyalinization was first studied by Hatakeyama and others (1966), who discovered this lesion to be present in nearly all adult testes. The characteristic deposits of this lesion may be small. They stand out as subendothelial nodules protruding toward the lumen or they may be large clumps. These deposits partially or completely collapse the arteriolar lumen; their structure is amorphous or fibrillar, with small vacuoles near the endothelium as well as near the smooth muscle cells. There are one or more vacuolated or pyknotic nuclei, which may or may not be surrounded by a clear zone on the inside of these clumps. Coinciding with these affected areas, the smooth muscle cells appear atrophied, are absent, or form a discontinuous layer. These lesions are PAS positive and resistant to diastase. Their distribution is fairly homogeneous. With oil-red-O stain, lipids are shown to be abundant, either in the form of small drops or in long crystals that show an acicular shape under polarized light. With Masson trichrome stain the small lesions—probably younger—stand out due to their affinity for the fuchsin stain. The more developed lesions are reddish stained, and alternate with other greenish or less stained zones. Alcian blue stains at different pH show little positivity either in small or in larger lesions. Using PTAH stain the whole range of colors, from ochre to intense red, is obtained. These lesions are not argyrophilic (Fig. 15–4A and B).

Immunological studies demonstrate the presence of plasmatic proteins in all cases, although the type of protein varies from one case to another. Not all of the

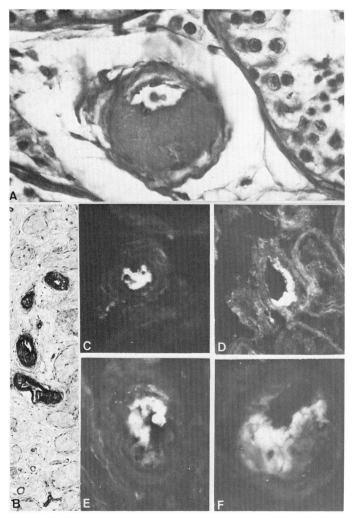

FIGURE 15–4. *Testicular arteriolar hyalinosis. A, Subendothelial hyaline deposits in an intertubular arteriole. Masson trichrome (x400). B, Multiple arteriolar hyalinosis lesions associated with tubular sclerosis. P.A.S. (x60). C and D, IgG deposits in testicular arterioles. E, IgM deposits in a testicular artery. F, Fibrin deposits in a testicular arteriole.*

arterial lesions show the same fluorescent intensity with the different antisera. The smaller lesions display greater intensity. The greatest intensities are obtained using IgM, fibrin, fibrinogen, and B_1C complement fraction antisera. Examination with most of the commonly used antisera is negative in some of the lesions (Fig. 15–4C, D, E, and F).

The arterioles studied with the electron microscope display alterations at different levels. The endothelial cells appear to be hypertrophic only occasionally, and contain abundant lipofuchsin granules in the cytoplasm. Electrodense deposits, which when extensive can envelop the basal lamina, are found below the latter. Seen at a low magnification, these deposits appear to be formed by an homogeneous material that is more electrondense than the basal lamina and are spotted by islets of some smooth muscle cell cytoplasms or very osmiophilic granules. At higher magnifications, these deposits show 200 Å granules, the presence of fibers with the collagen periodicity, fibrin, or amyloid may not be confirmed. The material extends from the proximity of the endothelial cells to the inner elastic sheath. In other arterioles the inner elastic sheath has completely or partially disappeared and the material has surrounded the smooth muscle cells of the tunica media (Fig. 15–5B and C).

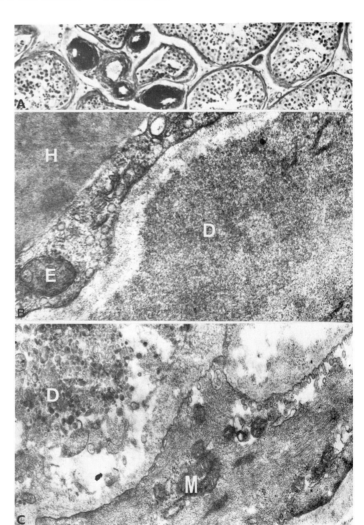

FIGURE 15–5. Testicular arteriolar hyalinosis. A, Arteriolar hyalinosis lesions associated with light spermatogenesis. P.A.S. (×125). B, Electron micrograph of fibrilar and granular subendothelial deposits (D), (E) Endothelium, (H) Hematie. (×35,000). C, Amorphous granular material deposits (D) among smooth muscle cells (M). (×25,000).

The lesions of testicular parenchyma that accompany hyalinosis are focal. They are characterized by a light, marked, or severe hypospermatogenesis, or by tubular sclerosis (Fig. 15–5A). The lesions generally develop near the rete testis and periseptal zones (Hatakeyama and others, 1979).

There is a certain parallelism between arteriolar hyalinosis and age. Toward the beginning of the third decade of life, the incidence distribution curve becomes sharply ascendent, reaching maximum values at around 30 years of age. The most affected blood vessels are arterioles with diameters between 50 and 100 microns. The material constituting the deposits is primarily glycoproteins and lipids. Much of the protein corresponds to immunoglobulin, fibrin, and fibrinogen. The lipids have been found to correspond to neutral fats and cholesterol. This composition coincides with that found in arteriolar hyalinosis in other organs (Dustin, 1962).

The accumulated material may have a serum origin. This hypothesis is supported by the finding of immunoglobulins, fibrin, and fibrinogen in the deposits. The initial lesion could consist of an alteration of endothelial cell permeability.

The repercussions of arteriolar hyalinosis on the testicular parenchyma are directly related to three factors: (1) the number of arteries with hyalinosis; (2) the degree of arteriolar affectation; and (3) the age. These factors are usually parallel. Testicular arteriolar hyalinosis is more frequent in those testes that display atrophic lesions. It is difficult to determine whether hyalinosis is always the cause of tubular sclerosis or whether it is a parallel lesion. Patients with the Klinefelter's syndrome have high incidences of testicular hyalinosis. Not less than half of the biopsies performed on these patients show arteriolar hyalinosis. Local factors in the arterial wall that facilitate hyalinosis deposits probably exist. The explanation is found, on the one hand, in the fact that not less than ten percent of these patients are diabetic and, on the other, in the anomaly of the basement membrane. This anomaly is probably not confined to the seminiferous tubules alone (Nistal and others, 1973).

TESTICULAR AMYLOIDOSIS

An amyloid is a fibrillar protein that is deposited in numerous tissues and organs causing different lesions in accordance to the different tissues damaged. Four types of amyloidosis are identified clinically: primary; secondary; macroglobulin-myeloma associated; and hereditary amyloidosis.

The testes are usually affected by secondary amyloidosis that has usually been anteceded by chronic pyogenic infections (including pyelonephritis; bronchiectasis; osteomyelitis; and empyema); chronic granulomatous infections (tuberculosis; leprosy; and Crohn's disease); chronic arthritis (rheumatoid; psoriasic; or ankylosing spondylitis); and some tumors (Hodgkin's disease, other lymphomas, renal and bronchogenic carcinomas).

The testicular lesions are preferentially vascular. The arteries and arterioles show subintima or transmural deposits that stained with H.E. are similar to those of arteriolar hyalinosis. This material is stained showing red-yellow birefringent dichroism using Congo-red stain. The seminiferous tubules lose size and a progressive atrophy of the germinal cell line is established. The interstitium may contain unspecific chronic inflammatory infiltrations (Fig. 15–3D).

SPERMATIC CORD TORSION

The hemorrhagic testis infarct, which is secondary to spermatic cord torsion, was first described by Delasiauve (1901). Spermatic cord torsion is a surgical emergency. If the operation is delayed for only a few hours, the testicular lesions will evolve into hemorrhagic necrosis or fibrosis and will destroy the testis.

The distribution curve by age shows two peaks of maximum incidence—one during neonatal period and the other at puberty. The ascending and descending curves of the latter are very gentle.

Spermatic cord torsion incidence is calculated at three to four patients per year in a general hospital (Skoglund and associates, 1970). We have found an average of nine to ten infarcted testes annually in our hospital. It is rare after 30 years of age (Altaffer, 1980). Bilateral torsions are very rare. Several intrauterine bilateral torsions have been described; however, the lesions, although characteristic, appeared to have occurred at different times. Intrauterine bilateral spermatic cord torsion could probably be the cause of anorchia (Aynsley-Green and others, 1976). The clinical symptoms, so marked in postnatal torsions, appear much more attenuated in intrauterine cases, in which the most important symptom is only the increase in testicular size. There is a slight predominance of the left side (60 percent) in the incidence of unilateral torsion.

There are a series of factors that predispose to torsion. The first are anatomic abnormalities in the insertion into the tunica vaginalis. The testis is fixed to the scrotal wall by three structures: the retroepididymal and retrovaginal surfaces in the posterior internal region; by the spermatic cord in the superior region; and by the scrotal ligament in the inferior region. The reduction of this attaching surface facilitates intravaginal torsion (Fig. 15–6).

A good number of children's and infants' testes present abnormally high reflections of the tunica vaginalis, so that much of the spermatic cord becomes ensheathed (Durand and Perrin, 1977). This situation confers exaggerated mobility to the testis, which may be responsible for the high frequency of funicular torsion in newborns (Campbell, 1948; Leach and Masih, 1980). From this fact, it is easier to explain cord torsions as being caused by sudden body movements or by energetic cremasteric contractions and the slightly higher incidence of the left sided torsion (Olivares and Tovar, 1976).

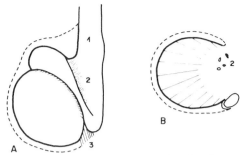

FIGURE 15–6. *The structures that fix the testis to the scrotal wall are: (1) spermatic cord; (2) retroepididymal surface; and (3) the scrotal ligament. Scheme A corresponds to sagittal section. Scheme B corresponds to a transverse section.*

Other predisposing factors are: nonexistant or very long gubernaculum testis; a long, or badly placed, epididymis; and spermatic artery anomalies. An abnormal testis position plays a decisive role in two different processes: retractile testis and cryptorchidism. In both cases the testes frequently undergo trauma and occasionally twist; but this occurs more frequently to the retractile testis. This feature is explained when we consider not only its abnormally high position, but also the hypermobility conferred by its vaginal implantation. If the testis is normally placed, torsion is very rare, and is nearly always the result of trauma of certain intensity.

Testicular torsion usually presents in two forms: low or intravaginal torsion; and supravaginal or extravaginal torsion. In the first case, the tunica vaginalis totally covers the testis and spermatic cord, with the former dangling as though hung from the latter, and the torsion is located in the superior portion. That is to say, the testis has rotated inside the tunica vaginalis, thereby twisting the cord from which it hangs. In the second case the twisting point of the spermatic cord, with respect to the tunica vaginalis that covers it, is very close to the inguinal canal; that is to say, the spermatic cord twists into a spiral. In this case, pain near the inguinal canal, in the proximal part of the cord is the first symptom, while these symptoms occur later and are not as intense in the testis.

The two presentations, intra- or extravaginal testicular torsion, appear at different ages, including the intrauterine period (Atallah and others, 1976). Extravaginal torsions, frequent during infancy, are rarely observed in older children or adults. On the contrary, intravaginal torsions occur primarily after puberty (Nistal and associates, 1971) (Fig. 15–7).

The most characteristic injury to the testicle, whether intra- or extravaginal torsion, is a hemorrhagic infarct. Macroscopically the testis is firm, red or blue in the first stages and black at the end. The veins, because of their thinner walls, collapse before the arteries stop supplying blood into the testis. The first ectasis is observable in the epididymis, followed by edema, and red infarct. The first phase usually lasts six hours; the germinal epithelium is rapidly destroyed by anoxia; this explains why most of the conservate attempts after this time produce poor results. This condition evolves to necrosis, possibly followed by calcification; fibrosis; or mummification. If the torsion is incomplete, or is produced in various stages, the seminiferous tubules slowly atrophy with-

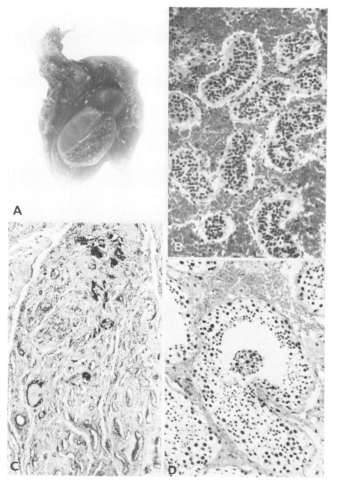

FIGURE 15–7. *Testicular torsion. A, Extravaginal torsion in 2-day-old infant. The dark color of the testis and epididymis corresponds to hemorrhagic infarct. B, Interstitial hemorrhage and seminiferous epithelium sloughing in a 18-hour-old spermatic cord torsion. H&E (x125). C, Testicular sclerosis with calcium salt deposits in a testis which 2 years earlier had suffered torsion and was surgically corrected. H&E (x60). D, Interstitial hemorrhage with relatively good tubular preservation in a 6-hour-long testicular torsion. H&E (x125).*

out symptoms other than hydrocele (Fig. 15–8A).

It has been noted with some frequency that a tumor may manifest itself through hemorrhagic infarct. Torsions of testes containing a tumor have been more frequently reported in undescended testes than in scrotal ones (Cos and others, 1983). Hemorrhagic infarct without torsion secondary to vena cava thrombosis has also been described (Waldbaum and others, 1976).

The differential diagnosis of a patient presenting with an acute scrotum must include not only spermatic cord torsion but also the following processes: strangled hernia, testicular tumor; testicular appendix torsion, traumatic hemorrhagic hydrocele; orchitis; and epididymitis.

The future of the twisted testis depends on the time elapsed from the onset to surgery. Skoglund and associates (1970) saved 83 percent of the testes operated on within 5 hours; 70 percent of those operated on within 10 hours; and only 20 percent of those in which the operation was performed after the first 10 hours had elapsed.

With the purpose of reducing the amount of time the testis suffers ischemia, it is recommended that an external manual reduction be attempted, which, although

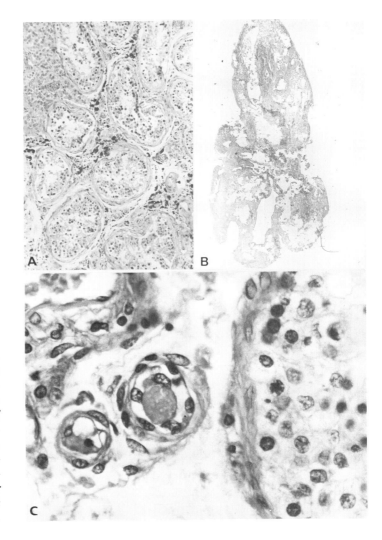

FIGURE 15–8. *A*, Hemosiderin laden macrophages in the intertubular space in a testis with history of an incomplete testicular torsion. H&E (x125). *B*, Hemorrhagic infarct in the testicular hydatid. H&E (x10). *C*, Partially reendothelized vascular thromboses located in intertubular arterioles of a patient with carcinomatosis. H&E (x400).

successful, must be followed by surgical fixation of the torsed testis. The prophylactic fixation of the contralateral testis is also recommended.

Regarding fertility, the prognosis for patients with testicular torsion, even when it has been promptly treated, is reserved. There are two reasons for this. From 33 percent to 68 percent of the testes that were considered to have been saved subsequently atrophy, which proves that the damage produced by the ischemia was underestimated. The second reason is more difficult to comprehend. From 50 (Bartsch et al, 1980) to 95 percent of the patients who had testicular torsion showed defective spermatogenesis. However in a large series of infertile patients none had a history of testicular torsion (Amelar and Dubin, 1973); this suggests that abnormalities of spermatogenesis found on semen analysis are not great enough to render a patient infertile (Scott et al, 1983). Whether the contralateral testis has a primary abnormality, as occurs in a large number of cryptorchid testes, or whether it is a secondary lesion due to unknown factors that operates negatively through the years is a question that still remains open to discussion (Krarup, 1978; Horica and others, 1982). Recent evidence suggests that immunologic factors stimulated by the torsion may effect and damage the contralateral testis.

TESTICULAR AND EPIDIDYMAL APPENDIX TORSION

Torsion of the appendices of the testis and epididymis are conditions that have been frequently observed since they were first described by Colt (1922). The etiologic factors are unknown. They have been related to intense physical activities as the majority of these lesions are observed in youths between 11 and 16 years of age during the months of July and August, which is when the most intense physical activity takes place (Skoglund and others, 1970) (Fig. 15–8B).

INTRAVASCULAR COAGULATION

This is a condition that may affect one or more organs and can present as chronic, subacute, and acute forms depending on the etiologic factors. Schematically it may be due equally to the activation of the intrinsic or extrinsic coagulation systems. Among the latter, coagulation induced by the massive release of thromboplastin (for example, pregnancy associated hypofibrinogenia; abruptio placentae; amniotic fluid embolism; toxemia; fetal respiratory distress) is a well-known feature. The high association between intravascular coagulation and carcinomatosis and acute promyelocytic leukemia, quite possibly due to the high cellular thromboplastin content, stand out among the cases observed in men. It has also been observed in infectious processes that give rise to bacterial septicemia and also activate the intrinsic coagulation system with damage to the vascular endothelium by antigen-antibody complexes. This has been observed in some anaphylactic reactions as well as in reactions to massive transfusions and surgical traumas, for instance in prostatic, pulmonary, or cardiac surgery (Fig. 15–8C).

ARTERITIS, POLYARTERITIS NODOSA

The inflammatory processes that affect the testicular and epididymal blood vessels can present clinically as epididymitis, orchitis, or tumors (Moward, 1971). The conditions that most commonly affect the testicular and epididymal blood vessels are polyarteritis nodosa, rheumatoid arthritis, and Henoch-Schönlein syndrome vasculitis. In all these conditions the vascular lesions present fibrinoid necrosis.

Polyarteritis nodosa is a systemic illness that preferentially affects middle-aged men. The clinical symptoms are secondary to the variable affectation of the different organs and structures. The middle-sized arteries are affected in decreasing order in the following: kidney, heart, skeletal muscle, skin, mesentery, digestive tract, mouth, pancreas, lung, liver, peripheral nerves, meninges, brain, and spinal cord.

The testes are affected so frequently that when it has not been possible to make a diagnosis by other means, spermatic cord exploration and testicular biopsy are indicated (Lee and co-authors, 1983). Testicular affectation varies from 20 to 85 percent. The lesions in the testis develop in the same manner as in the arteries of the other organs, according to this outline:
1. Fibrinoid reaction: The elements forming the tunica media fuse into an eosinophilic mass in which the ultrastructural details are lost. The greater part of this material is fibrin. This necrosis affects different areas along the length of the blood vessels, and includes a complete sector as seen in a transverse section (Fig. 15–9A and B).
2. Inflammatory reaction: first by netro-

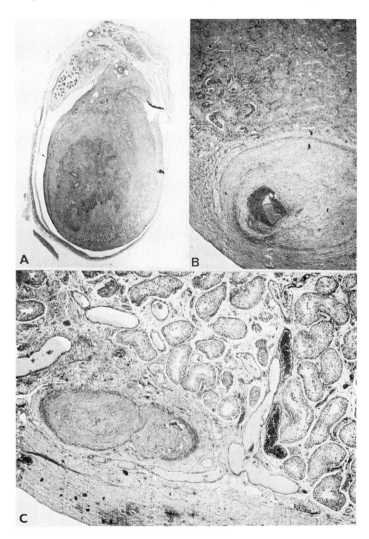

FIGURE 15–9. *Panarteritis nodosa. A, Hemorrhagic infarct affecting over two thirds of the testicular parenchyma. H&E (x4). B, Fibrinoid necrosis of a testicular artery wall and necrosis of neighboring testicular parenchyma. H&E (x60). C, Testicular vessels with long-standing thrombi, which are partially recanalized. H&E (x60).*

philic leukocytes, later by lymphocytes, plasma cells, and histiocytes. The inflammatory reaction around the necrotic areas is stronger.

3. Thrombosis: this is very frequent. It is total in the medium- and small-sized arteries (Fig. 15-9C).

4. Aneurysm formation: this is more frequent when larger vessels are affected. It is produced by a thinning of the tunica media and loss of the elastic fibers while the blood circulates under great pressure through the lumen.

The testicular parenchyma displays total or partial necrosis depending on the affected vessels' caliber. The lesions, when they only affect a few arteries, adopt a pyramidal form with the base located peripherally over the tunica albuginea.

Henoch-Schönlein purpura is a systemic vasculitis that principally affects the skin, joints, intestinal tract, and kidneys. The testis and scrotum are affected in over 15 percent of patients. Sometimes it appears with testicular torsion, and other times with edema and eccymoses of the spermatic cord, testis, testicular appendix, epididymis or scrotal wall, and other times with orchitis or testicular infarct (O'Regan and Robitaille, 1981). Small vessel vasculitis accompanies this condition. In addition to fibrinoid necrosis it presents infiltrations with abundant eosinophilic leukocytes.

Thromboangitis of the distal part in the spermatic cord has been described many years ago by Buerger (1924) and Abercrombie (1965). The histological pattern is similar to that of the other locations.

VARICOCELE

Varicocele is a clinical pathological condition characterized by dilatation, elongation, and increase in sinuosity of the blood vessels of the spermatic plexus, secondary to a venous hypertension. The pathogenetic mechanisms involved in varicocele genesis are multiple and probably, differ from one patient to another. The testicular lesions are progressive and, in the absence of proper treatment, can lead to conditions of testicular atrophy. It is frequently responsible for characteristic spermiogram abnormalities and testicular lesions (Turner, 1983).

Incidence

Varicocele is found in between 8 and 23 percent of the general population (Clarke, 1966; Uehling, 1968). It is more frequent in smokers than in nonsmokers (Klaiber and associates, 1980).

The incidence of varicocele among patients who have consulted for infertility ranges from 10 percent (Horstein, 1973) to 39 percent (Dubin and Amelar, 1975). The left testis is affected much more frequently (70 to 100 percent) than the right. Bilateral varicocele exists (0 to 23 percent), and exclusively right side presentation is rare (0 to 9 percent) (Jecht, 1977). It is observed during the prepuberty as much as during puberty (Pozza and coworkers, 1983). The highest incidence of these cases occurs at about 15 years of age (Hienz and others, 1980).

Clinical Classification

We have followed Dubin and Amelar's (1970) classification from among the multiple clinical classification available. The difficulty of exactly measuring of the degree of venous insufficiency is well known, so that the routine practice of phlebography is advisable. Dubin and Amelar (1970) distinguish the following degrees of varicocele:

First degree: Small varicocele. The size is not more than 1 cm under Valsava maneuver palpation.
Second degree: Moderate varicocele. Size between 1 to 2 cm.

Third degree: Large varicocele. A venous plexus larger than 2 cm in diameter. The venous package fills the hemiscrotum, and is easily visible from a distance.

A fourth degree of varicocele can be added to this classification: A subclinical varicocele or 0 degree, for the cases of spermatic vein reflux, without pampiniform plexus dilatation being present.

When palpated, the testis on the same side as the varicocele is soft and small; it is less descended than the normal contralateral testis (Fig. 15-10).

Anatomical Bases

Testicular venous drainage is primarily by three deep veins: the internal spermatic (testicular vein); the deferential vein, and the external spermatic vein (cremasteric vein); and secondly by a superficial venous system, which drains the scrotum and is constituted by the anterior and posterior scrotal veins, which go to the saphenous vein. There are abundant anastomoses between the superficial and profundus venous systems.

The route of the internal spermatic veins is different on the right and left. The right spermatic vein leads into the cava

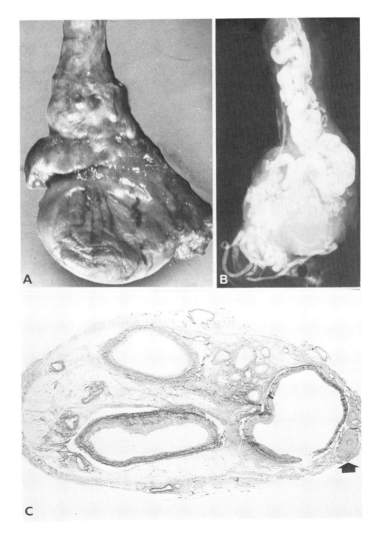

FIGURE 15-10. *Varicocele. A, Surgical specimen showing numerous protrusions produced by venous dilations at the level of the spermatic cord. B, Phlebography of the left spermatic vein showing numerous twisted and dilated vessels of the spermatic plexus. C, Spermatic cord transverse section showing three thick spermatic vein branches with intense lumen dilation and wall fibrosis. Compare the size of the dilated vessels with that of the ductus deferens (arrow). Masson trichrome (x6).*

below the renal vein at an angle of between 30 to 40°. The left spermatic vein is longer (over 42 cm in length) and leads into the left renal vein at nearly right angles. The ostium of its opening is usually opposite the left adrenal vein ostium. Besides its greater length and different angle of opening into the renal vein, the left spermatic vein differs from the right spermatic vein in several structural aspects. While the right spermatic vein has a pair of ostial valves, 40 percent of left spermatic veins lack them, and in a further 10 percent, though present, the ostial valves are insufficient. These facts permit us to deduce that one out two men will experience reflux at some point in their lives, although this does not necessarily imply varicocele. Anastomoses among various spermatic veins are not infrequently observed on the left side. Along its course, the internal spermatic vein may anastomose—as has been demonstrated in phlebographic studies—with renal capsular veins, the ascendent lumbar vein, abdominal wall veins, the external pudendal vein, and through it, to the iliac and its contralateral veins. The deferential vein leads to the vesical veins, and these to the hypogastric (internal iliac) vein. The external spermatic vein (cremasteric vein) drains via the inguinal canal into the inferior epigastric vein, which in turn, drains near the end of the femoral vein (Fig. 15–11).

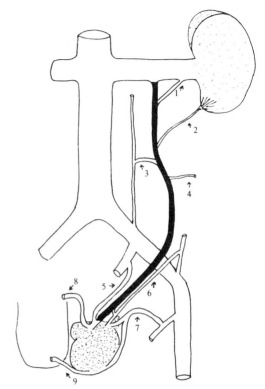

FIGURE 15–11. *Venous drainage of the left testis. (The spermatic vein is drawn in black.) 1, colateral vein from renal vein, 2, renal capsular vein, 3, ascending lumbar vein, 4, abdominal wall vein, 5, deferential vein opening into the hypogastric (internal iliac) vein, 6, external spermatic vein opening into the inferior epigastric vein, which, in turn, opens into the femoral vein, 7, anterior and posterior scrotal veins opening into the saphenous, 8, prepubic vein, 9, scrotal vein.*

Etiology

Due to the peculiarities of the left spermatic vein, it is precisely this side that presents the greater number of varicoceles. The possible causes for *left side varicocele* are:

1. Congenital absence of the valves or inadequate closing of the valves.
2. Inherited or congenital weakness of the blood vessel wall connective tissue that predisposes the venous ectasia.
3. High hydrostatic pressure of the left spermatic vein due to its great length.
4. The poor drainage condition of left spermatic vein created by the right-angle junction with the renal vein.
5. An alteration of the fascio-muscular pump in the spermatic cord.

The following causes may be added to those just listed: higher renal vein pressure than in the cava; extrinsic pressure originated by enlarged lymph nodes; defective cremaster muscle development or congenital scrotal atony.

Different causes may act in each case.

Varicocele may easily occur in the following manner: the lack or insufficiency of the ostial valve gives rise to reflux in the spermatic vein, which is aggravated by the adrenal vein flow since the opening of the adrenal vein faces that of the spermatic vein.

The reversed blood flow dilates and elongates the pampiniform plexus. If this dilation is persistent, changes are produced in the blood vessel walls. The number of elastic fibers decreases and hypertrophy of the tunica media in vessel vein walls is produced. Fascio-muscular pump atrophy superimposes upon the previous changes. The fascio-muscular pump is a physiological unit composed of cremasteric fascia and internal and external spermatic fasciae surrounding the spermatic cord (Shafik, 1983). The final result is venous dilatation and its effect on testicular and epididymal function.

Until a few years ago the only etiologic factor contributing to varicocele formation was the pathogenetic mechanism based on spermatic vein reflux. However, the ever increasing practice of phlebography associated with the failure of spermatic vein ligature in a number of cases has lead to the belief that some varicoceles are due more to iliospermatic reflux than to renospermatic reflux (Frang and others, 1978). The numberous anastomoses between the deferential and hypogastric veins, the scrotal and saphenous veins, and so forth. (Ponthieu and Huget, 1976; Chatel and associates, 1978) support this hypothesis. In the absence of renospermatic reflux, iliospermatic reflux can be produced. The mechanisms for this kind of varicocele are more hypothetical than in the earlier case. Relatively speaking, it has been observed frequently that the left external iliac artery distally compresses the iliac vein. The repeated microtraumas would give rise to fibrosis in its wall and the development of venous stenosis.

The possible causes for *right side varicocele* are:

1. Renal or other organ tumor growing in a retroperitoneal direction.
2. Abnormal opening of the right spermatic vein into the renal vein.
3. Situs inversus.

The possible causes for *bilateral varicocele* are:

1. Association between either a right side symptomatic varicocele or an abnormal opening of the right spermatic vein into the renal vein, and a left side varicocele.
2. Anastomoses between the left and right pampiniform plexus via suprapubic veins.

Physiopathology of the Testicular Lesions

The pathogenetic mechanisms that have been implicated in the development of testicular lesions in varicocele are: scrotal thermoregulation alterations; mechanical obstruction of the intratesticular spermatic pathways; reduced oxygen tension; and the toxic effects of renal and/or adrenal metabolites.

Thermoregulation Alterations

Many authors believe that the lesions found in patients with varicocele are secondary to increases in scrotal temperature. Many studies examining the damaging effect of heat on the testes have been carried out in men as well as animals (see heat atrophy in Chapter 14). In humans, the scrotal temperature is approximately 2.5°C below rectal temperature; there are no appreciable differences between testes. This temperature difference is notably diminished in patients with varicocele. According to Zorgniotti and MacLeod (1973) patients with varicocele and low-quality semen have a testicular temperature between 0.6°C and 0.8°C above that of normal men. Among these patients the testis affected by varicocele may reach 0.3°C above the contralateral testis temperature.

Mechanical Obstruction of the Intratesticular Pathways

The testicular mediastinum houses the intratesticular spermatic pathways (rete testis and tubuli recti), and is a zone of passage for veins and lymphatic vessels. The venous branches are not parallel to the arterial branches. Over two thirds of the testicular parenchyma closest to the rete testis drain to the rete testis veins.

In varicocele, besides the intense dilation of the pampiniform plexus blood vessels, there is also a marked dilation of the intraparenchymatous veins, which is appreciable not only in the vessels of the tunica vasculosa, but also in those that pass through the rete testis. These vein's walls have lesions that are characteristic in varicose veins: lumen dilation; wall fibrosis; hyalinization; and so forth. Since the relation to the seminiferous tubules is quite close on this level, it is quite possible that some tubuli recti, or even the seminiferous tubules themselves, may be compressed. The frequently found focal lobulillar atrophy in the testicular biopsies of patients with varicocele may have this pathogenetic origin.

Reduced Oxygen Tension

Since in varicocele patients the testis is bathed in venous blood, it has been supposed that the oxygen levels would be low, creating a permanent condition of hypoxia. The measurements of oxygen and CO_2 pressure, as well as pH, taken from the internal spermatic vein in the direction of the kidney and in the direction of the testis, do not clearly show that low oxygen concentration exists, but, on the contrary, the oxygen concentration is always high. This fact, a paradox at first inspection, has a physiological justification if we accept that most of the spermatic reflux originates in the renal vein. The kidney receives approximately 25 percent of the blood pumped by the heart; and the rate of tissue-oxygen-extraction per unit of volume is very low. The renal vein's oxygen concentration is high, being surpassed only by that of the pulmonary veins.

Toxic Effects of Adrenal and/or Kidney Metabolites

The proximity of the renal, adrenal, and spermatic vein openings suggested to MacLeod (1965) that adrenal secretions might pass into the spermatic vein and damage spermatogenesis, namely adrenal cortical hormones.

Later studies, carried out by Comhaire and Vermeulen (1974) arrived at a different conclusion. These authors investigated the origin of the spermatic vein blood flow, using controls and patients with varicocele, and measured cortisol and cathecolamine concentrations. In the controls, the rate of blood flow in the renal vein was 300 ml/min, and that of the adrenal vein was 2 ml/min. Given the reduced quantity of adrenal blood flow, its mixture with the renal vein flow would be greatly delayed. Cortisol levels registered in the spermatic veins are generally equal to those registered in the peripheral veins. Nevertheless, catecholamine levels are slightly elevated (Fig. 15-12).

The following schemes can be found in the spermatic veins of patients with varicocele:

1. Low cortisol and high catecholamine levels. In this case the blood flow preferentially proceeds the renal vein.
2. Cortisol and catecholamine levels similar to those of other peripheral veins. The blood flow is probably from iliospermatic vein reflux.
3. Higher cortisol and catecholamine concentrations than in the other peripheral veins. There is probably a

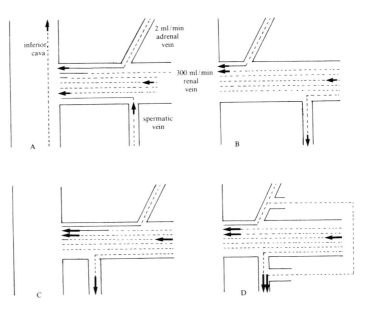

FIGURE 15–12. *Schematic drawing of the left renal vein flow. A, Normal renal vein flow. B, C, and D, in varicocele. B and C, Facing dispositions of adrenal and spermatic vein openings. In both cases the spermatic vein reflux is only of renal vein origin. D, Anastomoses between the adrenal and the spermatic veins, via the renal capsular veins, will determine a high corticoid and catecholamine concentration in the spermatic veins (Modified from Comhaire and Vermeulen, 1974).*

shunt—via the renal capsular veins—between the adrenal and spermatic veins.

Since in most of the cases studied, the catecholamine concentration is higher in the spermatic vein than in peripheral blood, it is logical to deduce that noradrenalin plays some role in the production of testicular lesions. It has been suggested that noradrenalin is transferred against the flow through the spermatic vein pampiniform plexus to the testicular arteries, which would provoke chronic testicular artery vasoconstriction giving rise to a decrease in testicular perfusion.

Histopathology of the Testis

Circulatory alterations have negative consequences for the epididymis and testis. The testis is damaged with long-standing varicocele, and the histological pattern produced is pathognomonic. So much so that even if clinical or laboratory data that lead to diagnose a varicocele are unknown, the varicocele may be suggested only by the histological study of the testis. The lesions affect, in varying degrees, all testicular structures: vessels; interstitial connective tissue; Leydig cells; and seminiferous tubules. The affectation is bilateral in a high percentage of patients.

Ipsilateral Testis

Vascular Lesions. The most characteristic lesion is not tubular atrophy, but rather interstitial tissue and venule wall changes. The testicular arterioles develop lesions in both the tunica intima and the tunica adventitia. Lesions in the tunica intima consist of endothelium cell hyperplasia while, in the tunica adventitia, a progressive hyalinization is observed.

The veins show lumen dilation, wall thickening, and sclerosis. These lesions are easily identified in the tunica vasculosa of the testis, and testicular mediastinum veins, as well as being relatively easily identified in the centrifugal and centripetal veins along the length of the testicular septa (Fig. 15–13A). The arterio-venous anastomoses show hyperplasia of myoepithelioid cells and perivascular fibrosis.

Interstitial Tissue Lesions. Interstitial tissue lesions are secondary to chronic congestion. In the initial stages, marked

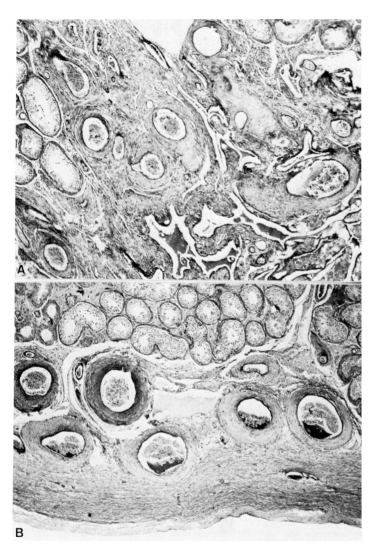

FIGURE 15–13. *Varicocele. A, Centripetal veins, with dilated lumen and irregular fibrosis of the wall, sectioned at the level of the rete testis. H&E (x60). B, Centrifugal veins, with the same lesions as in A, but sectioned at the level of the tunica vasculosa testis. H&E (x60).*

edema is added to the small vein and venule lesions, and is followed by a progressive increase in the reticular and collagen fibers that leads to sclerosis. The blood vessels are surrounded by fibrous rings and the small Leydig cell clusters break down. Each Leydig cell is surrounded by a fine fibrillar ring and many become vacuolated and hyperchromatic. These pictures suggest Leydig cell hypoplasia (Dubin and Hotchkiss, 1969). Clusters of Leydig cells with a larger amount of cells than normal appear in approximately a third of the testicular biopsies and probably represent compensating hyperplastic foci (Weissbach and others, 1975; McFadden and Mehan, 1978).

Tunica Albuginea Lesions. Tunica albuginea thickening along with intense tunica vasculosa edema; an increase in the amount of veins showing typical varicose lesions; lymphatic vessel dilation; Leydig cell clusters; and muscle cell hyperplasia have all been observed in patients with varicocele (Fig. 15–13B).

Seminiferous Tubule Lesions. In the beginning stages of varicocele, tubular diameter is not affected and the lesions are localized only in the adluminal compartment of the tubules, while the basal compartment remains normal for a time. Studies carried out with tracers like *lanthanum* have shown that the blood-testis barrier is not altered in patients with varicocele (Cameron and Syndle, 1980).

The Sertoli cell is considered to be the target cell through which the most severe germinal process lesions are produced. Perhaps the apical vacuolization lesions in the Sertoli cell cytoplasm, the disintegration of the periluminal cytoplasm covering the spermatids, and the degeneration of the spermatid-Sertoli cell junctions may be expressions of these lesions.

The diffuse lesions observed in spermatids consist of maturative anomalies, abnormal disposition, and early sloughing of immature germinal cells. In relation to the abnormal spermatid maturation, these cells have been observed to show a marked decrease in thiaminopyrophosphatase (TPPase), a selective Golgi complex marker. The most frequently observed maturative anomalies are the presence of thin, extremely long nuclei in most seminiferous tubules (Fig. 15–14A). Germinal cell sloughing is precocious and intensive, affecting principally spermatids, even giving rise to the appearance of giant cells within the lumen of the seminiferous tubules. These cells correspond to spermatids that have not completed cytokinesis. Spermatocyte sloughing is not infrequent. The intense adluminal compartment alterations contrast with the relative normal preservation of the basal compartment. This is in agreement with the different names that have described this condition—incomplete spermatogenetic element maturation; maturation arrest; and premature sloughing of immature spermatogenetic elements (Horstein, 1964).

The basal compartment is eventually damaged and, according to Hoffman and associates' (1982), cytological and histometric studies, the process should occur in this manner: The number of dark A spermatogonia decreases, although not as much as in other processes that affect germinal cell development. The decrease is bilateral, even with only left varicocele. In the early stages pale A spermatogonia may give numbers even higher than normal. This type of spermatogonia survives even in long-standing varicoceles. In the advanced stages an even more intense hypospermatogenesis occurs (Scott, 1958), in which spermatogonia are lost and only a few Sertoli cells remain. The tubules with hypospermatogenesis show a drop in primary spermatocytes that parallels the drop in dark A spermatogonia (Fig. 15–14B). Parallel to seminiferous epithelium depopulation, tubular wall fibrosis and lumen retraction develop (Fig. 15–14C and D).

There is also a series of focal lesions that always accompany the diffuse alterations, especially in testes with long-standing varicocele. The focal lesions adopt a lobular pattern. The most frequently observed are: focal hypoplasia of the spermatogenetic process; regressive Sertoli cell alterations (athrocytosis, cytoplasmic vacuolation, oncocytic transformation); and an increase in PAS positive material. Spermatocele and spermatid granulomas can also be found. Spermatocele is relatively frequent in patients with varicocele, in contrast to what occurs in testes with another disorder.

Contralateral Testis

In 90 percent of patients, the contralateral testis presents alterations similar to those on the side with varicocele; although usually these lesions are not so intense (Etriby and others, 1967; Agger and Johnsen, 1978). There are seminiferous epithelium sloughing and/or spermatid maturation anomalies in 60 percent of patients. A testicular mosaic pattern (tubules with only Sertoli cells, or associated with germinal hypoplasia, or maturation arrest, or normal spermatogene-

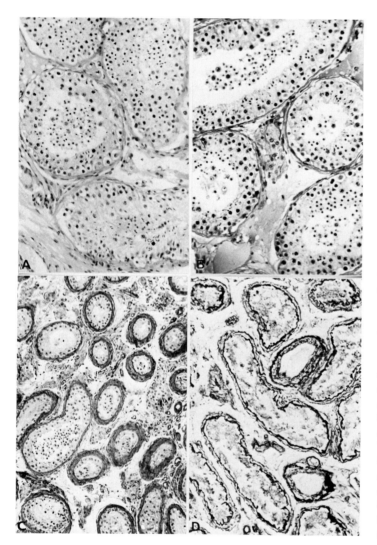

FIGURE 15–14. *Varicocele. A, Seminiferous tubules with good germinal cell line development showing tapered nucleus spermatids (asterisks). H&E (x125). B, Seminiferous tubules with light hypospermatogenesis and marked sloughing of young spermatids. Leydig cells containing numerous Reinke's crystals are seen. H&E (x125). C, Seminiferous tubules with severe hypospermatogenesis and marked peritubular fibrosis. Masson trichrome (x60). D, Silver impregnation showing a bilayered basement membrane, secondary to peritubular fibrosis (x60).*

sis) in 20 percent of patients. In the remaining 10 percent of patients, lesions are minimal; this contrasts with the moderately intense lesions found in the testis with varicocele (spermatid maturation anomalies and seminiferous epithelium sloughing) (Ibrahim and associates, 1977).

Spermiogram

A marked alteration of semen quality is produced in varicocele, which, for unknown reasons, is only observed in 50 percent of the patients. In 1965 MacLeod called attention to the decrease in spermatozoon number and the increase in tapering and amorphous forms. These alterations observed in patients with varicocele are identical to those of the stress pattern which MacLeod had previously described as occurring under different circumstances: during infectious diseases; following acute allergic reaction; the administration of antispermatogenetic agents; and so forth.

Subsequent comparative studies carried out in patients with and without varicocele who were studied for reduced semen quality (Rodríguez-Rigau and others, 1981; Jecht and associates, 1982) revealed that there were no great differences between the two groups, although a higher percentage of abnormal spermatozoon forms were observed in patients with varicocele. Specifically, degenerative, immature, and amorphous forms were more abundant in the patients with varicocele. The tapering forms were rather scarce in both groups and the difference was not significant.

Therefore the spermiogram is not pathognomonic, and its diagnostic value is very inferior to the clinical radiological methods. However, its importance increases in the selection of varicocelectomy candidates and in the establishment of a prognosis following surgery.

Hormonal Regulation

Varicocele may occur along with a pituitary alteration. Since the Sertoli cells are considered to be the target cells in varicocele, any alteration of them gives rise to not only seminiferous epithelium sloughing, but also an insufficient inhibin secretion, which gives rise to an increase in basal FSH levels and a marked increase in FSH secretion when stimulated by LH-RH. This alteration is found in over 10 percent of patients (Hudson and McKay, 1980).

Leydig cell dysfunction may determine either a decrease in the intratesticular testosterone concentration and secondarily, a germinal cell line lesion (Weiss and others, 1979), or else a decrease in peripherical testosterone levels and a rise in LH. This pattern appears in patients over 40 years of age and recalls Leydig cell insufficiency, which normally appears in males in their sixth and seventh decades.

Testosterone levels are usually normal in most patients (Mićić and others, 1983), but they are associated with minimally elevated LH levels in over half the cases. This increase is probably a compensating effect (Hudson and McKay, 1980).

Diagnosis and Treatment

Aside from the value of the spermiogram, which, as has been mentioned, is not pathognomonic, several studies are employed. These can be divided into non-invasive and invasive examinations. Scrotal thermography and sonography, Doppler flow measurements, and testicular perfusion studies using radioisotopes are of little value in diagnosing subclinical varicoceles but are among the principal non-invasive techniques used (González and co-authors, 1983; Wolverson and associates, 1983). Spermatic vein retrograde phlebography is the invasive technique most commonly used (Coolsaet, 1980). The most important value of phlebography is not so much in varicocele diagnosis, but rather in locating venous drainage anomalies, which is useful information when planning proper treatment.

Treatment not only improves spermiogram parameters, but also prevents the development of more serious lesions. In addition to the classical technique of high spermatic vein ligation (Bernardi, 1942; Palomo, 1949; Ivanissevich, 1960) others have appeared. The techniques of spermatic vein obliteration with different materials such as sclerotherapy (Iaccarino, 1977; Zeitler and others, 1980), and embolization (Thelen and associates, 1979; Weissbach and others, 1981; Barth and colleagues, 1982) have had success as alternatives to surgical treatment. The advantage of the latter two procedures over spermatic vein ligation is that they can be carried out on an out-patient basis.

Surgical Results

The following results have been found after internal spermatic vein ligation:

Spermiogram

Improvement is noted in 70 percent of patients. This improvement does not equally affect all parameters of the spermiogram. There is no change in volume. Sperm density and motility increases substantially. Even after several months there is little improvement in anomalous spermatozoon shape. The stress pattern does not completely disappear (Lindholmer and others, 1975).

Effect on Pregnancy Rate

The percentage of pregnancies increased in 20 to 50 percent of couples. The highest pregnancy rates are obtained from men whose sperm count was over 10 million/ml before the operation.

Postoperative Complications. There are two types: hydrocele and varicocele. Hydrocele appears in two percent of the operated patients. Either ligation of lymphatic vessels near the spermatic vein or venous flow suppression are considered to be possible causes. Varicocele persistence or varicocele relapse is interpreted as being secondary to the presence of an aberrant spermatic vein that was not ligated or to iliospermatic reflux. It has been suggested that patients whose spermiogram does not improve after varicocelectomy be treated with clomiphene as in idiopathic oligospermia (Check, 1980).

REFERENCES

1. Abercrombie GF: Thrombo-angitis obliterans of the spermatic cord. Brit J Surg 52:632, 1965
2. Agger P, Johnsen S: Quantitative evaluation of testicular biopsies in varicocele. Fertil Steril 29:52, 1978
3. Altaffer LF: Testicular torsion in men. J Urol 123:37, 1980
4. Amelar RD, Dubin L: Male infertility: current diagnosis and treatment. Urology 1:1, 1983
5. Atallah MW, Ippolito JJ, Rubin BW: Intrauterine bilateral torsion of the spermatic cord. J Urol 116:128, 1976
6. Aynsley-Green A, Zachmann M, Illig R, Rampini S, Prader A: Congenital bilateral anorchia in childhood: a clinical and therapeutic evaluation of twenty one cases. Clin Endocrinol 5:381, 1976
7. Barth KH, Kaufmann SL, Kadir S, White RI: Treatment of varicoceles by embolization with detachable balloons. In Jecht EW and Zeitler E (eds) Varicocele and male infertility Berlin: Springer-Verlag, 1982, p. 153
8. Bartsch G, Frank S, Marberger H, Mikuz G: Testicular torsion: late results with special regard to fertility and endocrine function. J Urol 124:375, 1980
9. Bernardi R: New incision for therapy of varicocele; semiologic and surgical concepts. Sem Med 2:165, 1942
10. Buerger L: The circulatory disturbances of the extremities. Philadelphia: Saunders Co., 1924, p. 311
11. Campbell MF: Torsion of the spermatic cord in newborn infants. J Pediatr 33:323, 1948
12. Cameron DF, Snydle FE: The blood-testis barrier in men with varicocele: a lanthanum tracer study. Fertil Steril 34:255, 1980
13. Chatel A, Bigot JM, Dectot H, Helenon C: Anatomie radiologique des veins spermatiques. A propos de 152 phlébographies spermatiques rétrogrades. J Chir 115:443, 1978
14. Clarke BG: Incidence of varicocele in normal men and among men of different ages. JAMA 198:1121, 1966
15. Check JH: Improved semen quality in subfertile males with varicocele-associated oligospermia following treatment with clomiphene citrate. Fertil Steril 33:423, 1980
16. Colt GH: Torsion of the hydatid of Morgagni. Brit J Surg 9:464, 1922
17. Comhaire F, Vermeulen A: Varicocele sterility: cortisol and catecholamines. Fertil Steril 25:88, 1974
18. Coolsaet BLRA: The varicocele syndrome: venography determining the optimal level for surgical management. J Urol 124:833, 1980
19. Cos LR, Peartree RJ, Descalzi M, Rabinowitz R: Torsion of intrascrotal malignant testis tumors. J Urol 130:145, 1983
20. Delasiauve LJF: Cited by Scudder CL: Strangulation of the testis by torsion of the cord. A review of recorder cases, together with the report of a recent case. Ann Surg 34:234, 1901
21. Dubin L, Hotchkiss RS: Testis biopsy in subfertile men with varicocele. Fertil Steril 20:50, 1969

22. Dubin L, Amelar RD: Varicocele size and results of varicocelectomy in selected subfertile men with varicocele. Fertil Steril 21:606, 1970
23. Dubin L, Amelar RD: Varicocelectomy as therapy in male infertility. Fertil Steril 26:217, 1975
24. Durand L, Perrin P: Les torsions du testicule. Ann Urol 11:15, 1977
25. Dustin P: Arteriolar hialinosis. In Richter GW and Epstein MA (eds): International Review of Experimental Pathology. New York: Academic Press 1962, p. 73
26. Etriby A, Saad M, Girgis SM, Hefnawy H, Ibrahim AA: Testicular changes in subfertile men with varicocele. Fertil Steril 18:666, 1967
27. Frang D, Rózsahegyi Than E: Operative management of varicocele by high retroperitoneal ligation of the spermatic vein. Int Urol Nephrol 10:131, 1978
28. González R, Reddy P, Kaye KW, Narayan P: Comparison of Doppler examination and retrograde spermatic venography in the diagnosis of varicocele. Fertil Steril 40:96, 1983
29. Hatakeyama S, Takizawa T, Kawahara Y: Focal atrophy of the seminiferous tubule in the human testis. Acta Path Jap 29:901, 1979
30. Hatakeyama S, Sengoku K, Takayama S: Histological and submicroscopic studies on arteriolar hyalinosis of the human testis. Bull Tokyo Med Dent Univ 13:511, 1966
31. Hienz HA, Voggenthaler J, Weissbach L: Histological findings in testes with varicocele during childhood and their therapeutic consequences. Eur J Pediatr 133:139, 1980
32. Hofmann N, Hilscher B, Passia D, Hilscher W, Haider SG: Histological, morphometrical, and enzyme histochemical studies on varicocele orchiopaty. In Jecht EW and Zeitler E (eds) Varicocele and Male Infertility. Berlin: Springer-Verlag, 1982, p. 27
33. Horica CA, Hadziselimovic F, Kreutz G, Bandhauer K: Ultrastructural studies of the contorted and contralateral testicle in unilateral testicular torsion. Eur Urol 8:358, 1982
34. Horstein D: Zur Klinik und Histopathologie des männlichen primären Hypogonadismus. Hodenparenchymschäden durch Varikozelen. Arch Klin Exper Dermat 218:347, 1964
35. Horstein OP: Kreislaufstörungen im Hoden-Nebenhoden-system und ihre Bedeutung für die männliche Fertilität. Andrologia 5:119, 1973
36. Hudson RW, McKay DE: The gonadotropin response of men with varicoceles to gonadotropin-releasing hormone. Fertil Steril 33:427, 1980
37. Iacarino V: Trattamento conservatio del Varicoceles: Flebographia selettiva e scleroterapia delle vene gonadiche. Riv Radiol 17:107, 1977
38. Ibrahim AA, Awad H, El-Haggar S, Mitawi B: Bilateral testicular biopsy in men with varicocele. Fertil Steril 28:663, 1977
39. Ivanissevich O: Left varicocele due to reflux. J Int Coll Surg 34:742, 1960
40. Jecht E: Varikozele und Fertilität. Zbl Haut Geschkrankh 138:177, 1977
41. Jecht EW, Müller R, Zieglwalner E: Varicocele and seminal cytology. In Jecht EW and Zeitler E (eds) Varicocele and Male Infertility. Berlin: Springer-Verlag, 1982, p. 35
42. Kaya M, Harrison RG: An analysis of the effect of ischaemia on testicular ultrastructure. J Pathol 117:105, 1975
43. Klaiber EL, Broverman DM, Vogel W: Increased incidence of testicular varicoceles in cigarette smokers. Fertil Steril 34:64, 1980
44. Krarup T: The testes after torsion. Brit J Urol 50:43, 1978
45. Krus S, Domaniewski J, Ryc K: Relationship between the intensity of atherosclerosis and histological appearance of testicles. Polish Med Sci Hist 14:83, 1971
46. Leach GE, Masih BK: Neonatal torsion of testicle. Urology 16:604, 1980
47. Lee LM, Moloney PJ, Wong HCG, Magil AB, McLoughlin MG: Testicular pain: an unusual presentation of polyarteritis nodosa. J Urol 129:1243, 1983
48. Lindholmer C, Thulin L, Eliasson R: Semen characteristics before and after ligation of left internal spermatic veins in men with varicocele. Scand J Urol Neprol 9:117, 1975
49. MacLeod J: Seminal cytology in the presence of varicocele. Fertil Steril 16:735, 1965
50. McFadden MR, Mehan DJ: Testicular biopsies in 101 cases of varicocele. J Urol 119:372, 1978
51. Mićić S, Illić, Iśvaneski M: Correlation of hormone and histologic parameters in infertile men with varicocele. Urol Int 38:187, 1983
52. Moward JJ: Periarteritis nodosa presenting as mass in testis. J Urol 105:109, 1971
53. Nistal M, Alcoba M, Contreras F: Torsión del cordón espermático a propósito de 87 nuevos casos. Revisión de la literatura. Arch Esp Urol 24:385, 1971
54. Nistal M, Potenciano J, Contreras F: La hialinización arteriolar del testículo. Arch Esp Urol 26:481, 1973
55. Olivares O, Tovar JA: Torsión testicular neonatal. An Esp Pediat 9:489, 1976
56. O'Regan S, Robitaille P: Orchitis mimicking testicular torsion in Henoch-Schönlein's purpura. J Urol 126:834, 1981
57. Palomo A: Radical cure of varicocele by a new

technique: preliminary report. J Urol 61:604, 1949
58. Ponthieu A, Huguet JF: Varicocele gauche et stase veineuse iliaque. J Urol Nephrol 3:187, 1976
59. Pozza D, D'Ottavio G, Masci P, Coia L, Zappavigna D: Left varicocele at puberty. Urology 22:271, 1983
60. Rodríguez-Rigau LJ, Smith KD, Steinberger E: Varicocele and the morphology of spermatozoa. Fertil Steril 35:54, 1981
61. Scott JH, Harty JI, Howerton LW: The management of testicular torsion in the acute pediatric scrotum. J Urol 129:558, 1983
62. Scott LS: The effect of varicocele on spermatogenesis. Stud Fertil 10:33, 1958
63. Shafik A: Venous tension patterns in cord veins. II. After varicocele correction. J Urol 129:749, 1983
64. Skoglund RW, McRoberts JW, Ragde H: Torsion of testicular appendages: presentation of 43 new cases and a collective review. J Urol 104:598, 1970
65. Steinberger E: In Johnson AD, Gomes WR, and Vandemar NL (eds) The Testis. New York: Academic Press, 1970, p. 313
66. Thelen M, Weissbach L, Franken T: Die Behandlung der idiopathischen Varikozele durch transfemorale Spiralokklusion der Vena testicularis sinistra. ROEFO 131:24, 1979
67. Turner TT: Varicocele: still an enigma. J Urol 129:695, 1983
68. Uehling DT: Fertility in men with varicocele. Int J Fertil 13:58, 1968
69. Waldbaum RS, Borden D, Cohen D, Naidich J, Oka M: Venous infarction of the testis owing to vena cava thrombosis. J Urol 116:259, 1976
70. Weiss DB, Rodrigues-Rigau LJ, Smith KD, Grotjan FH, Steinberger E: Leydig cell density and function and their relation to gonadotropins in infertile oligospermic men with varicocele. Isr J Med Sci 15:556, 1979
71. Weissbach L, Hienz HA, Rodermund OE: Spermatologische und histologische Befunde bei Patienten mit Varikozele. Urologe A 14:277, 1975
72. Weissbach L, Thelen M, Adolphs HD: Treatment of idiopathic varicoceles by transfemoral testicular vein occlusion. J Urol 126:354, 1981
73. Wolverson MK, Houttuin E, Heiberg E, Sundaram M, Gregory J: High-resolution real-time sonography of scrotal varicocele. AJR 141:175, 1983
74. Zeitler E, Jecht E, Richter EI, Seyferth W: Selective sclerotherapy of the internal spermatic vein in patients with varicoceles. Cardiovasc Intervent Radiol 3:166, 1980
75. Zorgniotti A, MacLeod J: Studies in temperature, human semen quality, and varicocele. Fertil Steril 24:854, 1973

16

MORPHOLOGICAL ABNORMALITIES OF THE SPERMATOZOA

Semen analysis constitute one of the habitual practices in infertility investigation (Schirren, 1983). These studies not only permit the estimation of the classical parameters—ejaculate volume and concentration; motility; and morphology of the spermatozoa present in the ejaculate—but also the biochemical analysis of the different components and enzymatic activities within the ejaculate (Lee and others, 1983; Mićić and Dotlic, 1983; Pleban and Mei, 1983). In addition, biological tests to evaluate the sperm fertilizing ability of penetration into zona-free Hamster oocytes can also be performed (Barros, 1979; Albertsen and others, 1983).

Volume, concentration, and spermatozoon motility can be measured by fairly objective techniques; however, the morphological evaluation of the spermatozoa is much more subjective. MacLeod (1964) specifies that although there are small variations in an individual's spermiogram during a long period of time, the differences between separate individual's spermiograms is quite marked. On the other hand it is well known that human spermatozoa display greater polymorphism than do those of other species, and that even a single spermatozoon may show several abnormalities, which implies a greater number of abnormal cells in the ejaculate.

The attempts to classify spermatozoa morphologically, based on the consideration of only one anomaly, are giving way to classifications that are in accordance with multiple-entrance criteria. This kind of classification permits the relationship between different defects occurring in the same ejaculate to be studied (Souchier and others, 1978; Roussel and others, 1983).

The system explaining the various morphological abnormalities of spermatozoa that we shall follow in this chapter is based on the one proposed by David and associates (1975) with some small modifications. The abnormalities are:

1. Head: microcephalic, macrocephalic, elongated, thin, irregular, and vacuolated heads.
2. Head and middle piece connection defect.
3. Middle piece: cytoplasmic droplets, bends, shortness, and excessive length.
4. Tail: short, coiled, multiple, absent, and various ultrastructural abnormalities.

Many of the malformations are detectable with a light microscope. Ultrastructural study, in addition to revealing more precise details of those abnormalities, has discovered other malformations, such as the lack of dynein arms in the peripheral axoneme doublets, or of the central pair of axial filaments. Some of the abnormalities we shall describe can be found in association with others.

HEAD ABNORMALITIES

Elongated Head

This term is applied to spermatozoa whose heads are over 6 microns in length. Some spermatozoa can reach 12 microns. There are seven major groupings, which include various subgroups.

Simple Elongation:

The width and outline are appreciable normal. This anomaly is accompanied by a middle piece lengthening.

Bell Clapper Elongation:

There is a subequatorial strangulation (Fig. 16–1**A**). It is observed in obstructive processes.

Tapering Head:

The elongation occurs principally at the base of the head, which is thinned (Fig. 16–1**B**). Other abnormalities such as bends or cytoplasmic droplets, are frequently present in the middle piece. The causes for a high proportion of this type of spermatozoa in the ejaculate are multiple. They can occur as follows: after testicular biopsy or irradiation; after the administration of antiandrogens such as cyproterone acetate or testosterone (MacLeod, 1974); as a result of infections (Rouy and Sentein, 1977); or due to varicocele (MacLeod, 1965; Anniballo, 1979). With the electron microscope, the majority of spermatozoa with an elongated nucleus show abundant foldings of the nuclear envelop at the base of the tail (Fig. 16–1**B**).

Thin Head

The head length is normal and the width is reduced.

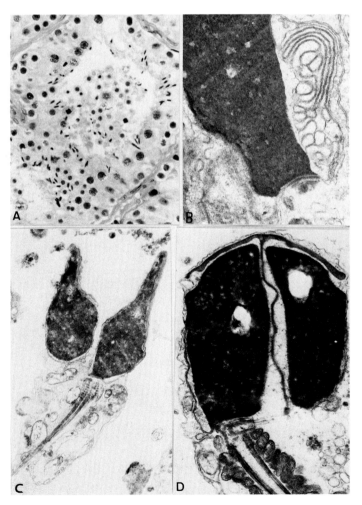

FIGURE 16–1. *A, Seminiferous tubule with numerous spermatids with bell-clapper lengthened nuclei. H&E (x250). B, Thin-based elongated spermatozoon. The nuclear envelope has many infoldings (x25,000). C, Bicephalous spermatozoon with only one tail (x9000). D, Binucleate spermatozoon. The acrosome, with a T-form at sectioning, penetrates between the facing nuclear surfaces (x25,000).*

Microcephalic Head

The head is small and there are two varieties of spermatozoa, with round head or with irregular head.

Round Head:

Completely spherical and lacking the acrosome; these details are clearly seen in the smears and in the semifine sections of Epon embedded material (Fig. 16–2). The chromatin is slightly condensed and shows a roughly granular appearance, although it also may show a normal degree of condensation. Nuclear vacuoles are frequent and they contain granular, filamentous, or membranous (mitochondria and myelin-like figures) material (Fig. 16–3) (Schirren and coworkers, 1971; Holstein and others, 1973; Pedersen and Rebbe, 1974; Anton-Lamprecht, 1976; Nistal and associates, 1978). The genesis of these spermatozoa has been studied in testicular biopsies. In some cases an acrosomic vesicle that is not in contact with the nuclear membrane has been observed (Fig. 16–4A); it sloughs off and is phagocytized by the Sertoli cells (Schirren and coworkers, 1971). In other cases the acrosomic vesicle forms in contact with the nucleus (Fig. 16–4B and C) but does not completely

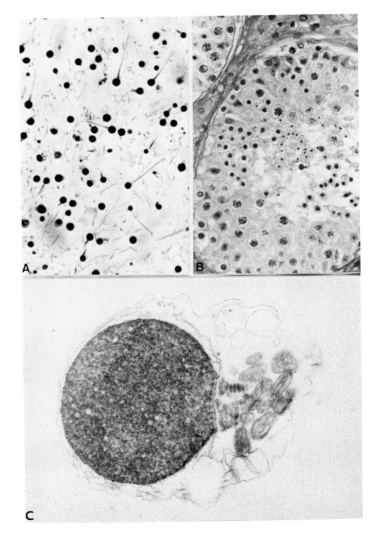

FIGURE 16–2. *Round headed spermatozoa. A, Microcephalic spermatozoa with spheric nuclei. One micron thick section. Toluidine blue (x450). B, Transverse section of a seminiferous tubule showing complete germinal cell line maturation. The nucleus remains round during spermiogenesis. H&E (x250). C, Lack of acrosome on a round headed spermatozoon (x19,000).*

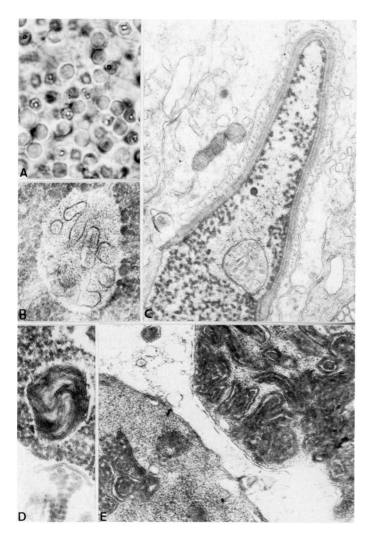

FIGURE 16–3. *Spermatozoon intranuclear inclusions. A, Vacuoles with refringent content in spermatozoon heads. Toluidine blue (x450). B, Membranous inclusions with a vesicular appearance in a spermatid in an advanced stage of maturation (x65,000). C, Intranuclear mitochondrial inclusion in a maturing spermatid with a low degree of chromatin condensation (x25,000). D, Pseudomyelinic laminar formation surrounded by a lightly condensed chromatin (x42,000). E, Nuclei from centrifugated semen containing numerous mitochondria with electrondense matrix (x15,000).*

differentiate and finally sloughs off (Nistal and Paniagua, 1978). The lack of acrosome has been suggested as the cause of the nucleus remaining spherical; however spermatozoa and otherwise normal heads lacking only the acrosome have been observed. It is more probable that the two features are not mutually dependent and are due to genetic defects, as is suggested by their familial presentation (Nistal and others, 1978).

Irregular Head:

Its outline is deformed. The nucleus may be lightly irregular, even pear-shaped. The amount of cytoplasm surrounding the nucleus can be ample. The chromatin condensation is appreciated as variable with an electron microscope and there may be nuclear vacuoles. The acrosome is very small and incomplete and between it and the nucleus (subacrosomic space), there is usually a larger than normal quantity of cytoplasm.

Macrocephalic Head

Generally the head is considerably enlarged with an irregular outline. The anomalies of the irregular headed spermatozoa can also be observed in these spermatozoa.

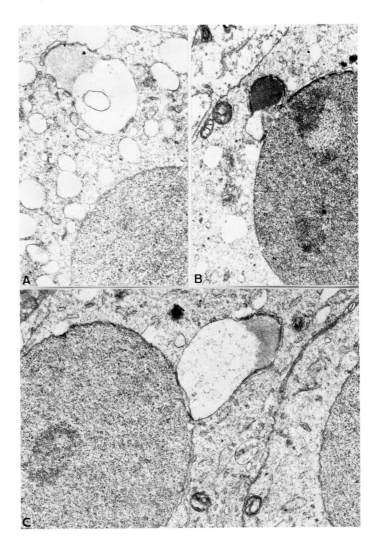

FIGURE 16-4. Morphogenesis of round headed spermatozoa. A, Acrosomic vesicle containing low electrondense material, located far from the nucleus. (x23,000). B, Small acrosomic vesicle partially in contact with the nuclear membrane (x23,000). C, The acrosomic vesicle contacts partially with the nucleus. Inside, the electrodense material corresponding to the acrosomic granule is observed. As with the former pictures, the habitual changes in nuclear configuration and in chromatin condensation are not observed. (x23,000).

Irregular Head

The head has normal dimensions, but the outline is irregular. The nucleus form is markedly variable, ranging from curved to having deep folds. Ultrastructural examination shows, in addition to the nucleus having an irregular form, that the nuclear membrane can present foldings and coilings that penetrate into the nucleus. These membranous formations affect the disposition to the acrosome, which may, in other respects, be completely normal. Nevertheless, on other occasions the principal abnormality affects principally the acrosome; so, one can see acrosomes with intraacrosomic vacuoles that are full of low electron dense material or membranous inclusions; lengthened acrosomes with a heterogeneous content; hypertrophic acrosomes; incomplete (nearly always without their postacrosomic sheath) or supernumerary acrosomes. Sometimes there is a wide subacrosomic space and, at other times, the acrosomes may remain notably separated from the nucleus and partially coiled. In all these cases, the malformations appear to be due to a genetic defect and since, more specifically, it is an acrosome defect, the fertility prognosis is bad.

Multiple Head

The presence of one or two percent of binucleated spermatozoa is considered to be normal. Two varieties exist.

Multiple Headed Spermatozoa:

There may be two, three, or even four clearly separate heads, each one surrounded by its corresponding plasma membrane, which join at the level of the middle piece. This may be partially split, but does continue in a single tail. Kojima (1973) found this anomaly in the boar. The only antecedent found in this animal in the days before the spermiogram study was a febrile status with temperatures over 40°C.

Multinucleate Spermatozoa:

There is a single head, but the plasma membrane surrounds two or more clearly individualized nuclei. There is also a single acrosome, which not only covers the nuclei's surface, but also insinuates itself between them, covering internal facing surfaces of the nuclei (Fig. 16–1D). The tail is single or double, at least in the initial region (Holstein, 1975; Sun and White, 1978). The cytokinesis may be the result of a failure of a rupture mechanism of the spermatid intercellular bridges. It has been suggested that the failure is in one of the heterochromosomes and that the affected system is the tubulin-actin filaments that regulate cytoplasm movement during the second meiotic division and the posterior spermatozoon configuration. This abnormality is frequent in cryptorchid testes (Vegni-Talluri and others, 1978), and after x-ray irradiation (MacLeod, 1974).

A variety of the multinucleate spermatozoa is the "double spermatozoa" (Baccetti and associates, 1979 a). These are spermatozoa with only one head that includes two nuclei sharing a single acrosome. The facing nuclear surfaces are separated by a laminar acrosome prolongation. These spermatozoa can have one or two tails. This abnormality is reversable and has been observed in hyperprolactinemia secondary to pituitary adenoma (Fig. 16–1D).

Vacuolated Head

In these spermatozoa it is not their nuclear configuration, but rather their nuclear tumefaction and scarce chromatin condensation that are the characteristic abnormalities. The nucleus is usually voluminous (Fig. 16–3A).

SPERMATIC HEAD AND MIDDLE PIECE CONNECTION DEFECT

A defect in the spermatozoon head-neck connection can be responsible for different spermiogram findings. In the less severe cases, only neck structural abnormalities, associated or not to others in the tail, can be identified. On other occasions, these abnormal spermatozoa break during their passage through the epididymis giving rise to loose sperm-heads and tails. Finally, in the most severe cases, the separation is produced in the seminiferous tubule itself. During spermiogenesis, the sperm head is phagocytized and the tails are expelled to constitute the only observable component in the spermiogram (Molnar and coworkers, 1978; Lannou, 1979).

Tail morphology is fairly well conserved in the instance of the decapitated spermatozoa. The proximal extreme begins at the proximal centriole, which is apparently covered by the plasma membrane, demonstrating it is not an artifact. A few tails have a rudimentary connecting piece, surrounded by a small amount of cytoplasm, while the middle piece is absent. Other tails are formed by a large cytoplasmic mass surrounding the connecting and middle pieces (Perotti and others, 1981). The abnormality probably has a genetic origin. Morphogenetic studies show a proximal centriole that is not attached to the nucleus, causing the tail to develop at a distance from the nucleus.

MIDDLE PIECE ABNORMALITIES

The middle piece is always thicker than the principal piece. In addition to the mitochondrial sheath, it carries some cytoplasm. But if the cytoplasmic droplets contribute a thickness of at least equal to 50 percent of that of the head, the spermatozoon should be considered anomalous. This abnormality can be accompanied by other malformations, especially in the tail (bends and shortness for example). It has been suggested that the presence of excessive cytoplasmic droplets implies a lack of spermatozoon maturation (Renieri, 1974). The following major patterns of cytoplasmic droplets are found:

Cytoplasmic Droplets Occupying Part or All of the Middle Piece and the Nuclear Base:

The spermatozoa usually display a certain degree of disorganization in the mitochondrial sheath and dense fibers. The following elements are found in the cytoplasmic droplets: variable sized vesicles containing granular material or myelin-like figures; nuclear envelope foldings; flattened cisternae similar to those of the Golgi complex; granules and fibers of material similar to that which constitutes the outer fibers and the fibrous sheath; microtubules; ribosomes; glycogen granules; and lipid droplets (Figs. 16–1B and C; 16–5C; and 16–6).

Cytoplasmic Droplets That Extend to the Head:

In these cases there is usually an ample subacrosomic space and the lack of the postacrosomic sheath. The alterations of the acrosome, which is also often covered by the cytoplasmic droplet, can explain the infertility that usually accompanies these spermatozoa. The contents of these cytoplasmic droplets are the same as the contents of the cytoplasmic droplets that do not reach the head.

Bent Middle Piece

When the angle formed by the sperm head and tail axis is less than 90°, one may speak of bent tails. These bends are usually found associated with other tail abnormalities such as the following: the loss of parallelism in the outer fibers; mitochondrial sheath distribution irregularities; a lack of some axoneme elements and cytoplasmic droplets at the middle piece level (Fig. 16–7).

An interesting bend observed in the boar (Kojima, 1975) is a hair-pin tail. The bend is produced in the distal extreme of the middle piece and is associated with cytoplasmic droplets persistence at the bent midpoint (Fig. 16–7D).

Some bends are not in the tail proper, which is straight, but are due instead to the tails's lateral implantation. In all cases motility is markedly reduced.

Elongated Middle Piece

This is associated with other anomalies of the head (cytoplasmic droplets and nuclear vacuolation) and the tail (lack of outer fibers and some axoneme element disorganization) (Pedersen and associates, 1971; Ross and co-workers, 1971). The middle piece can even measure about three times longer than normal. A hereditary cause has been suggested.

Short or Absent Middle Piece

This abnormality is the opposite of the defect just mentioned. It is associated with an excess of fibrous sheath material and a partial, or total, mitochondrial absence (Ross and others, 1973; Holstein, 1975; Alexandre and associates, 1978). A

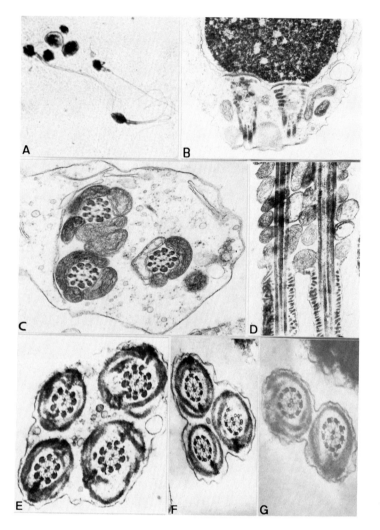

FIGURE 16–5. *A*, Spermatozoa with multiple tails. H&E (x800). *B*, Two tails implanted in independent connecting pieces (x19,000). *C*, Spermatozoon middle piece, which shows a transverse section of three tails included in the same cytoplasm (x41,000). *D*, The splitting of two tails at the beginning of the principal piece (x26,000). *E*, Spermatozoon with four tails sectioned at the level of the principal piece (x41,000). *F*, The three tails of a spermatozoon that are sectioned at the level of the principal piece. Fibrous sheath splitting is observed. One of the tails shows loss of peripheral doublets (x41,000). *G*, Principal piece transverse section of a spermatozoon showing intracytoplasmic tail coiling. In this case the coiling can be distinguished from the double tail because the dynein arm orientation is opposite in each section. Fibrous sheath splitting is also seen (x56,000).

hereditary cause has been suggested for this abnormality.

TAIL ABNORMALITIES

These abnormalities are different from those that only affect the middle piece. We shall now discuss the following: abnormalities that affect the tail in general; those concerning only the principal tail piece; or, what occurs most frequently, abnormalities involving the principal and middle pieces of the tail.

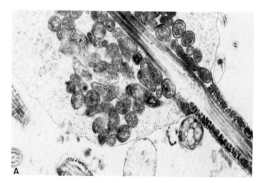

FIGURE 16–6. *A*, Mitochondrial sheath disorganization with mitochondrial proliferation in an abundant cytoplasmic droplets (x32,000).

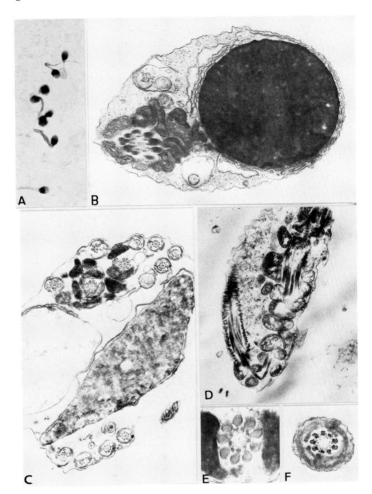

FIGURE 16–7. *A, Semen smear in which spermatozoa with short and thick tails, coiled and bent tails, and lack of tails are observed. H&E (x450). B, Bending at middle piece level in a round headed spermatozoon (x14,000). C, Perinuclear coiling of various tails which are sectioned at the levels of both the middle and principal pieces (x10,000). D, Hairpin bend at the level of the middle piece distal extreme (x13,000). E and F, Absence of the pair of central microtubules in the axoneme at the level of the middle piece (E) and the level of the principal piece (F) (x55,000).*

Lack of Sperm Tail

This malformation should be observed in a fresh smear and in a certain number of spermatozoa without loose tails being observed on the slide, so that it may not be interpreted as tail loss during manipulation. Observed with the electron microscope the connecting piece is seen to be sharply interrupted. This abnormality may be due to a primary defect, which implies an incapacity of the striated columns to organize themselves (Aughey and Orr, 1978) (Fig. 16–7A).

Short and Thick Sperm Tail

This defect constitutes a teratospermic syndrome characterized by the presence of tails, that are irregularly thick and do not reach half of the normal length; or spermatozoa whose tails are replaced by a cytoplasmic droplet of variable size; or spermatozoa without tails (Fig. 16–7A).

Below this light microscopic appearance, profound alterations of the majority of the structures that form the sperm tail can be observed in electronmicrographs. The middle piece is very short (Ross and others, 1973). In addition, mitochondria are scarce and are peripherally located in the abundant cytoplasmic droplet. The principal piece also contains ample cytoplasmic droplets and presents the following abnormalities: fibrous sheath duplication or splitting; outer fiber disorganization; a lack of parallelism in the structures of the fibrous sheath and outer fibers; irregular proliferation of outer fibers and fibrous sheath (Pedersen and Hammen, 1982); a loss of outer fiber elements or of the axoneme filaments; and lack of the dynein arms in the axoneme peripheric doublets (Afzelius and associates, 1975; Baccetti and coworkers, 1975). These abnormalities have been observed in different individuals of the same family and are proportionately more frequent in North African subjects (Bisson and others, 1979).

Coiled Sperm Tail

Sometimes the tail displays a simple loop, which, if it were not observed in such a high proportion, could be considered to be caused by the position of the tails during fixation. But at other times the coiling is intracytoplasmic and occurs within a thick cytoplasmic droplet. In this case, transverse sections observed with the electron microscope permit the observation, within the same section, of a tail that has been cut at different levels. (Figs. 16–7C and 16–5G). Frequently the tail shows a certain disorganization or loss of some elements. The habitual components of cytoplasmic droplets are found in these coiled tails (Bisson and others, 1974).

Sometimes the tail wraps itself around the nucleus within a perinuclear cytoplasmic droplet (Renieri and associates, 1974) (Fig. 16–7C).

In some cases microtubules are missing from the axoneme. The defect may have hereditary or dietary causes (Afzelius and Eliasson, 1979). Experimentally, zinc and selenium deficiencies are known to give rise to these abnormalities. Zinc is a normal component of outer fibers, as is selenium in microtubules.

Multiple Sperm Tails

A few spermatozoa showing double tails are commonly found in most spermiograms; but patients showing a high percentage of spermatozoa with three and four tails have also been discovered (Nistal and others, 1977) (Fig. 16–5). These spermatozoa usually have two or more connecting pieces, with their respective tails, attached to a single nucleus that is usually large and little condensed (Fig. 16–5B). The tails separate just at the end of the middle piece in some spermatozoa (Fig. 16–5D), but in others this separation is produced along the principal piece at a variable distance from the middle piece (Fig. 16–5E and F). The spermatozoa have been observed to contain an abnormal and excessive amount of DNA (German and associates, 1981). Studies done with fibroblast culture from patients with these spermatozoa have found cells with up to 92 chromosomes. This suggests that the cause of this abnormality would be a mitotic regulation defect that would affect the cells of the spermatogenetic process as well as the somatic cells.

Ultrastructural Sperm Tail Abnormalities

There are tail structure abnormalities that, as we have seen, can only be detected at an ultrastructural level. These abnormalities are generally not specific and can be found in association with other defects, which may or may not be visible under the light microscope. The most frequent are:

Axoneme

1. Absence of the central pair of microtubules (9 + 0 sperm syndrome) has been observed in some infertile patients. These tails are immobile and rigid. The morphology of the spermatozoa that carry this defect may be normal (Baccetti and others, 1979b; Afzelius and Eliasson, 1979) or else they are spermatozoa with short tails (Nistal and associates, 1979) (Fig. 16–7E and F). The lack of the central pair may be associated with: absence of the projections that form the central sheath

of the axoneme or the lack of one of the dynein arms, for example

2. The absence of both dynein arms is also seen in infertile patients (Afzelius and co-authors, 1975; Pedersen and Rebbe, 1975; Eliasson and others, 1977). The absence of dynein arms of the peripheral doublets is responsible for the lack of spermatozoon motility. An identical anomaly has been detected in the cilia of these patients, suggesting a genetic origin for this abnormality.

The term "immotile cilia syndrome" (Afzelius, 1976; Camner and others, 1979) refers to the association of this spermatozoon abnormality with chronic respiratory disease, which is present from childhood and is probably secondary to an air-pathway clearing defect caused by deficiencies in the respiratory tract cilia. Immotile cilia syndrome, in most cases, is identified with Kartagener's syndrome (chronic sinusitis; situs inversus; and bronquiectasis). The spermatozoon tails as well as the respiratory tract cilia both lack the peripheral doublet arms. This morphological defect is related to a dynein deficiency (Baccetti and others, 1981). The normal electrophoretic pattern of this polypeptide in human spermatozoa consists of 4 major bands with a molecular weight of 300,000 to 350,000 daltons. Only band 1 is present in these patients while Triton resistant ATPase activity is $1/5$ to $1/10$ of that encountered in normal spermatozoa. Kartagener's syndrome is associated with other sperm defects, such as complete axoneme absence, or radial-spoke defects, consisting in total or partial absence of interconnections between the central pair of microtubules and the peripheral doublets (Lungarella and associates, 1982).

3. The absence of the external or internal dynein arm or of the spoke heads of the axoneme (Afzelius and Eliasson, 1979) are abnormalities observed in infertile patients. The absence of internal arms seems to be more important than external arm absence because it is more frequently associated with immobile spermatozoa (Camner and co-authors, 1979).

4. Complete axoneme absence (Baccetti and others, 1980) is another rare abnormality found in spermiograms. The spermatozoa are immobile, flattened, and have tail incurvations.

5. Axoneme disorganization (Fig. 16–8B) and loss of some elements (Fig. 16–8C and D) are also seen in some patients (McClure and others, 1983).

Outer Fibers

An increase in the number of elements; complete fiber duplication or duplication of only some fibers; disorganized fiber production; and loss of outer fibers (Fig. 16–8A) are found in sperm tail abnormalities.

Fibrous Sheath

In this defect there is disorganization, duplication, or proliferation of the structures which form the fibrous sheath (Figs. 16–5E, F, and G, and 16–8B and C). In some cases the sheath may be absent entirely (Pedersen and co-authors, 1971; Ross and others, 1971).

Mitochondrial Sheath

In this kind of sperm tail defect there is: an increase in the number of mitochondria (Fig. 16–6); mitochondrial sheath duplication; a loss of some mitochondria; or total mitochondria absence (Eyden and Maisin, 1978).

The causes for spermatozoon morphological abnormalities are only known in part and, as we have seen in some cases, are the result of physical or chemical agent activity—heat; food additives; cadmium salts; mercury or arsenic; drugs; radiation; benzopyrene; insecticides; pesticides; pollution; lead compounds; or different types of treatments. It should be noted that different species or different individuals from the same species have different reactions

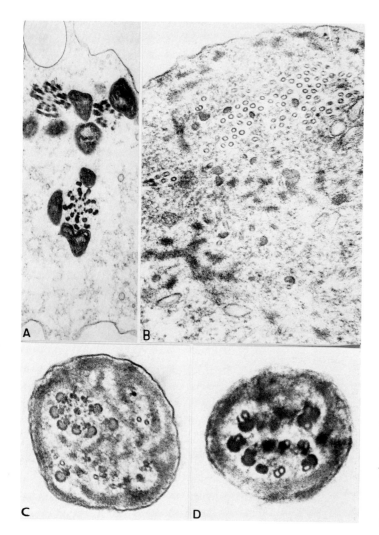

FIGURE 16-8. *A*, Outer fiber duplication and mitochondrion number decrease in a three-tailed spermatozoon (x31,000). *B*, Total disorganization of principal piece components observed in a tailless spermatozoon. Unordered microtubule and outer fiber proliferation is appreciated (x101,000). *C* and *D*, Partial disorganization of the outer fibers and of the axoneme, with a fibrous sheath and microtubule proliferation in a spermatozoon with short and thick tail (x152,000).

to the just-mentioned agents (ElJack and Hrudka, 1979; Hrudka and ElJack, 1979). An increase in morphological spermatozoon abnormality proportions is found at the onset of spermatogenesis in mice (Krzanowska, 1972 and 1981); in males who smoke heavily (Viczian, 1969; Raboch and Mellan, 1975); in chronic alcoholics (Semczuk, 1978); and in lead intoxications (Lancrajan and co-authors, 1975; Eliasson, 1978). An increase in the proportion of immature cells with spermatocytes and spermatids and spermatozoa with incompletely condensed nuclei appearing in the ejaculate are frequent responses to psychological stress (MacLeod, 1964). A genetic cause is thought to be responsible in other cases, such as round headed spermatozoa without acrosomes; complete lack of the fibrous sheath; short, multiple, or double tails; the absence of the central pair of microtubules; decapitated spermatozoa; and the absence of one or both dynein arms.

REFERENCES

1. Afzelius BA, Eliasson R, Johnsen O, Lindholmer C: Lack of dynein arms in immotile human spermatozoa. J Cell Biol 66:225, 1975
2. Afzelius BA: A human syndrome caused by immotile cilia. Science 193:317, 1976
3. Afzelius BA, Eliasson R: Flagellar mutants in man: On the heterogeneity of the immotile cilia syndrome. J Ultrastr Res 69:43, 1979
4. Albertsen PC, Chang TSK, Vindivich D, Robinson JC, Smyth JW: A critical method of evaluating testes for male infertility. J Urol 130:467, 1983
5. Alexandre C, Bisson JP, David G: Asthenospermie totale avec anomalie ultrastructurale du flagelle chez deux frères steriles. J Gyn Biol Rep 7:31, 1978
6. Anniballo R: Excessive ratio of tapering forms of spermatozoa as a distinctive feature in the presence of varicocele. Fertil Steril 32:704, 1979
7. Anton-Lamprecht I: Rundkopfspermien. Dermatologica 155:99, 1976
8. Aughey E, Orr PS: An unusual abnormality of human spermatozoa. J Reprod Fert 53:341, 1978
9. Baccetti B, Burrini AG, Pallini V, Renieri T, Rosati F, Menchini-Fabris GF: The short-tailed human spermatozoa. Ultrastructural alterations and dynein absence. J Submicr Cytol 7:349, 1975
10. Baccetti B, Fraidli F, Paolucci D, Selmi G, Spera G, Renieri T: High prolactin level and double spermatozoa. Gamete Research 2:193, 1979 a
11. Baccetti B, Burrini AG, Maver A, Pallini V, Renieri T: "9 + 0" immotile spermatozoa in an infertile man. Andrologia 11:437, 1979 b
12. Baccetti B, Burrini AG, Pallini V: Spermatozoa and cilia lacking axoneme in an infertile man. Andrologia 12:525, 1980
13. Baccetti B, Burrini AG, Pallini V, Renieri T: Human dynein and sperm pathology. J Cell Biol 88:102, 1981
14. Barros C, González J, Herrera E, Bustos-Obregón E: Human sperm penetration into zona-free hamster oocytes as a test to evaluate the sperm fertilizing ability. Andrologia 11:197, 1979
15. Bisson JP, Auroux M, David G: Ultrastructure des spermatozoïdes dans deux cas d'asthénospermie avec tératospermie. J Gyn Obst Biol Rep 3:65, 1974
16. Bisson JP, Leonard C, David G: Caractère familial de cértaines perturbations morphologiques des spermatozoïdes. Arch Anat Cytol path 27:230, 1979
17. Camner P, Afzelius BA, Eliasson R, Mossberg B: Relation between abnormalities of human sperm flagella and respiratory tract disease. Int J Androl 2:211, 1979
18. David G, Bisson JP, Czyglick F, Jouannet P, Gernigon C: Anomalies morphologiques du spermatozoïde humain. Propositions pur un système de classification. J Gyn Obst Biol rep 4, suppl 1:17, 1975
19. ElJack AH, Hrudka F: Pattern and dynamics of teratospermia induced in rams by parenteral treatment with ethylene dibromide. J Ultrastr Res 67:124, 1979
20. Eliasson R, Mossberg B, Camner P, Afzelius BA: The immotile-cilia syndrome. A congenital ciliary abnormality as an etiologic factor in chronic airway infections and male sterility. New Engl J Med 297:1, 1977
21. Eliasson R: Semen analysis. Environmental Health Perspectives 24:81, 1978
22. Eyden BP, Maisin JR: Observations on the structure and levels of expression of murine spermatozoon abnormalities with special reference to tail deformations. Arch Anat Microsc 67:19, 1978
23. German J, Rasch EM, Huang CY, MacLeod J, Imperato-McGinley J: Human infertility due to production of multiple-tailed spermatozoa with excessive amounts of DNA. Am J Hum Gen 33:64 A, 1981
24. Holstein AF, Schirren C, Schirren CG: Human spermatids and spermatozoa lacking acrosomes. J Reprod Fert 35:489, 1973
25. Holstein AF: Morphologische Studien an abnormen Spermatiden und Spermatozoen des Menschen. Virchows Arch A Path Anat and Histol 367:93, 1975
26. Hrudka F, ElJack AH: The effect of ethylene dibromide on differentiation of the acrosome, nucleus, and transient nuclear appendages in ram spermatids. J Ultrastruct Res 67:135, 1979
27. Kojima Y: Boar spermatozoa with multiple heads. J Reprod Fert 35:537, 1973
28. Kojima Y: Fine structure of boar sperm abnormality: hairpin curved sperm. J elect microsc 24:167, 1975
29. Krzanowska H: Influence of Y chromosome on fertility in mice. In Beatty RA and Gluecksohn-Walsch S (eds) The Genetics of the Spermatozoa. University of Edinburgh, Scotland: Department of Genetics 1972, p. 370
30. Krzanowska H: Sperm head abnormalities in relation to the age and strain of mice. J Reprod Fert 62:385, 1981
31. Lancrajan I, Popescu HI, Gavanescu O,

Klepsch I, Serbanescu M: Reproductive ability of workmen occupationally exposed to lead. Arch Envir Health 30:396, 1975
32. Lannou D: Le Teratospermie consistant en l'absence de tête spermatique par défaut de connexion tête-col, chez l'homme. J Gyn Obst Biol Rep 8:43, 1979
33. Lee JN, Lian JD, Lee JH, Chard T: Placental proteins (human chorionic gonadotropin, human placental lactogen, pregnancy-specific beta$_1$-glyco-protein, and placental protein 5) in seminal plasma of normal men and patients with infertility. Fertil Steril 39:704, 1983
34. Lungarella G, Fonzi L, Burrini AG: Ultrastructural abnormalities in respiratory cilia and sperm tails in patients with Kartagener's syndome. Ultrastructural Pathology 3:319, 1982
35. MacLeod J: Human seminal cytology as a sensitive indicator of the germinal epithelium. Int J Fertil 9:281, 1964
36. MacLeod J: Seminal cytology in the presence of varicocele. Fertil Steril 16:735, 1965
37. MacLeod J: Effects of environmental factors and of antispermiogenic compounds on the human testis as reflected in seminal cytology. In: Male Fertility and Sterility Mancini RE, and Martini L (eds) New York: Academic Press, 1974, p. 123.
38. McClure RD, Brawer J, Robaire B: Ultrastructure of immotile spermatozoa in an infertile male: a spectrum of structural defects. Fertil Steril 40:395, 1983
39. Mićić S, Dotlić R: Patterns of hormones in the seminal plasma correlated with sperm count and motility. Arch Androl 11:9, 1983
40. Molnar J, Bacsi E, Rappai G: Ueber Samenzellen aus Spermatozelen. Dermat Monasch 164:35, 1978
41. Nistal M, Paniagua R, Herruzo A: Multitailed spermatozoa in a case with asthenospermia and teratospermia. Virchows Arch B Cell Path 26:111, 1977
42. Nistal M, Paniagua R: Morphogenesis of round-headed human spermatozoa lacking acrosomes in a case of severe teratoospermia. Andrologia 10:234, 1978
43. Nistal M, Herruzo A, Sánchez-Corral F: Teratozoospermia absoluta de presentación familiar. Espermatozoides microcéfalos irregulares sin acrosoma. Andrologia 10:234, 1978
44. Nistal M, Paniagua R, Herruzo A: Absence de la paire centrale du complexe axonémique dans une tératospermie avec flagelles courts et épais. J Gyn Obst Biol Rep 8:47, 1979
45. Pedersen H, Hammen R: Ultrastructure of human spermatozoa with complete subcellular derangement. Arch Androl 9:251, 1982
46. Pedersen H, Rebbe H, Hammen R: Human sperm fine structure in a case of severe asthenospermia-necrospermia. Fertil Steril 22:156, 1971
47. Pedersen H, Rebbe H: Fine structure of round-headed human spermatozoa. J Reprod Fert 37:51, 1974
48. Pedersen H, Rebbe H: Absence of arms in the axoneme of immobile human spermatozoa. Biol Reprod 12:541, 1975
49. Perotti ME, Giarola A, Gioria M: Ultrastructural study of the decapitated sperm defect in an infertile man. J Reprod Fert 63:543, 1981
50. Pleban PA, Mei DS: Trace elements in human seminal plasma and spermatozoa. Clin Chim Acta 133:43, 1983
51. Raboch J, Mellan J: Smoking and fertility. Brit J Sex Medic 2:35, 1975
52. Renieri T: Submicroscopical observations of abnormal human spermatozoa. J Submicr Cytol 6:421, 1974
53. Ross A, Christie S, Kerr MG: An electron microscope study of a tail abnormality in spermatozoa from a subfertile man. J Reprod Fert 24:99, 1971
54. Ross A, Christie S, Edmond P: Ultrastructural tail defects in the spermatozoa from two men attending a subfertility clinic. J Reprod Fert 32:243, 1973
55. Roussel F, Bastit P, Delaville A, Bisson JP: Paramètres morphologiques du sperme Syndromes. J Gyn Obst Biol Repr 12:363, 1983
56. Rouy S, Sentein P: Particularités ultrasturales des spermatozoïdes humains a tête allongée. Pathol Biolg 25:691, 1977
57. Schirren CG, Holstein AF, Schirren C: Ueber die Morphogenese rundköpfiger Spermatozoen des Menschen. Andrologia 3:117, 1971
58. Schirren C: Was ist ein Spermiogramm? Andrologia 15:404, 1983
59. Semczuk M: Further investigations on the ultrastructure of spermatozoa in chronic alcoholics. Zeitschrift für mikroskopisch-anatomische Forschung 92:494, 1978
60. Souchier C, Czyba JC, Grantham R: Difficulties in morphologic classification of human spermatozoa. J Reprod Med 21:245, 1978
61. Sun CN, White HJ: The variety of abnormal spermatozoa from patients with fertility problems, an ultrastructural study. Mature forms. Cytologia 43:551, 1978
62. Vegni-Talluri E, Bigliardi A, Soldani P: Unusual incidence of binucleate spermatids in human cryptorchidism: a quantitative light and electron microscope study. J Submicr Cytol 10:357, 1978
63. Viczian M: Ergebnisse von Spermauntersuchungen bei Zigarettenrauchern. Zeitschrift für Haut- und Geschlechtskrankheiten 44:183, 1969

17
GONADAL DYSGENESIS: TRUE HERMAPHRODITISM AND MALE PSEUDOHERMAPHRODITISM

Gonadal Dysgenesis

These disorders are characterized by the presence of amenorrhea and streak gonads in phenotypic females. Various types of gonadal dysgenesis can be distinguished depending on the karyotype and whether or not somatic malformations are present:

1. XY gonadal dysgenesis. It can be present in two varieties: pure XY gonadal dysgenesis (both gonads are streak gonadas) and mixed XY gonadal dysgenesis (one is a streak gonad and the other is a testis).
2. XO gonadal dysgenesis or Turner's Syndrome
3. XX gonadal dysgenesis

This chapter will only study XY gonadal dysgenesis in its pure and mixed forms.

Pure gonadal dysgenesis is found in patients whose phenotype is female and who have primary amenorrhea; a hypoplastic uterus; streak gonads; very sparse axillary and pubic body hair; normal body stature or eunuchoid habitus; and 46,XY karyotype.

The histological pattern of streak gonads can vary widely from one patient to another. In some cases it is not possible to even identify gonadal vestiges, either because it may have precociously involuted or because it appears to have been destroyed by a tumor. Other times the structure of streak gonads is similar to the cortical stroma in the ovary with varying degrees of fibrosis. Finally it is also possible to observe a somewhat more complex organization. In these cases one can recognize: cylindrical epithelium perihiliar tubules, which if they are very abundant, can extend up to the cortical layer; solid nests of polyhedric cells surrounding one or various PAS positive hyalin eosinophil globules that are similar to Call-Exner bodies in the ovarian follicles, and are separated from the stroma by a basal membrane; and accumulations of Leydig cells or theca-luteinic cells in the hiliar region, among the tubular formations or in the fibrous stroma.

Some patients with pure gonadal dysgenesis are HY antigen negative (Hersch and co-authors, 1980) while others are HY antigen positive (Pickartz and others, 1980). The absence of testicular development of this second group may be due to the lack of a specific HY antigen gonadal receptor. This defect may be variable as to the time of appearance, duration, and severity.

The differential diagnosis between pure XY gonadal dysgenesis and Turner's syndrome and complete testicular feminization is not difficult. It is not possible to histologically distinguish between the first two, since both cases present streak gonads, but clinically the diagnosis is simple because the characteristic somatic anomalies of Turner's syndrome are not present in the other two disorders. As opposed to complete testicular feminization, pure gonadal dysgenesis patients display uterus, cervix, and a failure of spontaneous pubertal development. The gonads of patients with testicular feminization are testes that usually display a characteristic histological pattern (tubular microadenomas and immature Leydig cell hyperplasia).

Mixed gonadal dysgenesis will be discussed later in this chapter in the section entitled Dysgenetic Male Pseudohermaphroditism.

True Hermaphroditism

True hermaphroditism can be defined as an intersex state in which both testicular and ovarian tissue coexist within the same individual, either within the same or opposite gonads, and with an independent degree of development of external or internal genitalia.

True hermaphrodites can be classified upon the basis of their pathological characteristics. Considering the nature and location of the gonads, the following varieties can be distinguished:

1. Alternating variety: Coexistence of a testis on one side and an ovary on the opposite side. It represents one third of the total cases. The ovary is more frequently found on the left side. More than 50 percent of the cases present a male phenotype, and more than one third, approximately, are chromatin negative.
2. Bilateral variety: On both sides there is testicular and ovarian parenchyma, either in the form of an ovotestis or separate gonads. It represents one fourth of all hermaphrodites. The phenotype is also male in more than half of the cases. The female karyotype is the most frequent and the sexual chromatin is positive (Fig. 17–1).
3. Unilateral variety: Patients presenting on one side testicular and ovarian tissue—either in the form of an ovotestis or separated male and female gonads—and on the other side a testis in some patients, an ovary in others; and, in still others, a gonad, the nature of whose tissues can not be determined in some cases. The variants of unilateral hermaphroditisms are: (a) ovary and ovotestis; (b) ovary and bilateral testes; (c) ovary and two ovotestes; (d) one testis and an ovotestis; (e) ovotestis and absence of gonad; and (f) ovotestis and nonexamined gonad. In all, this group includes almost half of all hermaphrodites.

In a two to one proportion, the *ovary* is located on the left side; it is hypoplastic with rare primordial follicles and the gonadal stroma is predominant. If the patient is postpubertal, a few cystic follicles or follicular cysts are evident, and one can even observe the presence of corpus luteum. A correlation between genetic sex and ovarian development and maturation has been established. When the sex is male, hypoplasia is intense and the number of secondary and maturating follicles is very low. If the genetic sex is female the ovary in postpubertal state presents all maturation stages including the Graafian follicle and the formation of a corpus luteum.

The *testis* can be found indiscriminately on the right or left sides, at any level of descent, from abdomen to scrotum. At birth, its size is within normal limits; as it is during the first or second childhood when the delay in the growth rate becomes noticeable. At the onset of puberty the testes are clearly hypoplastic. The seminiferous tubules demonstrate a thickened basement membrane and have been compared to those observed in testicular dysgenesis; they are also similar to those found in abdominal cryptorchidism. The Sertoli cells may be the only cell type found inside the tubular epithelium. In some cases there is a germinal epithelium capable of producing spermatozoa. Finally, in some 2.5 percent of the cases, numerous spermatozoa can be observed (Fig. 17–2).

The *ovotestis* can be found on the right side twice as often as on the left. It is a bilobulate ovoid structure with two

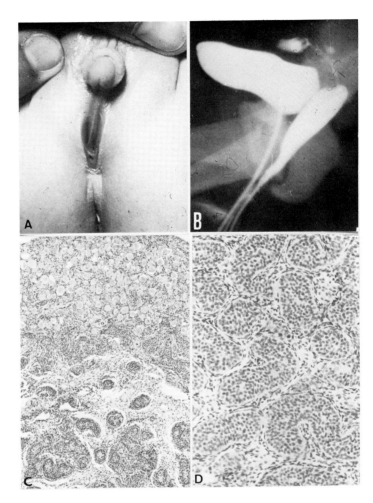

FIGURE 17–1. *A true hermaphrodite. A, External genitalia showing a penile clitoris, hypoplastic labia, and vaginal vestibule. B, Genitograph. Uterus and Fallopian tubes are shown. C, Ovotestes. The superficial ovarian zone contains numerous primordial follicles and is clearly separated from the testicular parenchyma H&E (×40). D, Ovotestes. Seminiferous tubules with Sertoli cell hyperplasia and an intense decrease in germinal cells. H&E (×125).*

different zones—ovarian and testicular—that can either be perfectly delimitated or that are united by a wide zone where primordial follicles and follicular cysts mix with seminiferous tubules. Another possibility is that the ovarian and testicular tissues constitute different structures (pelvic ovary, and inguinal or scrotal testis), placed at different levels (Fig. 17–3).

The differentiation of external genitalia and the degree of development of the secondary sex characteristics do not correspond to the chromosomal findings. This makes it impossible to distinguish clinically between hermaphrodites and other kinds of intersex states, and even more impossible to distinguish between the different variants of true hermaphrodites.

The external genitalia usually develop in accordance with the ipsilateral gonad type; they are very frequently ambiguous, but can be either male or female. The majority present with hypospadias (incomplete fusion of the labioscrotal folds) and cryptorchidism. If a scrotum can be distinguished on one side, even if it is hypoplastic and presents few transverse folds, usually a testis can be found ipsilaterally. If on the other hand, a well developed labium is found, it is to be presumed that the gonad is an ovary.

The differentiation of the internal genitalia follows the direction set by the

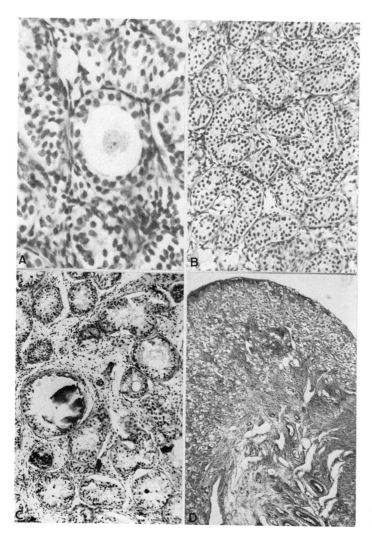

FIGURE 17-2. *A true hermaphrodite. A, Ovotestes. Oocyte inside a seminiferous tubule. H&E (x125). B, Seminiferous tubules with decreased mean tubular diameter, and marked decrease in Sertoli cell number, in a hermaphrodite of the alternating variety. H&E (x125). C, Testicular parenchyma from a two-year-old hermaphrodite, showing seminiferous tubules with central lumen, megatubules, and intratubular calcifications. H&E (x80). D, vary in a three-year-old hermaphrodite in which numerous primordial follicles can be seen. H&E (x10).*

gonads. In patients with a testis on one side and an ovary on the other, the differentiation of the ducts corresponds to the gonad on its respective side. The uterus is more developed in the unilateral variety and in that in which the gonad is an ovary. In the bilateral variety, the uterus is generally not present. In half of the patients, a bilateral inguinal hernia can be found.

Attempts have been made to explain the coexistence of both testicular and ovarian tissue in the same individual by the presence of a double cell line, one with male determinants, and the other with female determinants. But only a small number of true hermaphrodites present with mosaicism (XX/XY; XX/XXY; XX/XXYY; XY/XXY; XX/XY/XXY). Seventy percent of hermaphrodites have a normal female chromosomal pattern (46,XX) and are sex chromatin positive. Twenty percent are 46,XY, with normal male pattern and negative sex chromatin (Park, 1975).

Hormone assays in hermaphrodites with ovotestes suggest that both testicular and ovarian structures are capable of synthesizing androgens (principally testosterone) and estrogens (principally E_1). Furthermore, it appears that the testicular structures have a greater capacity for es-

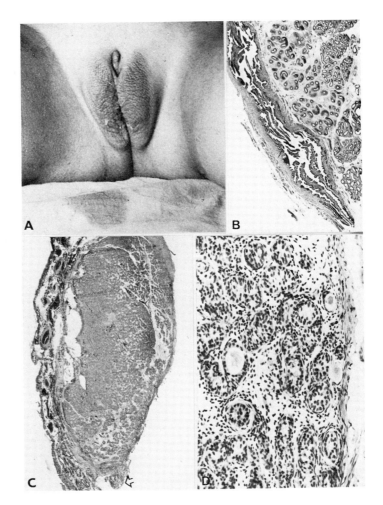

FIGURE 17-3. *A true hermaphrodite. A, External genitals showing transverse scrotal folds and slightly hypertrophic clitoris. B, Müllerian differentiation (Tube) and Wolffian differentiation (epididymis), corresponding to the right hand gonad in the hermaphrodite described above. H&E (x20). C, Ovotestes. Except for the zone designated by the arrow, the development of the gonad is toward the testis, although a loose seminiferous tubule distribution can be observed. H&E (x80). D, Ovotestes. A few oocytes are located both at the alluginea level and inside the seminiferous tubules. H&E (x60).*

trogen synthesis than do the ovarian structures (Gallegos and others, 1976).

Most true hermaphrodites are sterile, so that the purpose of surgical correction is to maintain the development of the predominant sex of the external genitalia, and to remove the opposite gonad.

MALE PSEUDOHERMAPHRODITISM

Male pseudohermaphroditism is caused by a disorder in normal male genitalia development in patients with testes and normal male karyotype. The genital abnormality can vary from external female genitalia to external male genitalia. This results from an alteration in testicular function during a critical period of fetal life. Three fundamental conditions are necessary for the formation of a male phenotype: fetal testicular differentiation; testicular hormone synthesis and secretion; and the peripheral action of these hormones on their target organs.

Testicular differentiation begins in the seventh week of gestation and is mediated by HY antigen (Ohno, 1978), a male histocompatibility protein produced by one or more genes of the short arm in the Y chromosome.

Testicular endocrine function begins during the eighth week of gestation. Leydig cells produce testosterone under HCG stimulation. Sertoli cells produce an antimüllerian hormone (Josso, 1977), a glycoproteic hormone that inhibits the development of Müllerian structures (Tran and Josso, 1982).

The virilization of the genitalia and suppression of the Müller ducts occurs during a critical period when the genital tissues are the most sensitive. The male genitalia are formed in the 14th week of gestation. The androgens produce the virilization of Wolffian's ducts and the external genitalia. With the presence of appropriate levels of testosterone, this is bound to an intracellular cytoplasmic receptor. Testosterone is converted intracellularly to dihydrotestosterone by the microsomal enzyme 5-alpha reductase. Testosterone is transferred to the nucleus where it does the following: it interacts with chromatin; it activates genetic transcription; and it augments the synthesis of specific proteins. While Wolffian development is testosterone dependent, the development of the external genitalia is dihydrotestosterone dependent. Penis growth continues throughout gestation while testicular descent does not occur until after the 28th week. Both of these processes are influenced by testosterone, which is controlled in turn by luteinizing hormone (LH) a pituitary hormone.

The classification of male pseudohermaphrodites is not final. The primitive anatomical classifications have not been found to correspond to any true cause. Similar genital appearances may be due to different etiologies. For this reason, groups tend more and more to be individualized on a biochemical or genetic basis. In spite of this, the inclusion of a determinate intersex form within any group must be done with the utmost care. In each case, the clinical findings as to external genitalia, the hormonal determinations, and the histological study must be evaluated (Imperato-McGinley and Peterson, 1976) (Table 17–1).

Based on these characteristics, patients with male pseudohermaphroditism can be classified into five groups:

1. Hereditary male pseudohermaphrodites due to deficiency in androgen synthesis
2. Hereditary male pseudohermaphrodites due to impaired metabolism of androgens by the peripheral tissues
3. Hereditary male pseudohermaphrodites due to deficiency in the regression of the Müllerian ducts
4. Male pseudohermaphroditism secondary to Leydig cell hypoplasia and
5. Male pseudohermaphroditism associated with other congenital anomalies.

Androgen Synthesis Defects

Congenital errors in the biosynthesis of testosterone give rise to an absent or inadequate virilization of the external genitalia. They are inherited as a recessive autosomic tract. In some cases Leydig cells are affected as much as the cells of the adrenal cortex developing an incomplete masculinization and a congenital adrenal hyperplasia secondary to a defect in the biosynthesis of cholesterol. The clinical variants which have been described are based on the following enzymatic defects in testosterone biosynthesis:

1. Pregnenolone formation deficiency
2. 3-β hydroxysteroid dehydrogenase deficiency
3. 17-alpha hydroxylase deficiency
4. 17.20 desmolase deficiency
5. 17-β hydroxysteroid dehydrogenase deficiency

Pregnenolone Formation Deficiency

In order to convert cholesterol into pregnenolone three microsonal enzymes are necessary: 20-alpha hydroxylase; 20.22 desmolase; and 22-alpha hydroxylase. A deficit of any of these gives rise to an alteration in the production of cortisol, aldosterone, and testosterone (Degenhart

TABLE 17-1. Classification of Male Pseudohermaphroditism.

Variant	Testes	Wolffian Ducts	Müllerian Ducts	Urogenital Sinus	External Genitalia	Feminization at Puberty	Defect
1. Androgen synthesis defects							
a) Pregnenolone formation	normal or cryptorchid	present	absent	blind-ended vagina or prostate	variable virilization	no	testosterone synthesis
b) 3-beta hydroxysteroid dehydrogenase							
c) 17-alpha hydroxylase							
d) 17.20 desmolase							
e) 17-beta hydroxysteroid dehydrogenase							
2. Defective androgen action							
a) Complete androgen insensitivity	cryptorchid	absent or present	absent	blind-ended vagina	female	yes	androgen receptor
b) Incomplete male pseudohermaphroditism type I (Reifenstein; Lubs; Rosewater; Gilbert-Dreyfus syndromes)	normal or cryptorchid	present	absent	blind-ended vagina or prostate	variable virilization	yes	androgen receptor
c) Incomplete male pseudohermaphroditism type II (pseudovaginal perineoscrotal hypospadias syndrome) (PPHS)	cryptorchid	present	absent	blind-ended vagina	female	no	17-ketosteroid reductase or 5-alpha-reductase or delay in fetal maturation
d) 5-alpha reductase deficiency	cryptorchid	present	absent	blind-ended vagina	female	no	5-alpha reductase deficiency
3. Müllerian structure regression defect							
a) Dysgenetic male pseudohermaphroditism	normal or cryptorchid	present	present	vagina, uterus, Fallopian tubes	intersex	no	Müllerian-inhibiting factor
b) Mixed gonadal dysgenesis	normal or cryptorchid	present	present	vagina, uterus	male or intersex	no	Müllerian-inhibiting factor
c) Persistant Müllerian duct syndrome	normal or cryptorchid	present	present	prostate	male	no	Müllerian-inhibiting factor
4. Leydig cell hypoplasia	cryptorchid	present	absent	vagina	female	yes	abnormal LH or LH receptor
5. Malformative pseudohermaphroditism	normal or cryptorchid	present	absent	variable	variable virilization	no	unknown

and co-authors, 1972; Summitt, 1972). The first case of this disorder was described by Prader and Gurtner (1955), in a male child with external female genitalia. The adrenal glands had a hyperplastic appearance and contained large amounts of cholesterol, which lead to this condition also being known as congenital lipoid hyperplasia. In spite of treatment, the majority of the children die at an early age. Some, who have survived longer show a feminine phenotype (Kirkland and others, 1973).

3-β-Hydroxysteroid Dehydrogenase Deficiency

This enzymatic defect gives rise to a virilization of the external genitalia in girls and an incomplete virilization of the male genitalia (Bongiovanni, 1961). The boys die of adrenal failure with large salt loss due to reduced aldosterone secretion.

The few surviving children show scarcely masculinized external genitalia, with the logical variations from one case to another in relation to the intensity of the enzymatic defect. During puberty, virilization increases, and gynecomastia appears (Parks and co-authors, 1971).

17-Alpha-Hydroxylase Deficiency

In this enzyme defect there is an equal fall in cortisol and testosterone synthesis. Low cortisol plasma levels stimulate ACTH secretion, which, in turn, results in an increase in aldosterone precursor production, which gives rise to hypertension and hypocalemia.

This defect was first described by Biglieri and others (1966) in a female, and by New (1970) in a 24-year-old male patient with perineal hypospadias who developed gynecomastia at puberty.

17.20 Desmolase Deficiency

The first cases of this defect in the male were published by Zachmann and associates (1972). Three pseudohermaphrodites from the same family evidenced—in addition to a minimal masculinization of the external genitalia—a marked increase in pregnanetriolone excretion. Pregnanetriolone is a 17-alpha-hydroxyprogesterone metabolite.

In other cases (Goebelsmann and co-authors, 1974), it has been demonstrated that the defect may also affect the adrenal cortex since ACTH stimulation is not followed by an increase of dehydroepiandrosterone and androstenedione.

17-β-Hydroxysteroid Dehydrogenase Deficiency

This enzyme is necessary in order to transform androstenodione into testosterone and estrone into estradiol. A marked androstenodione elevation along with low testosterone levels is discovered in the plasma of these patients. The hormonal pattern does not vary after HCG stimulation. The patients show a feminine phenotype at birth and are raised as girls. At puberty they develop marked virilization (Forest, 1981) and sometimes gynecomastia (Virdis and others, 1978).

The clinical features of androgen synthesis defects vary from partial to complete male pseudohermaphroditism, depending on the intensity of the anomaly and the biological activity of the steroid precursors that accumulate as the result of specific enzymatic defects. The testes may be cryptorchid; on occasion the seminiferous tubules show germinal line development, with varying degrees of spermatogenesis, and the Leydig cells may be increased in number (Goebelsmann and co-authors, 1975).

Impaired Metabolism of Androgens by the Peripheral Tissues

It is a hereditary form of male pseudohermaphroditism characterized by the presence of a female phenotype in patients with testes. The chromosomal pattern is 46,XY and the sex chromatin is negative. Rarely the karyotype may be 47,XXY (Gerli and others, 1979). These patients represent from 15 to 20 percent of all intersex forms. Their frequency is estimated at 1:20,000 (Fig. 17–4).

During childhood the development is similar to that of a normal girl. The diagnosis is therefore very difficult, unless examination for a hernia, a tumor, or family history induces suspicion (Fig. 17–5). The testes may be located in the abdomen, inguinal canal, or labia. The seminiferous tubules can, in some cases, be of a normal diameter; the tubular fertility index is decreased; and the interstitium shows a large number of fetal Leydig cells during the first two years. In some patients, the seminiferous tubules consist of solid cellular cords in which germinal cells can hardly be distinguished.

Patients with this type of pseudohermaphroditism have a great tendency to present female development after puberty. Due to this phenotype, this disorder is also known as "Syndrome of testicular feminization." However, there have also been cases of testicular feminization in which complete feminization is never achieved.

The complete androgen insensitivity form is characterized by a female phenotype who displays well-developed breasts with small nipples and areolae—the latter being lightly pigmented; infantile female external genitalia; an absence of facial and pubic hair; scarce or absent axillary hair (hairless women), a hypoplastic vagina, which is shallow and ends in a blind sac; the absence of a uterus, Fallopian tubes, and ovaries; and a ureteral orifice that is usually anomalous. The complaint leading the patient to seek physical examination is most often amenorrhea or sterility (Botella and Nogales, 1952; Morris, 1953). Another group of patients differs from the form of feminization described previously in that they exhibit normal axillary and pubic hair; hypertrophy of clitoris and labia; mammary hypoplasia; and eunuchoid appearance. Intermediate forms (similar to complete feminization, but with clitoromegalia and hypertrophic labia) are also observed (Turksoy and co-authors, 1976).

The testes may present two different patterns that correlate rather well with the

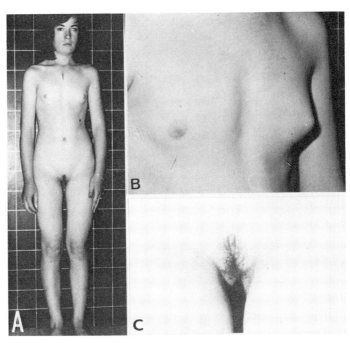

FIGURE 17–4. *Testicular feminization syndrome. 16-year-old patient with 46, XY karyotype and negative sex chromatin (A). Mammary gland development is clearly observed. (B), as well as deficiency in pubic and axillary hair development (C).*

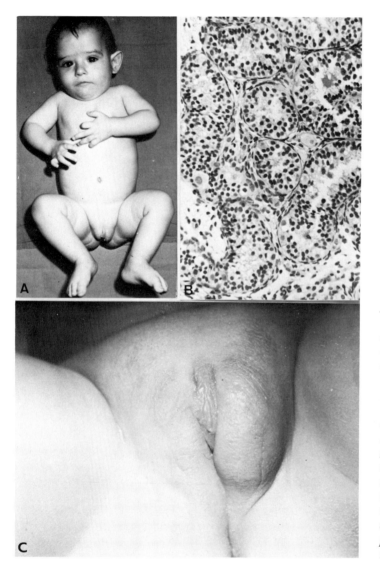

FIGURE 17-5. *Testicular feminization syndrome. A, 8-month-old patient. During surgery for an inguinal hernia on the left side, a gonad located in that region was removed. Karyotype 46, XY and negative sex chromatin. B, Testicular parenchyma of the same patient, showing normal mean tubular diameter, a good tubular fertility index, and involuting fetal Leydig cells. H&E (x125). C, External genitalia in the same patient presenting female characteristics. Observe the presence of transversal folds in labia.*

clinical forms of testicular feminization just described.

In the complete form, the development of the testicular parenchyma is greatly delayed. The seminiferous tubules that present infantile or fetal development, are clustered together forming "microadenomas." Among them, Leydig cells can be found. The nuclei of the Sertoli cells are spherical, without folds, and contain a small nucleolus. The Leydig cells are also immature, similar in many ways to fetal Leydig cells. They have numerous lipid inclusions, abundant smooth endoplasmic reticulum and the mitochondria contain polymorphous lipid inclusions. In other areas of the testes, and in the "microadenomas" one can frequently observe fibrosis and hyalinization of the stroma. The peritubular elastic tissue is absent (Gordon and others, 1964) (Fig. 17-6). In patients in whom the diagnosis was reached late in life (after the sixth decade), the seminiferous tubules appear sclerosed, and the Leydig cells marked hyperplastic (Khodr, 1979). In these gonads, smooth-muscle cell proliferation and a similar ovarian stroma have also been found.

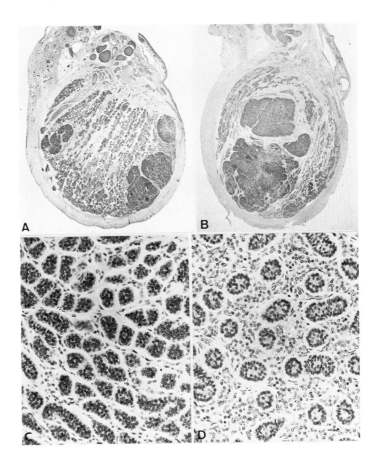

FIGURE 17-6. *Complete testicular feminization syndrome. Patient of 22 years with 46, XY karyotype. A and B, Transverse sections of the right (A) and left (B) testes, showing various microadenomas. H&E (x2.5). C, Seminiferous tubules of a microadenoma, containing only immature Sertoli cells. The basal membrane is markedly hyalinized. H&E (x125). D, Microadenoma with immature seminiferous tubules and immature-looking Leydig cells. H&E (x125).*

In the variety of testicular feminization syndrome that exhibits cliteromegaly and hypertrophic labia, the testes show postpubertal development. The seminiferous tubules contain spermatogonia and spermatocytes, but lack spermatozoa. The Sertoli cells show a more advanced stage of maturation and the interstitium shows diffuse Leydig cell hyperplasia (Fig. 17-7).

Frequently, in either group of patients with testicular feminization, cystic formations—which sometimes resemble Fallopian tube fimbria—can be observed in the proximity of the testis. The epididymis and vas deferens are not present in most cases.

The testicular pattern in the complete testicular feminization syndrome may require to be distinguished from a well-differentiated Sertoli cell tumor. Testicular microadenomas are characteristic of the testicular feminization syndrome and are formed by seminiferous tubules of identical diameter and cellularity. They are generally multiple. The cells forming the tubules show the same degree of differentiation, conditions that are not present in Sertoli cell tumors. On the other hand, the latter are not associated with genital tract disorders, are frequently functional, and present foam cells in the interstitium (Nistal and associates, 1979).

The testes of patients with testicular feminization syndromes are predisposed to malignant degeneration. In 82 patients, 7 cases of malignancy have been observed. Among 50 patients above 30 years of age, 11 presented malignant tumors. For all these reasons, the removal of these testes immediately after puberty is strongly recommended.

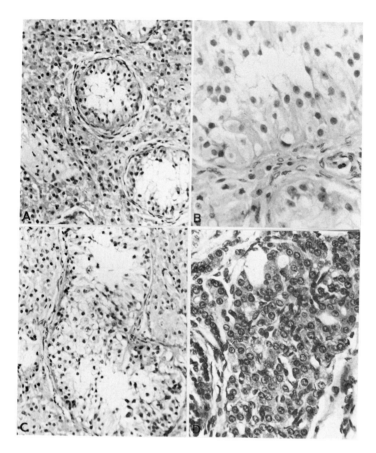

FIGURE 17-7. Incomplete testicular feminization syndrome. Patient of 28 years. A, Testicular parenchyma showing postpubertal development in which Leydig cell hyperplasia is evident. H&E (x125). B, Seminiferous tubules with incompletely matured Sertoli cell hyperplasia (nonindented spherical or ovoid nuclei with small nucleoli). H&E (x250). C, Seminiferous tubules with spermatogenesis up to the spermatid stage. H&E (x125). D, Clumps of Leydig cells with abundant lipofuchsin granules. H&E (x250).

The exact pathogenesis of testicular feminization has only been explained in some cases. In general terms the hypothesis suggested by Wilkins (1957), that a peripheral insensitivity to testosterone existed, is still believed to be correct, and has been proved in some cases. This insensitivity accounts for female differentiation of the external genitalia which occurs during the fetal stage. Fetal testes produce a normal amount of Müllerian duct inhibiting factor, causing their complete regression, thus impeding the development of the uterus and Fallopian tubes. The pubertal feminization is due to the action of testicular estrogens. Since the testes are removed after puberty, substitute estrogen therapy is required.

Cases with normal androgen receptor capacity have been described (Amrhein and others, 1976), which has lead to suggestions concerning the possibility of a qualitative deficit of the receptors (Pinsky and co-authors, 1981; Griffin and Durrant, 1982) or of the existence of a receptor anomaly (Brown and others, 1982).

In patients with complete testicular feminization, the testis also present an insensitivity to androgens, reflected at the tubular level by the absence of both nuclear indentation and prominent nucleolus in the Sertoli cells.

The testicular feminization syndrome is a familial pseudohermaphroditism. The heredity may imply a recessive sex-linked gene. Studies of family histories show that half of the male descendants are feminized, and female descendants are normal. It is also known that the mothers of some of these patients may present deficient axillary and pubic hair.

Type I Incomplete Male Pseudohermaphroditism

Incomplete male pseudohermaphroditism affects genetically male patients who have normal regression of Müllerian structures, but show variable degrees of masculinization of the external genitalia, probably secondary to a partial insensitivity to androgens.

Genetically, incomplete male pseudohermaphroditism can be divided into two groups: Type I, with recessive X chromosome-lined heredity (Wilson and others, 1974), and Type II, with autosomal recessive heredity.

Type I male pseudohermaphroditism includes patients who exhibit a variable degree of virilization, ranging from almost complete testicular feminization to an advanced degree of virilization. Within this range, the syndromes that follow have been described.

Lubs, Vilar, and Bergenstal syndrome (1959). Four of the five members of the same family that were affected had grown up as females. They can be differentiated from testicular feminization patients in that they present partial development of the Wolffian derivatives; partial labioscrotal fusion; pubic and axillary hair; and a male skeletal development.

Gilbert-Dreyfus, Sebaoun, and Belasich syndrome (1957). This syndrome represents a more advanced step towards a male phenotype. The patients have a small hypospadiac penis, incomplete Wolffian derivatives, and gynecomastia.

Reifenstein syndrome (1947). This syndrome is even one step closer to being a normal male. It present with perineoscrotal hypospadias which is frequently associated with incomplete fusion of the scrotal folds and gynecomastia at the onset of puberty.

Rosewater, Gwinup, and Hamwi syndrome (1965). This syndrome can be considered a minimum expression of male pseudohermaphroditism. While these patients present with sterility and gynecomastia, they exhibit no apparent defect in the development of the internal and external genitalia.

All Type I male pseudohermaphrodites are known to represent a variable spectrum of the same clinical entity, produced by a mutation of a single gene, with variable expressivity.

In both Type I male pseudohermaphroditism and testicular feminization, peripheral resistance to androgens can be demonstrated (Pérez-Palacios and others, 1975). Plasma testosterone and LH are high, which is indicative of proper Leydig cell function as well as failure of the feedback mechanism (Wilson and co-authors, 1974).

Sterility in Type I patients could be due to a defect in spermatogenesis or to anatomical alterations of the spermatic ducts. Some of the patients are able to produce spermatozoa.

Type II Incomplete Male Pseudohermaphroditism

Patients with PPSH syndrome (pseudovaginal perineoscrotal hypospadias), described by Opitz and associates (1972), belong to this group. This syndrome refers to patients presenting the following elements: a female phenotype at birth, with a 46,XY karyotype; perineal hypospadias; clitoromegaly; posterior labial fusion; small vagina ending in a blind sac; evident testes, epididymis, and spermatic cords; and an absence of Müllerian elements. At puberty the patients develop male characteristics with little or no mammary development. The syndrome has a familial presentation, probably due to a recessive gene.

Concerning etiology, at least three different mechanisms can account for this syndrome:

1. 17-ketosteroid reductase deficiency. These patients usually develop male characteristics during puberty. The

deficiency is a congenital defect in testicular steroidogenesis (Givens and co-authors, 1974)
2. 5-alpha reductase deficiency. All the patients with this disorder develop male characteristics during puberty (Walsh and others, 1974)
3. A delay in the onset or a partial inhibition of fetal maturation. This condition may be caused by: a delay in testicular maturation or testosterone synthesis; the inhibition of testosterone synthesis by extragonadal substances; a delay in the appearance of the necessary factors for a normal response to testosterone (Meyer and others, (1978).

In this group of patients, the prepubertal testes show a slight decrease in the tubular fertility index. In the postpubertal patients, one can appreciate testicular mosaicism comprised of: tubules containing adult Sertoli cells only; tubules with complete spermatogenesis; tubules in which maturation reaches only the spermatocyte or spermatid stage; and areas in which tubules are hyalinized or have a thickened basement membrane. These features have been interpreted as a primary testicular failure. The Leydig cells are generally hyperplastic. The patients have a markedly elevated serum androstenodione with low or nearly normal serum testosterone. FSH and LH levels are normal or slightly high. More the 70 percent of plasma testosterone derives form blood androstenodione (Leinonen and co-workers, 1983).

Male Pseudohermaphroditism Secondary to 5-Alpha Reductase Deficiency

The first cases of this variety of male pseudohermaphroditism were described by Imperato-McGinley and co-authors (1974) and Walsh and others (1974). Imperato-McGinley studied 24 patients from 13 families who lived in a rural community in the Dominican Republic. Walsh studied two black siblings with similar characteristics.

This syndrome (Peterson and associates, 1977) can be observed in males with a normal karyotype who exhibit at birth a clitoriform penis; a failure in fusion of the scrotal folds; a urogenital sinus; and testes located in the inguinal ducts or labioscrotal folds. The structures derived from Müllerian elements are absent. At puberty the patients develop male habitus, including: growth of penis and scrotum; ejaculations and libido; scarce body hair and beard; no temporal hair-line recession; and small prostate.

Testicular biopsy reveals varying tubule development. There are cases in which the seminiferous tubules have a small diameter, lack a germinal cell line; and have immature Sertoli cells. In other cases the seminiferous tubules show maturation or complete spermatogenesis arrest. Leydig cells are present in normal numbers or show clear hyperplasia.

FSH, LH, and testosterone levels are higher than normal in patients with this syndrome, yet dihydrotestosterone levels are clearly lower than normal. Metabolic clearance levels for testosterone and dihydrotestosterone are normal, but the conversion of testosterone to dihydrotestosterone is very low. There is an excessively elevated gonadotropin response to LH-RH stimulation and, on occasion, there is hyperprolactinemia (Okon and co-authors, 1980).

The disorder is due to a marked decrease in the biotransformation of testosterone into dihydrotestosterone, secondary to a decrease in the steroid hormone 5-alpha reductase. This decrease prevents dihydrotestosterone-dependent structures from developing in a male manner (Fig. 17–8). The effect of 5-alpha reductase, however, is probably much wider and can affect structures other than the classically androgen-dependent organs (Kutten and

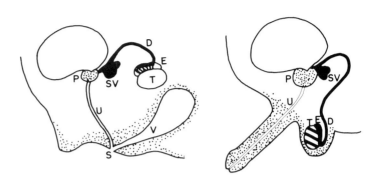

FIGURE 17–8. *Differentiation of the genitalia due to androgenic hormonal action. Testosterone dependent structures (black), and dihydrotestosterone and androsterone dependent structures (dotty) are represented. T: testis; E: epididymis; D: vas deferens; SV: seminal vesicle; P: prostate; U: urethra; S: urogenital sinus; V: vagina ending in a blind sac.*

others, 1979). This defect is transmitted as an autosomic recessive tract.

This syndrome is easily distinguished from the testosterone biosynthesis disorder and androgen insensitivity because male characteristics develop at puberty—along with an absence of gynecomastia—with normal development in the structures derived from the Wolffian ducts, which in some cases even include spermatogenesis.

Müllerian Structure Regression Defect

This group of pseudohermaphrodites have in common a testicular dysgenesis that can be either uni- or bilateral. The patients may present with either male external genitalia or variable degrees of virilization. Testicular dysgenesis can be characterized by the presence in the testes of a peripheral zone that is similar to the ovarian stroma. Jirasek (1970) points out that the following findings are necessary in order to diagnose testicular dysgenesis: thin and lightly collagenized tunica albuginea; imprecise delimitation or separation between the testicular parenchyma and the albuginea; and presence of epithelial cords or seminiferous tubules within the albuginea. This defect in albugineal structure, along with the simultaneous persistence of Müllerian structures, is interpreted as a result of the insufficient action of the Müllerian inhibitor factor because of lack of synthesis, because of asynchronism between the time of synthesis and the time of receptivity of the Müllerian structures, or because of an alteration in the receptivity of the Müllerian structures to this factor.

Three types of male pseudohermaphroditism with deficiency in the regression of Müllerian structures can be distinguished: (a) dysgenetic male pseudohermaphroditism; (b) mixed gonadal dysgenesis (Sohval's syndrome); and (c) persistant Müllerian duct syndrome.

Dysgenetic Male Pseudohermaphroditism

This defect is defined by the presence of abnormal bilateral testes and the persistence of Müllerian structures in sexually ambiguous patients who have a Y cell line.

These patients frequently present with cryptorchidism and Turner's stigmata. The karyotype can be either 46,XY or 46,XY/XO. In addition to the abnormal albugineal differentiation, testicular biopsy reveals a reduced tubular fertility index. In the postpubertal testes, complete spermatogenesis is not attained. The Leydig cells are increased in number (Grumbach and Van Wyck, 1974; Rafjer and associates, 1978) Müllerian and Wolffian derivatives coexist in the same patient. The vas deferens follow the lower edge of the fallopian tube from the broad ligament, along the lateral wall of the uterus,

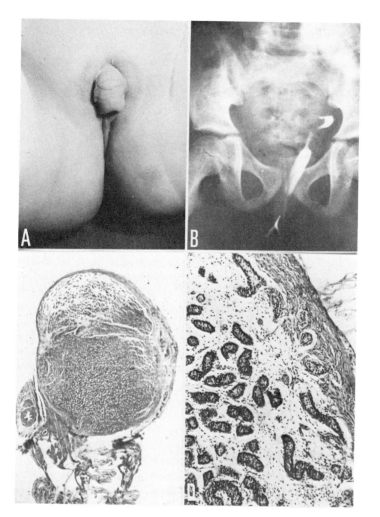

FIGURE 17-9. *Male pseudohermaphroditism with bilateral testicular dysgenesis. A, Patient of one and a half years with clitoromegaly and hypoplastic labia. B, Genitograph of the same patient showing uterus and tubes. C, Sagital section of the gonad in the same patient. A peripheral crescent with seminiferous tubules presenting a more loose distribution than in the rest of the testicular parenchyma is observed. H&E (x8). D, Thin and lightly collagenized albuginea in which small seminiferous tubules can be seen. H&E (x60).*

to the vagina where it opens into. (Fig. 17-9).

Mixed Gonadal Dysgenesis

Male pseudohermaphrodites with mixed gonadal dysgenesis (Sohval, 1963) have a karyotype that is frequently 46,XY/45,X. Clinically they can have stigmata of Turner's syndrome. The short stature is an expression of the 45,X cellular line. Other habitual clinical data are cryptorchidism, incomplete virilization, and infertility. Most patients are raised as males and manifest spontaneous virility with puberty (Davidoff and Federman, 1973).

Laparotomy reveals a testis, epididymis, and vas deferens on one side and a streak gonad, or gonadal absence, on the opposite side associated with a Fallopian tube. A hypoplastic uterus communicates with a poorly developed vagina.

The testes demonstrate typical testicular dysgenetic lesions (Robboy and co-authors, 1982). During infancy the seminiferous tubules can show normal cellularity, or more frequently, a low tubular fertility index (Fig. 17-10) and absent or deficient spermatogenesis during adulthood. These abnormal testes are incapable of: inhibiting Müllerian development; achieving complete differentiation of mesonephric duct structures; adequately

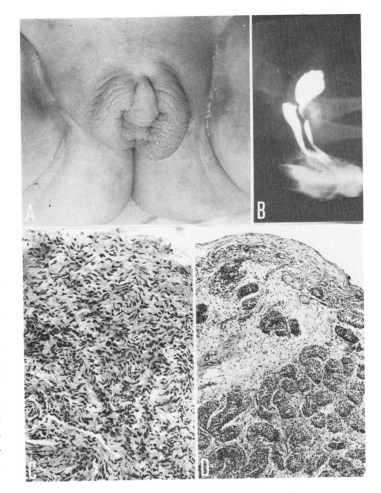

FIGURE 17–10. *Male pseudohermaphroditism with mixed gonadal dysgenesis. A, Ambiguous external genitalia in a three-year-old patient in whom a laparotomy revealed the presence of a hypoplastic uterus and a streak gonad on the right hand side, and a testis on the left hand side. B, Genitograph in the same patient showing the imprint of the cervix and the fully repleted vagina. C, Whorled stroma similar to the ovarian cortex, visible in the streak gonad. H&E (x125). D, Testicular parenchyma including two regions: the superficial region presents an albuginea with typical features of testicular dysgenesis; the deeper region shows seminiferous tubules with low fertility index. H&E (x60).*

masculinizing external genitalia and, in the majority of cases, do not descend properly (Josso and others, 1983).

If we consider the histologic pictures of the gonads in true hermaphrodites and in these two types of male pseudohermaphrodites, a whole sequence of intermediate pictures can be observed between the classical ovotestis and testicular dysgenesis, on one hand, and between the ovary and the fibrous streak gonad on the other. If to this we add the tendency for ovarian tissue in dysgenetic gonads to degenerate, it is not surprising that, depending on the age at which the patient is examined, some cases can first be diagnosed as true hermaphrodites, and years later as male pseudohermaphrodites with a deficiency in the regression of Müllerian structures and testicular dysgenesis.

Persistent Müllerian Duct Syndrome (Male with Uterus)

Most patients with male pseudohermaphroditism with persistence of Müllerian structures show alterations, either in androgenic function or antimüllerian hormone. A male with a uterus constitutes the typical example of an isolated antimüllerian hormone deficiency. The external genitalia are male, the phenotype is normal male, and the patients behave as males. Some have married and have been evaluated because of infertility. In others, the finding of a uterus is incidental, during surgery for a hernia; this condition is known as "hernia uteri inguinalis." There are cases with unilateral cryptorchidism and contralateral inguinal hernia containing Müllerian structures.

In addition, males with uteri may have other structures derived from the Müllerian ducts, namely fallopian tubes and the upper third of a vagina. The testes usually show reduced mean tubular diameter and tubular fertility index during childhood, and hypospermatogenesis with Leydig cell hyperplasia in adult life. The albuginea covering the ipsilateral testis to the persistent Müllerian structures is thin, minimally collagenized, with whorled formations and tubular structures within its limits (Nistal and others, 1980), all features that are characteristic of testicular dysgenesis (Fig. 17-11).

The Wolffian structures are identified in most cases. Although the majority of cases published on males with uteri correspond to isolated observations, the affectation of various members of the same family has been reported (Brook and coauthors, 1973; Weiss and associates, 1978).

The capacity for malignant degeneration of dysgenetic testes is high. In 25 percent of patients with mixed gonadal

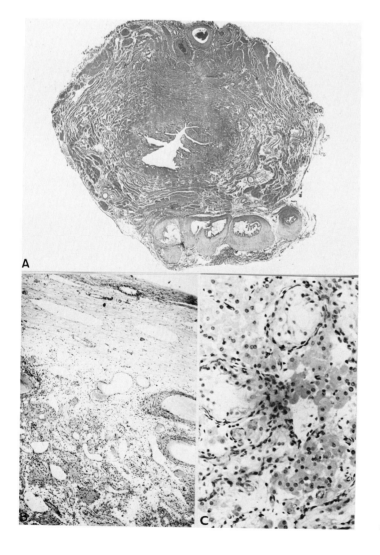

FIGURE 17-11. *Male with uterus. Patient of 27 years with right abdominal cryptorchidism, who developed a tumor in the contralateral testis. The resected tissue included, in addition to the testis, a uterus located within the inguinal duct. A, Transverse section in which a hypoplastic uterus next to a winding spermatic cord can be seen. H&E (x3.5). B, Left testis with thin and lightly collagenized albuginea, in which seminiferous tubules can be observed. H&E (x60). C, Seminiferous tubules in the same testis with only Sertoli cells in which the nucleus lacks indentations and in which the nucleolus is small. In the interstium a marked Leydig cell hyperplasia is visible. H&E (x125).*

dysgenesis, and in 15 percent of male pseudohermaphrodites with bilateral testicular dysgenesis, gonadoblastomas develop. In 30 percent of the patients with gonadoblastoma, dysgerminomas appears (Scully, 1981; Aarskog, 1970), so for this reason a prophylactic gonadectomy is indicated.

In one male with a uterus, we observed in both testes the presence of a diffuse intratubular germinal-cell tumor. The testis on the uterus side showed, in addition, a combined tumor (seminoma, embryonal carcinoma, and teratoma). The experience of other authors that this kind of patient does not tend to develop malignant testicular tumors (Potashnik and others, 1977) is being reviewed (Melman and associates, 1981).

Male Pseudohermaphroditism Secondary to Leydig Cell Hypoplasia

Leydig cell hypoplasia as a cause of male pseudohermaphroditism has been described in nonrelated patients having: a female phenotype without gynecomastia; ambiguous external genitalia; vagina; fusion of the inferior labial region; and testes in the inguinal ducts. The uterus and Müllerian structures are absent and the karyotype is 46,XY (Berthezéne and co-authors, 1976; Brown and associates, 1978).

In this kind of abnormality testosterone levels are low and fail to respond to HCG stimulation. The LH levels, however, are very high and the FSH levels are normal. No deficiency in the enzymatic activity responsible for testosterone synthesis can be found.

The size and shape of the testes are normal except for a grayish and mucoid appearance when sectioned. Microscopically, immature seminiferous tubules with reduced diameter, Sertoli cells, and spermatogonia can be observed. The basement membrane is found to be thick and hyalinized. The interstitium is edematous and contains few Leydig cells, which contrasts with the Leydig cell hyperplasia frequently observed in the majority of pseudohermaphrodites. The epididymis and the spermatic cord are nearly normal.

The Leydig cell deficiency is responsible for the low testosterone levels, the absence of spermatogenesis, and the defect in the male external genitalia conformation; the absence of Müllerian derivatives must however be attributed to the normal development of the Sertoli cells that secrete Müllerian duct inhibiting factor at the appropriate moment. This disorder is considered to be a consequence of the testicular insensitivity to LH, or to the presence of biologically inactive LH.

Male Pseudohermaphroditism Associated with Other Congenital Anomalies

This group includes a variety of disorders (Bakarat and others, 1974) in which the intersex state in the male is only an additional expression of the malformative syndrome. Many examples of this group can be cited in the following syndromes: Patau's; Edward's; Ellis-Van-Creveld's; Smith-Lemli-Opitz's; Robinow's; and Aarkog's. The cause of the genital ambiguity; the constant or inconsistant hormonal alterations, and the histological lesions in these cases are not well known.

The association of Wilm's tumor (with or without aniridia) and male pseudohermaphroditism merits special mention (Turleau and others, 1981). Of 10 intersex patients who developed Wilm's tumor (Rajfer and Walsh, 1981), 7 had gonodal dysgenesis (5 mixed gonadal dysgenesis, one dysgenetic male pseudohermaphroditism, and one 46,XY pure gonadal dysgenesis). Since all these gonads have a predisposition to develop tumors, a common defect located on the urogenital ridge, the embryonic kidney, and gonad precursor has been suggested.

REFERENCES

1. Aarskog D: Clinical and cytogenetic studies in hypospadias. Acta Pediatr Scand Suppl 203, 1970
2. Amrheim JA, Meyer WJ, Jones HW, Migeon CJ: Androgen insensitivity in man: evidence for genetic heterogeneity. Proc Nat Acad Sci USA 73:891, 1976
3. Bakarat AY, Papadopoulou ZL, Chandra RS, Hollerman CF, Caleagno PL: Pseudohermaphroditism. Nephron disorder and Wilm's tumor: a unifying concept. Pediatrics 54:366, 1974
4. Berthezéne FF, Forest MG, Grimaud JA, Claustrat B, Mornex R: Leydig cell agenesis. A cause of male pseudohermaphroditism. N Engl J Med 295:969, 1976
5. Biglieri EG, Herron MA, Brust N: 17-alpha-hydroxylation deficiency in man. J Clin Investig 45:1946, 1966
6. Bongiovanni AM: Unusual steroid pattern in congenital adrenal hyperplasia: deficiency of 3-beta-hydroxydehydrogenase. J Clin Endocrinol Metab 21:860, 1961
7. Botella-Llusiá J, Nogales F: Seudohermafroditismo masculino con feminización total. Acta Ginecol 3:379, 1952
8. Brook CG, Wagner H, Zachmann M, Prader A, Armendares S, Frenk S, Aleman P, Najjar SS, Slim MS, Genton N, Bozic C: Familial occurrence of persistent Müllerian structures in otherwise normal males. Brit Med J 1:771, 1973
9. Brown DM, Markland C, Dehner LP: Leydig cell hypoplasia: a cause of male pseudohermaphroditism. J Clin Endocrinol Metab 46:1, 1978
10. Brown TT, Maes M, Rothwell SW, Migeon CJ: Human complete androgen insensitivity with normal dihydrotestosterone binding capacity in cultured skin fibroblasts: evidence for a qualitative abnormality of the receptor. J Clin Endocrinol Metabol 55:61, 1982
11. Davidoff F, Federman DD: Mixed gonadal dysgenesis. Pediatrics 52:725, 1973
12. Degenhart HJ, Visser HK, Boon H, O'Doherty NJ: Evidence for deficient 20-alpha-cholesterol-hydroxylate activity in tissue of a patient with lipoid adrenal hyperplasia. Acta Endocrinol 71:512, 1972
13. Forest MG: Inborn errors of testosterone biosynthesis. In Josso N (ed) The intersex child. Pediatric Adolescent Endocrinology 8, 133. Karger: Basel 1981
14. Gallegos AJ, Guizar E, Armendares S, Cortés-Gallegos V, Cervantes C, Bedolla N, Parra A: Familial true hermaphrodism in three siblings: plasma hormonal profile and "in vitro" steroid biosynthesis in gonadal structures. J Clin Endocrinol Metab 42:653, 1976
15. Gerli M, Migliorini G, Bocchini V, Venti G, Ferrarese E, Donti E, Rosi G: A case of complete testicular feminization and 47,XXY karyotype. J Med Genet 16:480, 1979
16. Gilbert-Dreyfus S, Sebaoun CIA, Belasich J: Etude d'un cas familial d'androgynoädisme avec hypospadias grave, gynécomastie et hyperoestrogènie. Ann Endocrinol 18:93, 1957
17. Givens JR, Wiser WJ, Summitt RL, Kerber IJ, Andersen RN, Pittaway DE, Fish SA: Familial male pseudohermaphroditism without gynecomastia due to deficient testicular 17-ketosteroid reductase activity. N Engl J Med 291:938, 1974
18. Goebelsmann U, Davajan V, Israel R, Mestman JH, Mishell DR, Zachmann M: Male pseudohermaphroditism consistent with 17.20-desmolase deficiency. Gynecol Investig 5:60, 1974
19. Goebelsmann U, Hall TD, Paul WL, Stanczyk FZ: In vitro steroid metabolic studies in testicular 17-beta-reduction deficiency. J Clin Endocrinol Metab 41:1136, 1975
20. Gordon GB, Miller LR, Bensch KG: Electron microscopic observations of the gonads in the testicular feminization syndrome. Lab Invest 13:152, 1964
21. Griffin JE, Durrant JL: Qualitative receptor defects in families with androgen resistance: failure of stabilization of the fibroblast cytosol androgen receptor. J Clin Endocrinol Metabol 55:465, 1982
22. Grumbach MM, Van Wyck JJ: In Williams RH (ed) Textbook of Endocrinology. Philadelphia: Saunders C, 1974
23. Hersch JH, Kable WT, Yen FF, Yussman MA, Weisskopf B: A case of familial XY gonadal dysgenesis. Fertil Steril 34:599, 1980
24. Imperato-McGinley J, Guerrero L, Gautier T, Peterson RE: Steroid 5-alpha-reductase deficiency in man: an inherited form of male pseudohermaphroditism.' Science 186:1213, 1974
25. Imperato-McGinley J, Peterson RE: Male pseudohermaphroditism: the complexities of male phenotypic development. Am J Med 61:251, 1976
26. Jirasek JE: In: Rosenberg E, Paulsen CA (eds) The Human Testis. New York: Plenum Press, 1970
27. Josso N, Fekete C, Cachin O, Nezelof C, Rappaport R: Persistence of Müllerian ducts in male pseudohermaphroditism, and its rela-

tionship to cryptorchidism. Clin Endocrinol 19:247, 1983
28. Josso N, Picard JY, Tran D: The antimüllerian hormone. Rec Progr Hormone Res 33:117, 1977
29. Khodr GS: An elderly patient with testicular feminization. Fertil Steril 32:708, 1979
30. Kirkland RT, Kirkland JL, Johnson CM, Horning MG, Librik L, Clayton GW: Congenital lipoid adrenal hyperplasia in an eight-year-old phenotype female. J Clin Endocr Metab 36:488, 1973
31. Kuttenn F, Mowszowicz I, Wright F, Baudot N, Jaffiol C, Robin M, Mauvais-Jarvis P: Male pseudohermaphroditism: A comparative study of one patient with 5-alpha-reductase deficiency and three patients with the complete form of testicular feminization. J Clin Endocrinol Metab 49:861, 1979
32. Leinonen P, Dunkel L, Perheentupa J, Vihko R: Male pseudohermaphroditism due to deficiency of testicular 17-ketosteroid reductase. Acta Paediatr Scand 72:211, 1983
33. Lubs HA, Vilar O, Bergenstal DM: Familial male pseudohermaphroditism with labial testes and partial feminization. J Clin Endocrinol Metab 19:1110, 1959
34. Melman A, Leiter F, Pérez JM, Driscoll D, Palmer C: The influence of neonatal ochiopexy upon the testis in persistent Müllerian duct syndrome. J Urol 125:856, 1981
35. Meyer WJ, Keenan BS, Lacerda L de, Park IJ, Jones HE, Migeon CJ: Familial male pseudohermaphroditism with normal Leydig cell function at puberty. J Clin Endocrinol Metab 46:593, 1978
36. Morris JM: The syndrome of testicular feminization in male pseudohermaphrodites. Amer J Obst Gynec 65:1192, 1953
37. New MI: Male pseudohermaphroditism due to 17-alpha-hyroxylase deficiency. J Clin Invest 49:1930, 1970
38. Nistal M, Dela Roza C, Cano J: Síndrome de feminización testicular completa. Patología 12:119, 1979
39. Nistal M, Paniagua R, Isorna S, Mancebo J: Diffuse intratubular undifferentiated germ cell tumor in both testes of a male subject with uterus and ipsilateral testicular dysgenesis. J Urol 124:286, 1980
40. Ohno S: The role of the HY antigen in primary sex determination. JAMA 239:217, 1978
41. Okon E, Livni N, Rösler A, Yorkoni S, Segal S, Kohn G, Schenker JG: Male pseudohermaphroditism due to 5-alpha-reductase deficiency: Ultrastructure of the gonads. Arch Pathol Lab Med 104:363, 1980
42. Opitz JM, Simpson JL, Sarto GE, Summitt RL, New M: Pseudovaginal perineoscrotal hypospadias. Clin Genet 3:1, 1972
43. Parks GA, Bermúdez JA, Anast CS, Bongiovanni AM, New MI: Pubertal boy with the 3-beta-hydroxysteroid dehydrogenase defect. J Clin Endocrinol Metab 33:269, 1971
44. Park IJ: An etiologic and pathogenetic classification of male pseudohermaphroditism. Am J Obst Gynec 123:505, 1975
45. Pérez-Palacios G, Ortiz S, López-Amor E, Morato T, Febres F, Lisker R: Familial incomplete virilization due to partial and organ insensitivity to androgens. J Clin Endocrinol Metab 41:946, 1975
46. Peterson RE, Imperato-McGinley J, Gautier T, Sturla E: Male pseudohermaphroditism due to 5-alpha-reductase deficiency. Am J Med 62:170, 1977
47. Pickartz H, Moltz L, Altenähr E: XY (H$^-$Y$^+$) gonadal dysgenesis. Virchows Arch A Path Anat and Histol 389:103, 1980
48. Pinsky L, Kaufman M, Summitt R: Congenital androgen insensitivity due to a qualitatively abnormal androgen receptor. Amer J Genet 10:91, 1981
49. Potashnik G, Sober I, Inbar I, Ben-Aderet M: Male Müllerian hermaphroditism: A case report of a rare cause of male infertility. Fertil Steril 28:273, 1977
50. Prader A, Gurtner HP: Das Syndrom des Pseudohermphroditismus Masculinus bei kongenitaler Nebennierenrinden-Hyperplasie ohne Androgenüberproduktion. Helvetica Paediatrica Acta 10:397, 1955
51. Rajfer J, Mendelsohn G, Arnheim J, Jeffs RD, Walsh PC: Dysgenetic male pseudohermaphroditism. J Urol 119:525, 1978
52. Rajfer J, Walsh PC: Mixed gonadal dysgenesis-dysgenetic male pseudohermaphroditism. In Jossa N (ed) The intersex child. Pediatric Adolescent Endocrinology 8:105, Basel, Switzerland: Karger, 1981
53. Reifenstein EC: Hereditary familial hypogonadism. Clin Res 3:86, 1947
54. Robboy SJ, Miller T, Donahue PK, Jahre C, Welch WR, Haseltine FP, Miller WA, Atkins L, Crawford JD: Dysgenesis of testicular and streak gonads in the syndrome of mixed gonadal dysgenesis. Hum Pathol 13:700, 1982
55. Rosewater S, Gwinup G, Hamwi GJ: Familial gynecomastia. Ann Intern Med 63:377, 1965
56. Scully RE: Neoplasia associated with abnormal sexual development and abnormal sex chromosomes. In: Jossa N (ed) The Intersex Child. Pediatric Adolescent Endocrinology 8:203. Basel, Switzerland: Karger, 1981.

57. Sohval AR: Mixed gonadal dysgenesis: a variety of hermaphroditism. Am J Hum Genet 15:155, 1963
58. Summitt RL: Differential diagnosis of genital ambiguity in the newborn. Clin Obst Gynec 15:112, 1972
59. Tran D, Josso N: Localization of anti-Müllerian hormone in the rough endoplasmic reticulum of the developing bovine Sertoli cell using immunocytochemistry with a monoclonal antibody. Endocrinology 111:1562, 1982
60. Turksoy RN, Mitchell GW, Safaii HS: Testicular response to exogenous gonadotropin in the syndrome of feminizing testes. Fertil Steril 27:670, 1976
61. Turleau C, De Grouchy J, Dufier JL, Hoang-Phuc L, Schmelck PH, Rappaport R, Nihoul-Fekete C, Diebold N: Aniridia, male pseudohermaphroditism, gonadoblastoma, mental retardation, and del 11p13. Human Genetics 57:300, 1981
62. Virdis R, Saenger P, Senior B, New MI: Endocrine studies in a pubertal male pseudohermaphrodite with 17-ketosteroid reductase deficiency. Acta Endocrinol 87:212, 1978
63. Walsh PC, Madden JD, Harrold MJ, Goldstein JL, MacDonald PC, Wilson JD: Familial incomplete male pseudohermaphroditism type 2 decreased dihydrotestosterone formation in pseudovaginal perineoscrotal hypospadias. N Engl J Med 291:944, 1974
64. Weiss EB, Kiefer JH, Rowlatt UF, Rosenthal IM: Persistent Müllerian duct syndrome in male identical twins. Pediatrics 61:797, 1978
65. Wilkins LM: The diagnosis and treatment of endocrine disorders in childhood and adolescence. Springfield, Illinois: Charles C Thomas, 1957, p. 276
66. Wilson JD, Harrod MJ, Goldstin JL, Hemsell DL, McDonald PC: Familial incomplete male pseudohermaphroditism, type 1. Evidence for androgen resistance and variable clinical manifestations in a family with the Reifenstein syndrome. N Engl J Med 290:1097, 1974
67. Zachmann M, Vollman JA, Hamilton W, Prader A: Steroid 17,20-desmolase deficiency. Clin Endocrinol 1:369, 1972

18

INFLAMMATORY DISEASES OF THE EPIDIDYMIS AND TESTIS

Infections produced by bacteria, fungi, protozoa, and parasites are included in this chapter. Inflammatory disorder of the epididymis, testis, and tunica vaginalis are considered separately. The term epididymo-orchitis is reserved for those cases in which the structures of both the testis and the epididymis are affected (Morgan, 1976).

Epididymitis

Acute Epididymitis

Before the era of antibiotics the etiology of most epididymitis was gonococcal. Today only nine percent of acute epididymitis are due to gonococci (Harnisch and others, 1977). When bacteriological examination of urine smears and epididymal aspirations were performed, an etiology has been found in 80% of the cases (Berger and others, 1979). *Chlamydia trachomatis* was the most frequently responsible in men less than 35 years old. *E. coli* was the principal cause of acute epididymitis in men over 35 years of age. The remaining cases show, for example, *Aerobacter aerogenes, Pseudomonas,* and *Trichomonas vaginalis.*

Acute gonococcal epididymitis affects one to four percent of gonorrhea cases. It appears during the second and third week of urethritis, preferentially affects the globus minor and is accompanied by hydrocele.

Acute epididymitis is caused by organisms that reach the testis through the following routes:

1. Hematic: Meningococcal and pneumococcal epididymitis, and those caused by *Hemophilus influenzae*, are transmitted by the blood vessel route.
2. Canalicular: This route follows the spermatic pathways from a focus located in the kidneys, prostate gland, seminal vesicles, or urethra (postcatheterization epididymitis).
3. Lymphatic: from urinary bladder, prostate, or seminal vesicle foci.
4. Direct: In the cases of direct trauma.

Epididymitis is generally unilateral and most frequently occurs on the right. The clinical manifestations are similar in all types of epididymitis, and are independent of the etiological agent.

Histopathology of the acute epididymitis: An increase in the size of the epididymis and in its vascularization is produced, as well as an increase in color intensity. On sectioning, microabscesses are sometimes observed. The tunica vaginalis is also affected in half of the cases.

The principal change is seen microscopically to occur in the cauda epididymis. Polymorphonuclear leukocyte deposits occur in the lumen of the ductus of epididymis and, sometimes, the tubules may become disrupted. The stroma appears markedly congested and contains polymorphonuclear leukocyte exudates (Fig. 18-1 **A**).

The evolution of the inflammatory process is usually positive toward healing, either "ad integrum" restoration or with fibrosis and obliteration of the ductus of the epididymis. Other cases evolve chronically, giving rise to suppurative epididymo-orchitis.

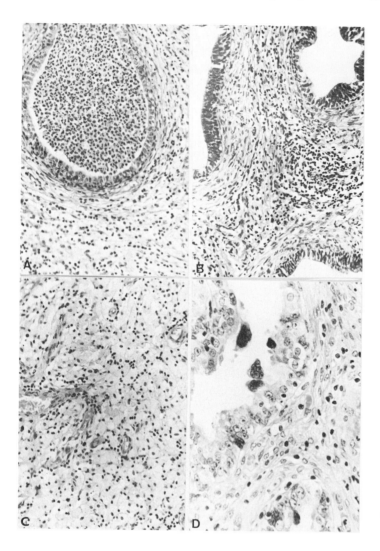

FIGURE 18–1. *Epididymitis A,* Acute epididymitis. Ductus of the epididymis full of polymorphonuclear leukocytes. The periductal connective tissue shows edema and inflammatory cells. H&E (x60). B, Non-specific chronic epididymitis. Infiltrate of plasma cells, lymphocytes and isolated histiocytes in the connective tissue of the epididymis. H&E (x60). C, Xhantomizated histiocyte accumulation and inflammatory infiltrates in a longstanding epididymitis. H&E (x80). D, Chronic epididymitis in a 36-year-old patient with a clinical history of chronic epididymitis. Giant multinucleate cells stand out in the lumen as well as the epithelial lining of the ductus of the epididymis. H&E (x250).

Chronic Non-specific Epididymitis

This form of epididymitis can present itself as a hardened epididymis without clinical evidence of acute inflammation. There is interstitial lymphocyte infiltration and moderate fibrosis. However, it can also appear clinically as acute inflammation (recurrent epididymitis). The histological picture show: chronic non-specific inflammation with lymphoid follicles; epidermoid metaplasia of the ductus of the epididymis; microabscesses with destruction of the ductus of the epididymis; spermatic granulomas; and xanthomatous histiocytes (Fig. 18–1 **B** and **C**).

Changes in the epididymal epithelium consisting of bizarre nuclei and syncytial transformation of the epithelial cells, similar to those notes by Kuo and Gómez (1981) in the epididymis as well as in the seminal vesicles, were associated with minimal inflammatory infiltrations in two patients with chronic epididymitis. Whether the nature of these changes was degenerative or viral has not be determinated (Fig. 18–1 **D**).

Orchitis (Epididymo-orchitis)

Acute Epididymo-orchitis

Simultaneous involvement of both the testis and the epididymides is produced in the course of some systemic diseases such as: pneumococcal meningitis; salmonellosis (paratyphic B); in Klebsiella pneumonia; and in erysipeas (Scott and Cosgrove, 1977) (Fig. 18–2 **A**).

Other types of epididymo-orchitis develop, for example, in the course of influenza (Thomas and co-authors, 1981); infectious mononucleosis; chicken pox, sandfly fever, typhus; and rickets. The most frequent forms in our habitat are epididymo-orchitis from the mumps virus and orchitis from coxackie B virus.

Epididymo-orchitis from the *mumps* virus is by far the most common condition in this group. It is a complication that occurs in 36 percent of the adult mumps patients and is bilateral in one of six cases. The clinical symptoms or orchitis usually appear during the first week of the disease. Histologically the initial lesions consist of an interstitial edema, vascular congestion, and a slight exudate, which is fibrinous and/or hemorrhagic. Next, inflammatory cells in the intertubular spaces as well as in the interior of the seminiferous tubules appear and the seminiferous epithelium degenerates. At the end of the third week, the seminiferous tubules collapse and atrophy; all the inflammatory cells disappear and the only aftereffect is a focal tubular sclerosis (Charny and Meranze, 1948) (Fig. 18–2 **B** and **C**). Fifty percent of the patients who develop unilateral or bilateral orchitis develop testicular atrophy (Werner, 1950). In 85 percent of the cases with testicular involvement the epididymis is also affected.

Mumps epididymo-orchitis is a frequent cause of sterility. Seventy-six percent of the unilateral cases usually normal normal semen analyses while only thirty percent of the bilateral cases do. Apart from testicular atrophy, some patients later develop gynecomastia. This feature has been related to a Leydig cell involvement, in which an incapacity to produce testosterone has been demonstrated (Aiman and others, 1980). This form of orchitis is very rare in children (one percent), but it can also lead to azoospermia in adults (Ballew and Masters, 1954).

Orchitis is a frequent complication in *coxackie B virus infection* (six percent). It is generally unilateral, appears in the second week of the disease and resolves in a few days. The testis shows interstitial inflammation, preferentially with monocytes; obliteration of some seminiferous tubules by cellular debris and polymorphonuclear leukocytes; and maturation arrest (Freij and associates, 1970).

The frequency of epididymitis in prepubertal patients is similar to that of spermatic cord torsion (Doolittle and co-authors, 1966). The etiology is by nonspecific organisms and does not appear to associate frequently with underlaying malformations (Gislason and others, 1980). The differential diagnosis is to be made between spermatic cord torsion, testicular appendix torsion, orchitis, and incarcerated hernia.

Chronic Epididymo-orchitis

Non-specific Chronic Epididymo-orchitis

The testis is affected in some suppurating epididymitis and *Escherichia coli* is usually the responsible agent. *Streptococcus, Staphylococcus, Pneumococcus,* and other Gram-positive cocci have also been isolated from testicular or epididymal abcesses. The testis can present two different histological patterns: in some cases there are microabcesses and even fistulization to the exterior; in other cases there is a focal tubular-interstitial occurrence. In these areas, the histological picture is sim-

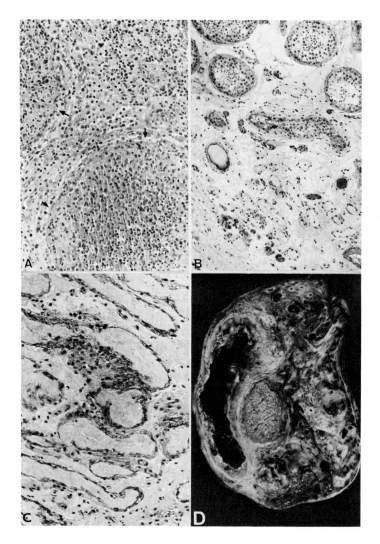

FIGURE 18–2. *A, Acute orchitis. Seminiferous tubules (arrows) showing an epithelium destroyed by polymorphonuclear leukocyte infiltrate. This infiltrate is also found in the testicular interstitium. H&E (x60). B and C, Mumps virus orchitis. B, Focal sclerosis in a group of seminiferous tubules of a patient who was evaluated for infertility with a previous history of orchitis coinciding with mumps. H&E (x60). C, Sclerosed seminiferous tubules from the same patient, in which the tunica propria elastic fibers still persist. Van Gieson elastic stain (x125). D, Chronic epididymo-orchitis Orchiectomy specimen from a 51-year-old patient who had displayed a right testis inflammation with a fistula to the skin. The epididymis and the testis show various microabscesses. The extremely thickened tunica vaginalis contained abundant purulent material.*

ilar to that of idiopathic granulomatous orchitis (Fig. 18–2 **D**).

Other suppurative orchytis is caused by actinomyces. Testicular actinomycosis appears in the form of orchitis, which is sometimes fistulized or recurrent and that evolves over a long time. The origin is unknown in most of cases, since actinomyces have not been found in the lungs, intestine, or teeth. It is well known, however, that the primary focus may be cured while the metastasis persist. Dissemination occurs through the blood stream. The histological pattern, showing multiple abcesses and actinomyces grains, is characteristic (Fig. 18–4**D**).

Granulomatous Epididymo-orchitis

There are many etiological agents that can induce an inflammatory reaction of the granulomatous type. The causal relationships are easily demonstrated in some cases such as: tuberculosis; syphilis; leprosy; fungi; specific parasites; and brucellosis; in other cases these relationships are difficult to define, such as in idiopathic granulomatous orchitis and in malakoplakia.

Tuberculosis. Tuberculosis of the epididymis and testis is secondary to: lesions in the lungs, bones, joints, and lymph nodes; or to lesions of the genitourinary tract. In the first case, the bacilli arrive via the blood stream and in the second, they arrive via the spermatic pathways. The age of greatest incidence coincides with the age of major sexual activity, namely between 15 and 45 years of age.

Clinically, a painful increase in scrotum size is noted. The affected epididymis is firm and thick, and the spermatic cord may also be thickened. Epididymitis is bilateral in a third of cases. Prostate gland and seminal vesicles involvement is very frequent (Fig. 18–3A). Isolated tuberulous epididymo-orchitis has been reported (Stein and Miller, 1983).

Numerous granulomas are observed between the epididymal ductus sections. Although in the beginning they can be observed in the cauda epididymis, they later affect wide areas of the epididymis. The granuloma are formed by a central area of necrosis and a bordering zone with Langhan-type giant cells, epithelioid cells, and lymphocytes. It is easy to observe the bacilli with the Ziehl's stain (Köhler, 1973).

The testis is affected in the advanced stages and only in a small number of cases.

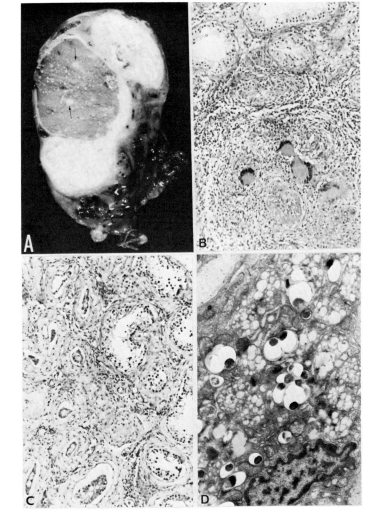

FIGURE 18–3. *A and B, Tuberculous epididymorchitis. A,* Longitudinal section of the testis and epididymis showing numerous caseous zones in the epididymis and a small whitish spot (arrows) in the testicular parenchyma. *B,* Tuberculoid granulomas surrounding a necrotic area in the testicular parenchyma. H&E (x60). *C and D, Lepromatous orchitis. C,* Tubular atrophy and interstitial inflammatory infiltrates formed by lymphocytes and histicocitary cells. H&E (x60). *D,* Histiocitary cells with numerous bacilli in their cytoplasm (Virchows' cells) present in the testicular interstitium (x14,000).

The tuberculosis granulomas develop over the seminiferous tubules as well as in the intertubular spaces. The lesions are focal and multiple (Fig. 18–3 **B**) (Kahn and McAninch, 1980).

Leprosy. Leprosy can clinically appear in three different forms: lepromatous, tuberculoid, and borderline. These forms express the patient's immune reaction capacity. In lepromatous leprosy there is a lack of immune response and the lesions are formed by large accumulations of macrophages with vacuolated cytoplasm (Virchows' cells); numerous bacilli are found within the vacuoles. In tuberculoid leprosy the defense mechanisms are good and resistance to the penetration of Hansen's bacillus is high; the lesions are formed by tuberculoid granulomas; bacilli are rare and the lesions are not accompanied by visceral lesions. In borderline leprosy the lesions are tuberculoid as well as lepromatous, and lower numbers of bacilli are observed (Fig. 18–3 **C** and **D**).

The types of leprosy that can affect the testis and epididymis are the lepromatous and borderline forms. Epididymal and testicular affectation is commonly observed in the former form. It usually develops clinically as an acute epididymoorchitis associated with gynecomastia (10 to 20 percent of patients). Macroscopically the testes are small and upon sectioning display whitish or yellowish spots.

The histological picture varies with the age of the lesion. In the beginning there is a perivascular lymphocyte infiltration and macrophage infiltrates containing a large number of bacilli in the interstitium. The next stage is a progressive testicular atrophy with seminiferous tubule sclerosis and marked Leydig cell hyperplasia. The blood vessels display obliterating endoarteritis lesions and the inflammatory infiltrate disappears, while a marked interstitial edema persists (Carayon and others, 1971). The epididymis usually shows a lesser degree of inflammation. The changes observed in borderline leprosy are similar to those observed in lepromatous leprosy.

The fertility of patients with lepromatous leprosy is reduced, and even more so among males. It has been said that the eradication of leprosy in seventeenth century France was the result of a law obliging lepers to marry among themselves or with their descendents. An indirect relation appears to exist between the duration of lepromatous leprosy and fertility.

Syphilis. Syphilitic orchitis can appear in two forms: congenital and acquired. Congenital syphilitic orchitis appears at birth and is associated with bilateral testicular enlargement, and a histological pattern similar to that of the interstitial form of acquired syphilis. In some patients the diagnosis is delayed until adolescence and, in these patients, the testes have already undergone marked fibrosis and retraction (Fig. 18–4 **A**).

Acquired syphilitic orchitis is a terciary complication and can adopt two different forms: the chronic interstitial inflammation type and the gummous type (Persaud and Rao, 1977).

The pathological pattern of chronic interstitial inflammation shows a testicular size increase of two or three times normal in the initial stages, which is not painful. Upon testicular sectioning grayish and translucid areas contrast with the areas of healthy yellowish seminiferous tubules that have been resected. In the initial stages inflammatory round cell infiltrations and endoarteritis lesions are frequent. The inflammatory infiltrations, which are more intense in the mediastinum and in interlobular septa, later surround each seminiferous tubule. Occasionally there are small gummas. The seminiferous tubules lose the germinal cell line, show peritubular fibrosis, and gradually disappear. In the final stages, the chronic inflammation regresses, areas of fibrosis lose cellularity, and the lesions

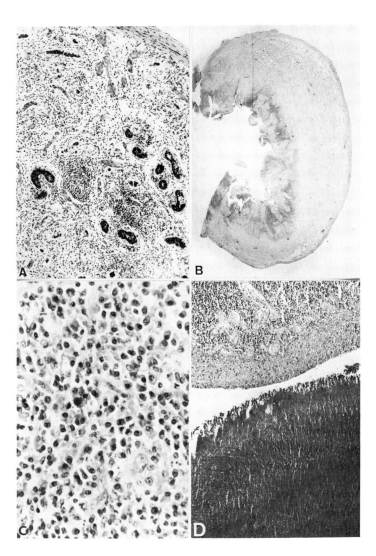

FIGURE 18–4. *A, B, and C, Syphilitic orchitis. A,* Congenital syphilitic orchitis. Dense plasma cell inflammatory infiltrates in the testicular interstitium, associated to signs of endoarteritis and tubular atrophy. H&E (x25). *B,* Longitudinal section of a testis with a gummous type of necrosis in the central part. Marked tubular atrophy is observable in the periphery. H&E (x3). *C,* Dense plasma cell infiltrates in the peripherical zone of the gummous necrosis. H&E (x250). *D,* Testicular actinomycosis. The section includes an abscess wall in which some seminiferous tubules are still recognizable. The abscess contains an actinomyces granule. H&E (x25).

adopt the appearance of scars. The epididymis is usually not affected.

The gummous type of syphilitic orchitis also develops with a painless increase in testicular size. Upon sectioning one can observe a large, well-outlined gummatous necrosis (or various small gummas) that is readily apparent due to its yellowish-grey coloration. Microscopically, the original tubular architecture is visible as imprecise lines within the necrotic zones. The peripheral zone is surrounded by lymphocytes, plasma cells, and a few giant cells. The pattern of the testicular parenchyma is similar to those of the interstitial form of acquired syphilis (Fig. 18–4 **B** and **C**).

Fungi. Infections caused by fungi are rare. The most frequent are: blastomycosis; coccidiomycosis; and histioplasmosis (Orr and co-authors, 1972).

Blastomycosis, the dissemination forms observed in North America, frequently affect the lungs, bones, urinary system, and genital tract. The prostate, epididymis, testis, and seminal vesicles are the parts of the genital tract affected in the order of respective frequency. Upon sectioning the testis or epididymis, small cavities appear, which have a purulent content that is occasionally caseous. Histologically there are granulomas with giant cells and numerous 8 to 15 microns diameter fungi, with a double refringent contour that is easily identified with PAS or silver-metenamine stains (Eickenberg and others, 1975). The standard therapy for blastomycosis is amphotericin B. A new oral antifungal agent, ketoconazole, with less adverse reactions, has been successfully used (Short and co-workers, 1983).

Coccidiomycosis, in those parts of America in which it is endemic, sometimes gives rise to dissemination in various organs including the epididymis. The histological lesions are granulomatous and similar to those observed in tuberculosis. With the PAS stain, 30 to 60 microns diameter sporangia and their spores are observed.

Histoplasma capsulatum has an ample worldwide distribution. Human infection begins in the lungs, following spore inhalation, and can be asymptomatic. Genital involvement has been observed in leukemia patients treated with steroids. The lesion can affect the prostate, seminal vesicles, testis and epidymis. Epididymitis by *Histoplasma* as the only manifestation of the disease have been described (Kauffman and associates, 1981). Histologically, a caseous necrosis, with or without granuloma, is observed. The etiologic agent measures from 1 to 5 microns in diameter and can be stained with silver metenamine. Amphotericin B is very useful in the treatment of this type of epididymitis.

Parasites. Parasite infections are frequent, even in the areas in which parasites are endemic. The most frequent are: phylariasis and eschistosomiasis.

Phylariasis is caused by the *Wucheria bancofti*, a nematode that lives in the tropical and subtropical regions of Asia, Africa, South America, the Pacific islands, and North Australia. The adult nematode develops in man and emigrates to the lymphatic vessels of the inguinal region. Acute funiculitis and epididymo-orchitis with hydrocele develops at the same time as does the infection (Das and others, 1983). The vascular endothelium proliferates, the lymphatic vessel lumen occludes, and eosinophilic infiltrates develop around the worm. These lesions cause the obstruction of the ductus of the epididymis. The subsequent lymphatic stagnation leads to lymphatic varicosities and scrotal elephantiasis. The worms surrounded by the inflammatory infiltrate die, and their debris are calcified or isolated by fibrosis. These lesions can be recognized as hard nodules along the length of the spermatic cord (Fig. 18–5A) (Michael, 1945).

Genital involvement by the *Schistosoma haematobium* affects the inhabitants of wide areas of the Middle East and Africa. Man is infected by bathing in water containing cercaria. The cercaria penetrate the body through the skin and develop in the liver. Later the worms emigrate to the pelvic and vesical veins, where they lay eggs and die. The eggs are large (150 × 50 μm), and have a lateral spur. The worms may pass to the epididymis or the spermatic cord, via the spermatic and deferential veins, but they do not usually enter the testis (Houston, 1964). Macroscopically, the lesions of the spermatic cord or the epididymis are nodular and yellow. Histologically, either the parasite or a granulomatous reaction with giant cells around the eggs can be observed. Spermatic vein thrombosis; sclerosing polypoid granulomatous phlebitis of the spermatic cord (Elbadawi and others, 1979); and testicular hemorrhagic infarction secondary to spermatic arteritis; are lesions that have been described as being associated with this condition (Fig. 18–5B).

Brucellosis. Epididymitis and orchitis used to be frequent complications of undulant fever or brucellosis (between 5 and

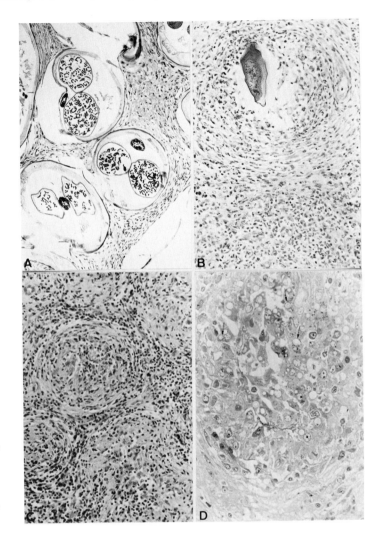

FIGURE 18–5. *A, Epididymal fillariasis. Epididymis parasitized by phylarias, several transverse sections of which containing numerous microphylaria can be seen. H&E (x25). B, Epididymal schistosomiasis. Granulomatous reaction with numerous eosinophilic leukocytes surrounding a Schistosoma haematobium egg. H&E (x100). C, Idiopathic granulomatous orchitis. Seminiferous tubules showing only Sertoli cells and macrophages can be recognized. The testicular interstitium contains abundant lymphocyte, plasma cell and monocyte infiltrates. The tubular wall has a concentric lamellar appearance due to inflammatory infiltrates. H&E (x100). D, Testicular malakoplakia. Case previously diagnosed as idiopathic granulomatous orchitis. Numerous concentric lamellar formations (arrows) in the cytoplasm of a macrophage located within a seminiferous tubule. Toluidine blue (x250).*

18 percent of the cases). *Brucella melitensis* is more frequent than *Brucella abortus*. Genital tract lesions can appear at any time during the course of the illness. Histological studies show a nonspecific chronic inflammatory process in the testis as well as in the epididymis, with occasional histiocyte accumulations. The inflammatory infiltrates are focal (Castro, 1946).

Idiopathic Granulomatous Orchitis. This is an inflammatory lesion of unknown origin that is characterized clinically by an increase in testicular size and which can simulate a malignant tumor.

The patients frequently have had previous trauma to the area and two thirds of the patients have a history of urinary infection. Cultures of the affected testicular tissues are generally negative. Forty percent of the patients have spermatic granuloma in the epididymis, which suggests an autoimmune etiology. The appearance of this abnormality in 50 to 70 year-old men is clinically notable. The most frequent symptoms are: an increase in testicular size; hardening; and pain. It may be bilateral. The clinical diagnosis includes: mumps virus orchitis; bacterial and tuberculosis epididymo-orchitis; spermatic granuloma; and testicular tumor. The definitve diagnosis is histological.

Macroscopically, an increase in testicular size is observed, which corresponds closely with the abundant amount of tunica vaginalis exudate. Upon sectioning, the testis is large and has a nodular appearance. Areas of necrosis and infarction are frequent. The epididymis is affected in half of the cases and may contain one or more spermatic granulomas.

Depending on the extension of the lesions, focal and diffuse forms are observed microscopically. There are two forms observed in the histological pictures: one that is primarily tubular and another that is initially interstitial, but the two forms may become similar in the advances stages.

Primary tubular granulomatous orchitis shows a histological pattern with the following characteristics: The most frequent tubular lesions are destruction of the germinal epithelium, the presence of Sertoli cells showing both a vacuolated cytoplasm and a vesiculous nucleus, and multinucleate giant cells in the seminiferous tubule lumen. The associated interstitial lesions consist of variably intense inflammatory infiltrates composed of lymphocytes, plasma cells, and monocytes. The inflammatory cells infiltrate the tunica propria forming concentric rings. Interstitial giant cells can be recognized in the final stages. The blood vessels show thrombosis and arteritis lesions.

In primary interstitial granulomatous orchitis there is a disproportion between the intensity of the interstitial inflammatory process and the comparatively lower degree of tubular atrophy during the initial stages, which persist for a long time. The composition of the inflammatory infiltrate is similar to that observed in primary tubular granulomatous orchitis.

The final condition of the testis, in both forms of idiopathic granulomatous orchitis, is one of tubular atrophy, with basement membrane disorganization, caused by the inflammatory infiltrate, and loss of the germinative epithelium. At no time during the evolution of this condition are phagocytated spermatozoa observed at either the tubular or interstitial levels (Fig. 18–5C).

The histological pattern of these two forms of idiopathic granulomatous orchitis correlates well with models of experimental allergic orchitis (Tung and associated, 1981).

Primarily tubular orchitis lesions can be experimentally reproduced by the injection of serum from the affected animals. The inflammation occurs secondarily to germinal cell lesions and develops around the affected tubules (Toullet and Voisin, 1976). Primarily interstitial orchitis can be transferred by the injection of immune cells (Bernard and others, 1978; Sato and associates, 1981).

When both testes develop idiopathic granulomatous orchitis in a metachronic manner, good results have been obtained using steroid therapy when the second orchitis occurs (Chilton and Smith, 1979).

During the course of chronic granulomatous orchitis, the epididymis can show different types of lesions such as spermatic granulomas and nonspecific chronic infiltration.

The tunica vaginalis is affected, in most cases, by chronic nonspecific inflammatory infiltrates and hydrocele.

Malakoplakia. Malakoplakia is a chronic inflammatory disease characterized by the accumulation of a large number of histocytes with eosinophilic and granular cytoplasm. The cytoplasm contains concentric lamellar bodies, known as Michaelis-Gutmann inclusions.

Malakoplakia was first described by Michaelis and Gutmann in 1902 as a lesion of urinary bladder mucosa. The morphological characteristics were detailed in 1903 by von Hansemann, who created the term malakoplakia, from the Greek words *malakos* (soft) and *plakos* (plaque), to describe the soft yellowish mucosal plaques of the urinary bladder. (Macroscopically, the lesions are cartilaginous in consistency, and drab brown with yellowish areas.) Although von Hansemann's report appeared a year after his former assistant Michaelis, it was the former who—while doing an autopsy on a sixty-year-old patient who had died of fibrocaseous pulmonary tuberculosis—found what he initially thought were urinary bladder tumors (Damjanov and Katz, 1981).

It has been observed that malakoplakia can affect not only different parts of the urinary tract: ureter; renal pelvis; kidney; and urethra, but also other organs or systems such as: the digestive tract (especially the colon and rectum); the female genital system (endometrium, vagina, parametrium, and ovary); the mesenterium; the adrenal glands; the skin, the cerebrum; the lymph nodes; the lungs; the bones; and the connective tissue of paranasal sinuses (Nistal and others, 1984) and oropharynx (Stanton and Maxted, 1981).

The first observation of testicular affectation was described by Haukohl and Chinchinian (1958), and the first isolated case of epididymal involvement was described by Green (1968). There are not more than 25 cases of only testicular or simultaneous (testicular and epididymal) involvement mentioned in the literature, and there are only 8 of exclusively epididymal involvement, although it probably is more frequent than has been reported (Waisman and Rampton, 1968; Montero and co-authors, 1977, McClure, 1980; Pérez-Barrios and associates, 1981). Simultaneous affectation of both testis and prostate has been reported (Saraf and others, 1983). When surgical material from epididymal and testicular inflammatory diseases is reviewed, it is not unusual to find new cases of malakoplakia from orchitis or epididymitis cases that were previously diagnosed as nonspecific or granulomatous.

When malakoplakia affects the epididymis, one can observe how the accumulates of von Hansemann histiocitary cells enlarge the intertubular spaces. A variable number of plasma cells, lymphocytes, and most cells are also found among the histiocitary cells in the intertubule connective tissue. The epithelium of the ductus of the epididymis can be atrophic or demonstrate reactive hyperplasia. (Fig. 18–6**A** and **B**).

The histological pattern of malakoplakia is similar to that of idiopathic granulomatous orchitis. The interstitium contains numerous histiocytes over an inflammatory background. The histiocytes show 3 to 15 microns of concentric, lamellated inclusions (Michaelis-Gutmann bodies), which are positive to: the PAS technique (before and after diastase digestion of glucose); to the von Kossa technique for calcium; and to the Perl technique for iron. Instead of the seminiferous epithelium, the seminiferous tubules show uni- or multinucleate macrophage aggregates, which may present Michaelis-Gutmann bodies (Fig. 18–5**D**).

Electron microscope studies have shown a great variety of lysosomic structures which can be classified into three types (McClure and others (1981): phagolysosomes; intermediate formations; and Michaelis-Gutmann bodies. All of the structures are surrounded by a unit membrane and its matrix is constituted by numerous membranous formations, layered like a finger print, forming whorls or loops. In addition, the intermediate forms show focal crystallization. The largest Michaelis-Gutmann bodies have a characteristic bull's eye structure composed of alternating concentric hydroxyapatite crystals and nonmineralized rings. (Fig. 18–6**C**) Hydroxyapatite crystal presence has been confirmed by X-ray diffraction (Price and associates, 1973) in a skin malaloplakia, and in the different components of the crystals that have been investigated by Rinaudo and others (1977) with quantitative microanalysis techniques.

Malakoplakia, like other inflammatory processes, evolves through time. At least this is what has been observed in

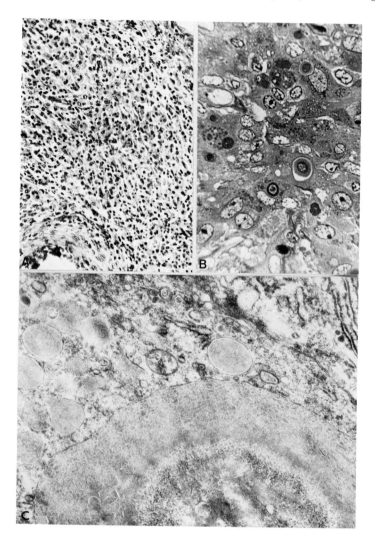

FIGURE 18–6. *Malakoplakia of the epididymis.* A, Inflammatory infiltrates of a chronic nature, preferentially formed by histiocitary cells with eosinophilic cytoplasm. H&E (x60). B, Histiocytes with numerous concentric lamellar inclusions (Michaelis-Gutmann bodies). Toludine blue (x450). C, Part of a Michaelis-Gutmann body surrounded by numerous lysosomes (x22,000).

urinary bladder malakoplakia. Smith (1965) has described three phases: the *initial phase*, which is preceeded by marked edema and congestion with an infiltrate rich in plasma cells, eosinophilic leukocytes, and some macrophages. These macrophages have ample, granular, and eosinophilic cytoplasm, but lack Michaelis-Gutmann bodies. The histologic pattern is not useful for diagnosis; the *classic phase* in which the infiltrate is predominantly formed by von Hansemann histiocytes and the Michaelis-Gutmann bodies are abundant; and the *fibrosis phase* during which the histiocitary infiltrate is conserved, but the lesion is criss-crossed by bundles of fibroblasts and bands of collagen fibres.

The pathogenesis of malakoplakia is unclear. Although the beliefs that it represents: a tumor; is a special tuberculosis complication; an alteration of the mast cells; or is related to erythrophagocytosis or sarcoidosis belong to history, the precise pathogenetic mechanisms remain unknown. Lewin and associates (1976) have suggested the following explanations: the causal agent could be an unusual strain of bacteria; the immune response to infection could be altered, abnormal, or inadequate; and/or it might be due to abnormal macrophage response.

Although electron microscope and culture studies have proven the presence of a great variety of bacteria, fungi and viruses, the frequency with which Gram negative germs, including *Escherichia coli* (alone or associated to *Klebsiella*, *Aerobacter*, or *Mycobacterium*) have been identified is significant. Malakoplakia has been reproduced experimentally without the presence of bacteria being necessary, requiring only some of their constituents, as in the Csapo and associates (1975) experiments employing a lipopolysaccharide extract obtained from pathogenic *Escherichia coli* strain.

Immune system anomalies have been observed in some patients with malakoplakia. They have also been found in patients with: tuberculosis; sarcoidosis; or cancer; in immunodepressed patients; and in some patients with low levels of serum immunoglobulins. However, many patients with malakoplakia do not present any detectable immune response alteration.

The most sensible pathogenic explanation is based on considering a possible macrophage function defect with an abnormal histiocitary response. It is suggested that the macrophages are able to phagocytize bacteria, but are unable to kill or digest them. Larger and larger quantities of these bacteria are accumulated in the phagolysosomes and calcium salts are subsequently deposited on them. The progressive transformation of phagolysosomes into Michaelis-Gutmann bodies, or the latters' posterior growth, would be produced by their fusion with new lysosomes. In this respect, the septate junctions described between different lysosomal structures (Nistal and co-authors, 1978) that would favor their union are noteworthy. Another important finding was made by Abdou and others (1977) in a patient with intestinal malakoplakia. These authors reported abnormal lysosomal function with low cyclic guanine monophosphate (GMP) levels and with monocyte incapacity to liberate beta glucosidase and other lysosomic enzymes. Cyclic GMP acts as a signal for microtubular assemblage and is necessary for lysosome enzyme liberation—low GMP levels would therefore lead to the formation of giant lysosomes. If this hypothesis is confirmed, the malakoplakia defect would have many points in common with the Chediak-Higashi anomaly (a syndrome characterized by low levels of cyclic GMP, giant lysosomes, deficit of bactericidal enzymes, and inadequate lysosome degranulation).

Patients with malakoplakia would be able to benefit from drugs such as cyclic GMP, cholinergic agonists, ascorbic acid, which promote microtubular assembly and have been used successfully in patients with the Chediak-Higashi syndrome.

Differential diagnosis with idiopathic granulomatous orchitis is based on the search for Michaelis-Gutmann bodies. Many inflammatory diseases that were previously diagnosed as idiopathic granulomatous orchitis are actually diagnosed as testicular malakoplakia. The presence of some giant cells in some cases of testicular malakoplakia has made it necessary to discount the possibility of granulomatous infections such as syphilis, atypical mycobacterium, fungi, and viruses, among others. Testicular malakoplakia can also be observed in association with abscessed orchitis.

REFERENCES

1. Abdou NI, Napombejara C, Sagawa A, Ragland C, Stechschulte DJ, Nilsson U, Gourley W, Watanabe I, Lindsey NJ, Allen MS: Malakoplakia: evidence for monocyte lysosomal abnormality correctable by cholinergic agonist in vitro and in vivo. New Engl J Med 297:1413, 1977
2. Aiman J, Brenner PF, MacDonald PC: An-

drogen and estrogen production in elderly men with gynecomastia and testicular atrophy after mumps orchitis. J Clin Endocrinol Metab 50:380, 1980
3. Ballew JW, Masters WH: Mumps: a cause of infertility. Fertil Steril 5:536, 1954
4. Berger RE, Alexander ER, Harnisch JP, Palsen SA, Monda GD, Ansel J, Holmes HK: Etiology, manifestations and therapy of acute epididymitis: prospective study of 50 cases. J Urol 121:750, 1979
5. Bernard CCA, Mitchell GF, Leydon J, Bargerbos A: Experimental autoimmune orchitis in T-cell-deficient mice. Int Arch Allergy Appl Immunol 56:256, 1978
6. Carayon A, Languillon J, Maydat L, Bronstein J, Fromantin M: Role du blocage lymphatique spermatique dans les lésions testiculaires de la lépre lepromateuse avec gynécomastie. Ann Endocr 32:39, 1971
7. Castro D: Brucelosis genital en el hombre. Arch Uruguayos de Medicina, Cirujía y especialidades 29:61, 1946
8. Charny CW, Meranze DR: Pathology of mumps orchitis. J Urol 60:140, 1948
9. Chilton CP, Smith JB: Steroid therapy in the treatment of granulomatous orchitis. Brit J Urol 51:404, 1979
10. Csapó Z, Kuthy E, Lantos J, Ormos J: Experimentally induced malakoplakia. Amer J Path 79:453, 1975
11. Damjanov I, Katz M: Malakoplakia. In Sommers SC, Rosen PP (eds). Pathology Annual. New York: Appleton-Century-Crofts, 1981, 2:16, p. 103
12. Das S, Tuerk D, Amar AD, Sommer J: Surgery of male genital lymphedema. J Urol 129:1240, 1983
13. Doolittle KH, Smith JP, Saylor ML: Epididymitis in the prepubertal boy. J Urol 96:364, 1966
14. Elbadawi A, Khuri FJ, Crockett, AT: Polypoid granulomatous and sclerosing endophlebitis of spermatic cord. New pathologic type of schistosomal funiculitis. Urology 13:309, 1979
15. Eickenberg H, Amin M., Lich R, Jr: Blastomycosis of the genitourinary tract. J Urol 113:650, 1975
16. Freij L, Norby R, Olsson B: A small outbreak of Coxackie B 5 infection with two cases of cardiac involvement and orchitis followed by testicular atrophy. Acta Med Scand 187:177, 1970
17. Gislason T, Noronha RF, Gregory JG: Acute epididymitis in boys: a 5-year retrospective study. J Urol 124:533, 1980
18. Green WO, Jr: Malacoplakia of the epididymis (without testicular involvement); the first reported case. Arch Path 86:438, 1968
19. Harnish JP, Berger RE, Alexander ER, Monda G, Holmes KK: Aetiology of acute epididymitis. Lancet 1:819, 1977
20. Haukohl RS, Chinchinian H: Malakoplakia of the testicle: Report of a case. Amer J Clin Path 29:473, 1958
21. Houston W: Bilharziasis of the testis. Brit J Urol 36:220, 1964
22. Kahn RI, McAninch JW: Granulomatous disease of the testis. J Urol 123:868 1980
23. Kauffman CA, Slama TG, Wheat LJ: Histoplasma capsulatum epididymitis. J Urol 125:434, 1981
24. Köhler H: Uebertragung einer Tuberkulose auf dem Genitalwege. Zschr Urol 66: 207, 1973.
25. Kuo T, Gómez LG: Monstruous epithelial cells in human epididymis and seminal vesicles. Am J Surg Pathol 5:483, 1981
26. Lewin KJ, Fair WR, Steigbigel RT, Winberg CD, Droller MJ: Clinical and laboratory study into the pathogenesis of malakoplakia. J Clin Path 29:354, 1976
27. McClure J: A case of malakoplakia of the epididymis associated with trauma. J Urol 124:934, 1980
28. McClure J, Cameron CHS, Garret R: The ultrastructural features of malakoplakia. J Pathology 134:13, 1981
29. Michael P: Filariasis: histopathologic study. United States Naval Medical Bulletin 45:225, 1945
30. Michaelis L, Gutmann C: Ueber Einschlüsse in blasentumoren. Z Klin Med 47:208, 1902
31. Montero J, Urrutia M, Parra T, Pino A: Testicle malakoplakia associated with aplastic anemia and cutaneous sarcoidosis. Act Urol Esp 1:227, 1977
32. Morgan AD: Inflammation and infestation of the testis and paratesticular structures. In Pugh RC (ed) Pathology of the testis Blackwell Oxford, England: Blackwell Scientific Publications, 1976, p. 124
33. Nistal M, Regadera J, Razquin S, Paniagua R, Gavilán J: Malakoplakia of the maxillary sinus. Anal Otol Rhinol Laryngol, 1984 (In press)
34. Nistal M, Rodríguez-Echandía EL, Paniagua R: Septate junctions between digestive vacuoles in human malakoplakia. Tissue & Cell 10:137, 1978
35. Orr W, Mulholland SG, Walzak MP, Jr: Genitourinary tract involvement with systemic mycoses. J Urol 107:1047, 1972
36. Pérez-Barrios A, Usera-Sárraga G, Navas-Palacios JJ: Malacoplaquia de testículo. Estudio

óptico y ultraestructural de un caso. Patología 14:143, 1981
37. Persaud V, Rao A: Gumma of the testis. Brit J Urol 49:142, 1977
38. Price HM, Hanrahan JB, Florida RG: Morphogenesis of calcium-laden cytoplasmic bodies in malakoplakia of the skin: An electron microscopic study. Hum Pathol 4:381, 1973
39. Rinaudo P, Damjanov I, Stoesser B: Malakoplakia of testis. Int Urol Nephrol 9:249, 1977
40. Saraf P, DiSant'Agnese P, Valvo J, Caldamone A, Linke C: An unusual case of malakoplakia involving the testis and prostate. J Urol 129:149, 1983
41. Sato K, Hirokawa K, Hatakeyama S: Experimental allergic orchitis in mice. Histopathological and immunological studies. Virchows Arch. A Path Anat 392:147, 1981
42. Scott MB, Cosgrove MD: Salmonella infection and the genitourinary system. J Urol 118:64, 1977
43. Short KL, Harty JI, Amin M, Short LF: The use of ketoconazole to treat systemic blastomycosis presenting as acute epididymitis. J Urol 129:382, 1983
44. Smith BH: Malakoplakia of the urinary tract: a study of twenty-four cases. Amer J Clin Pathol 43:409, 1965
45. Stanton MJ, Maxted W: Malakoplakia: a study of the literature and current concepts of pathogenesis, diagnosis and treatment. J Urol 125:139, 1981
46. Stein AL, Miller DB: Tuberculous epididymo-orchitis: a case report. J Urol 129:613, 1983
47. Thomas D, Simpson K, Ostojic H, Kaul A: Bacteremic epididymo-orchitis due to hemophilus influence type B. J Urol 126:832, 1981
48. Toullet F, Voisin GA: Passive transfer of autoimmune spermatogenetic orchiepididymitis (AITO) by antispermatozoa sera. Clin Exp Immunol 26:549, 1976
49. Tung KSK, Teuscher C, Meng AL: Autoimmunity to spermatozoa and the testis. Immunol Rev 55:217, 1981
50. Von Hansemann D: Ueber Malakoplakie der Harnblase. Virchows Arch (Pathol Anat) 173:302, 1903
51. Waisman J, Rampton JB: Malakoplakia of the testis and epididymis. Arch Path 86:431, 1968
52. Werner CA: Mumps orchitis and testicular atrophy. I. Occurrence. Ann Intern Med 32:1066, 1950

19

DISORDERS SECONDARY TO OBSTRUCTION OF THE EPIDIDYMIS AND VAS DEFERENS

Spermatic duct obstructive lesions are responsible for 7.4 percent (Dubin and Amelar, 1971) to 14.3 percent (Wong and Straus, 1973) of male infertility. The causes for the obstruction can be either congenital or acquired (White and Paulson, 1977). The congenital causes have been reviewed in Chapter 6.

The acquired causes are due either to inflammatory or surgical processes. The inflammation that most frequently produces epididymal and vasal blockage is gonorrhea. Gonococcic epididymitis preferentially affects the cauda epididymis and the proximal portion of the vas deferens. Since the affectation is usually bilateral, the result is azoospermia.

Tuberculosis of the epididymis is a frequent cause of spermatic duct obstruction. The resulting sterility is not always due to a bilateral epididymal lesion, but rather to the concomitant involvement of the prostate and seminal vesicles.

The surgical causes of the blockage can be voluntary—as in birth control measures—or iatrogenic as in the ligature of the vas deferens while repairing, for example, a hernia (Friberg and Fritjofsson, 1979), a hydrocele, or varicocele.

It is interesting to note that there are patients with azoospermia or severe oligospermia whose testicular biopsy is normal or shows few alterations whereas spermatic duct radiological exploration show that these ducts are patent. These "obstructive" conditions without actual obstruction can be explained in two ways. The spermatozoa along the length of the epididymis may be absorbed when they are produced in a small number, and only reaching the ejaculate when they attain a certain number (Makler and Geresh, 1979). The second possibility would be a partial obstruction of the spermatic ducts. In these cases the diagnosis can be suggested by a quantitative analysis of the testicular biopsy (Silber and Rodríguez-Rigau, 1981). A partial obstruction definitely exists if the number of immature spermatids in each seminiferous tubule is over 20, and the sperm count is lower than 10 million. This method also appears to be useful in the prediction of the expected spermatozoon number after surgical correction of an obstruction.

Young's syndrome (Young, 1970) refers to the association between obstructive azoospermia (some patients can have a few spermatozoa in the ejaculate) and sinusitis, bronchitis, and/or bronchiectasis. The frequency of this syndrome has been estimated to be 50 percent of all obstructive azoospermias. The vasogram is normal but the caput epididymis appears to be intensely distended. The ductuli efferentes histologically prove to be intensely dilated and contain large accumulations of spermatozoa, cellular debris, and cholesterol clefts. As this is associated with respiratory system illness, and the efferent ductules also contain ciliated cells, an abnormality in the cilia has been suggested. The nature of this abnormality is unknown (Hendry and others, 1978).

SPERMATIC DUCT ECTASIS

The obstruction of the spermatic ducts causes ectasis of the flow of spermatozoa with the subsequent dilatation of all the anatomical structures located between the point of obstruction and the seminiferous tubule.

Both epididymis and proximal vas deferens expand due to the increase in intratubular pressure when an obstruction is produced at the level of the vas deferens. The dilatation is significant during the year following the obstruction and causes ductal wall thinning, (Schmidt and Brüschke, 1976). If a sperm granuloma is present at the level of the obstruction, the vas luminal diameter is normal (Belker and associated, 1983). The most sensitive structures are the ductuli efferentes, which are converted into large cavities full of spermatozoa. The epithelium of the epididymis and vas deferens becomes thin while cellular specialized junctions remain intact. Numerous racket-shaped crystals appear within the lysosomal vacuoles in the cytoplasm of the epithelial cells. These crystals can resemble spermatozoa when seen with the light microscope. Actually they are indicative of a great increase in the absorptive functions these cells usually perform (Fig. 19–1A and B).

Enormous amounts of spermatozoa can be seen inside the lumen of the vas deferens, the ductus of the epididymis, and ductuli efferentes in long-standing ectasis. Electron microscopy, performed at the same time as vas deferens re-anastomosis

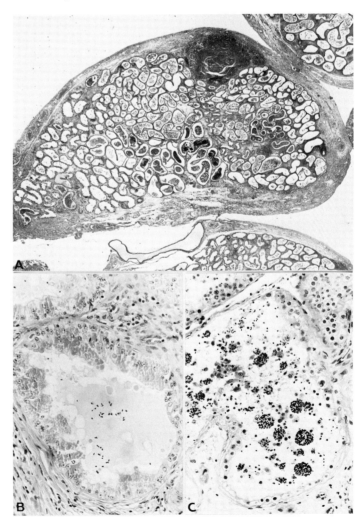

FIGURE 19–1. Spermatic duct ectasis. A, Intense dilatation of caput epididymis ducts, secondary to cauda epididymis obstruction. A spermatic microgranuloma has developed beside the tunica albuginea. H&E (x10). B, Section of a ductulus efferens showing few spermatogonia in the lumen and numerous spherical granulations in the apical portion of the epithelial cell cytoplasm. H&E (x250). C, Abundant spermiophages in a seminiferous tubule lumen. H&E (x250).

in vasectomy patients, has revealed that many of the spermatozoa were in an advanced stage of degeneration. Numerous macrophages with cytoplasm containing dozens of spermatozoa are found in the lumen of these spermatic ducts and, as an exception, in the seminiferous tubules (Phadke, 1975). The macrophages are derived from blood monocytes that have crossed the epithelium and completed a phagocytic activation process. Later some of these may possibly return to the testicular interstitium. The authors who accept this believe this is the manner in which B and T lymphocytes are instructed to begin the process of antisperm antibody production (Fig. 19-1C).

The obstruction also has a detrimental effect on the testis, which differs according to the point of the obstruction. When it is situated far from the testis, as in some vasectomized patients, after the obstruction a marked decrease in spermatogenesis can be observed, the number of spermatid decreases and an incomplete maturation arrest is established. Later, spermatogenesis is restored at a slower rate, with tubular lumen dilatation reaching, on the one hand, an equilibrium between: spermatogenesis; increased epididymal size; and spermatic flow, and the storage and reabsorption of the spermatic flow on the other. In some cases the lesions are irreversible. Spermatogenesis completely returned to normal in vasectomized subjects in whom re-anastomosis was performed within 10 years of the first operation. This was not true of the 50 percent who submitted to re-anastomosis at a later date (Fig. 19-2).

When the obstruction is located in the caput epididymis or an alteration in the testis-epididymis union exists, the lesions are more severe. The seminiferous tubules progressively atrophy until they show complete sclerosis, similar to what is seen in chromatin negative Klinefelter's syndrome (Makler and Hampel, 1975).

Sperm Granuloma

The chronic inflammatory lesion induced by spermatozoon extravasation is known as a sperm granuloma. The causes are multiple: a previous history of epididymal inflammation (Glassy and Mostofi, 1956); traumas (Rovinescu and Reid, 1966); epididymal or vas deferens obstruction; or ischemia (Povysil, 1976). However, the cause is unknown in 40 percent of cases. It is an incidental finding in autopsies or surgical specimens obtained from patients with epididymitis or chronic orchitis. Nevertheless, sperm granuloma represents a complication in no less than 15 percent of vasectomies (Fig. 19-3).

Macroscopically, nodules can be found that range in size from microscopic up to several centimeters and that, upon sectioning, show a yellowish or cream color. They may be multiple or single. Their histological pattern varies with the age of the granuloma. During the initial stages, the spermatozoa spread into the tissue near the broken duct. They then break up and the extravasation zone becomes a necrotic area surrounded by leukocytes, epithelioid cells, and some giant cells. The nearby histiocytes phagocytize the fatty acids that have been released. Later, this material oxidizes and can be observed as yellowish granulations in the cytoplasm. Long after the spermatozoa have disappeared, groups of histiocytes with this pigment in their cytoplasm (ceroid granuloma) can be found. In the final stages, the granuloma transforms into a fibrotic area with or without calcification. Kennedy and Heidger (1980) experimentally followed the development of these granulomas.

Sperm granuloma are present in 2.6 percent of autopsy epididymides, most of which had been asymptomatic. Contrary to clinical spermatic granuloma, which is more common in young men than older ones, the incidence of asymptomatic

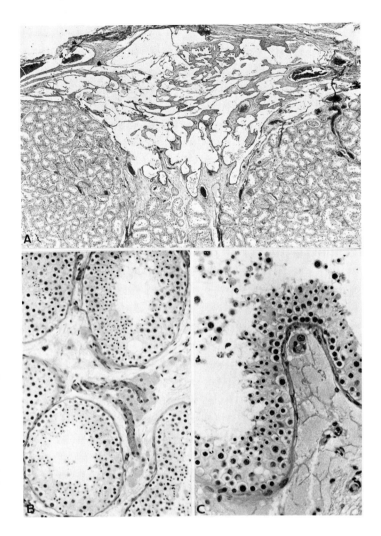

FIGURE 19-2. *Spermatic duct ectasis. A, Intense dilatation of rete testis and tubuli recti. Some cavities contains numerous spermatozoa and spermiophages. H&E (x25). B, Testicular biopsy of a patient with azoospermia produced by bilateral obstruction of the initial segment of the vas deferens. A slight seminiferous tubule dilation as well as some Sertoli cell vacuolation can be observed. H&E (x125). C, Testicular biopsy of a patient with an obstructive type of sterility showing marked sloughing of the seminiferous epithelium. The saw-toothed appearance acquired by the apical portion of the seminiferous epithelium suggests that each Sertoli cell, along with its corresponding germ cells, has separated from each other. H&E (x250).*

sperm granuloma increases with age. Sperm granuloma is also associated with idiopathic granulomatous orchitis.

Autoimmune responses are frequently produced in addition to the local granulomatous reaction caused by the spermatozoa when the ductuli efferentes disrupt. Spermatozoa, which do not appear until puberty—many years after the establishment of the immune tolerance—are a source of varied antigenic material. This material does not normally come in contact with the immune system due to the cellular barrier formed by the Sertoli cells or spermatic duct epithelium. Antigens that agglutinate or immobilize spermatozoa have been identified in the blood serum of these patients.

Vasitis nodosa is a variety of sperm granuloma that is observed in vasectomized patients or in those whose vas deferens has been involuntarily sectioned. It is noted for numerous interconnected or blind-ended ducts that occasionally produce spontaneous vas deferens re-anastomosis (Schmidt and Morris, 1973). A similar microscopic lesion, has been considered to be congenital and designated as mesonephric hamortoma (Tamayo and Ruffolo, 1967; Warner and other, 1983).

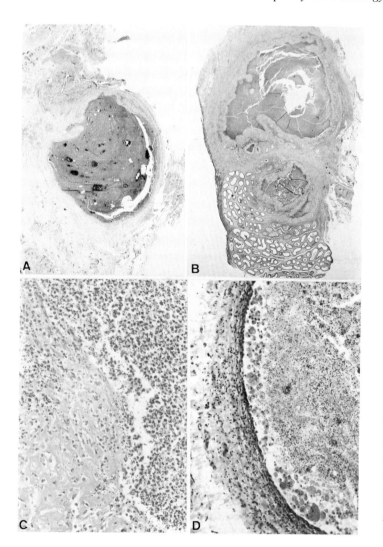

FIGURE 19-3. *Sperm granuloma. A, 1 cm diameter sperm granuloma observed in autopsy epididymis. H&E (x4.5). B, Sperm granuloma associated with epididymal tuberculosis. H&E (x6). C, Spermatozoa infiltrating the disrupted wall of the ductus of the epididymis. H&E (x60). D, Histiocyte accumulation, with abundant cytoplasmic pigmentation, surrounding a long-standing spermatic granuloma. H&E (x60).*

SPERMATOCELE

This term refers to cysts containing spermatozoa that are located: in the ductus of the epididymis; in the ductuli efferentes of the caput epididymis; in the rete testis; or in aberrant ducts. Spermatocele appears after puberty and reaches its maximum incidence during the fourth and fifth decades of life. It has been suggested that spermatocele develops following obstruction of a segment of the spermatic ducts (one or more ductuli efferentes or aberrant ducts) that are consequently isolated from the remaining spermatic duct system. In spite of the spermatocele, spermatozoa flow persists normally. Vasectomy has no influence upon the cyst size.

The cysts can be uni- or multilocular. They are covered by a pseudostratified, cubic, or flat epithelium that is supported by a thin fibrous layer. The interior holds a liquid containing numerous spermatozoa, spermiophages, and sloughed cells. The cysts may not show spermatozoa in older men. On occasion they may be large enough to provoke local discomfort and require extirpation (Fig. 19–4A).

A study of the contents of 28 spermatoceles performed by Molnar and associates in 1978 showed 20 to 25 percent

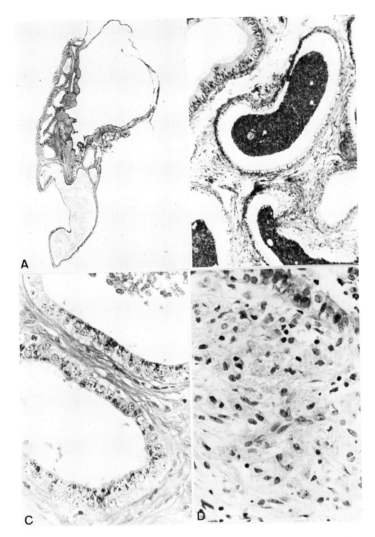

FIGURE 19-4. *A*, Longitudinal section of the caput epididymis showing two cystic dilations, one of which is full of spermatozoa. H&E (x8). *B, C,* and *D:* Brown patches in the epididymis. *B,* Granular material and spermatozoon deposits in the ductuli efferentes. H&E (x125). *C,* Lipofuchsin granule accumulations in the apical region of the epithelial cells of the ductuli efferentes. H&E (x125). *D,* Numerous histiocytes near a ductulus efferens showing abundant cytoplasmic granules. H&E (x250).

of the spermatozoa to be immotile; 7 cases showed marked neck- or middle-piece malformations (thickening or thinning). Patients with spermatocele frequently show sperm agglutinating antigens. The intraluminal pressure probably favors the absorption of spermatozoon-derived products and sets off the appearance of antibodies (Bandhauer, 1963). These antibodies rarely disappear after corrective surgery. At times, 50 percent of the vasograms performed after spermatocelectomy show a decrease in the preoperative amounts of spermatozoa, which may be caused by epididymal duct stenosis after cicatrization. These features counsel against spermatocele extirpation when the patient has been seen because of infertility (Chiari and Drujan, 1980).

Spermatocele and hydrocele can coincide in some patients when the former has broken the tunica vaginalis cavity causing spermatic hydrocele.

BROWN PATCHES IN THE EPIDIDYMIS

Brown patches in the epididymis are present in half of adult autopsies (one fourth of epididymides). The lesions are round or oval (0.5 cm in diameter) and yellow or brown. Characteristically they present some or all of the following features (Mitchinson and co-authors, 1975) (Fig. 19–4**B**, **C**, and **D**).:

1. Marked variation of the ductuli efferentes diameters: dilated ductuli efferentes areas alternate with areas of atrophied ductuli, the latter being more closely placed to the ductus of the epididymis.
2. Abnormal content of the ductuli efferentes: The dilated ductuli contain spermatozoon masses and a spermiophage excess. The stenosed ductuli contain eosinophilic material or packed accumulations of spermatozoa. All intermediate conditions exist between both ductulus types. The eosinophilic material is PAS positive and shows cholesterol clefts.
3. Abnormal pigmentation of tubular epithelium: Present in both the stenosed and dilated ductuli, particularly the former. The pigment is granular, PAS positive, and oil-red-o positive like has lipofuchsin granules. The epithelial cells show no spermatozoa in their cytoplasm.
4. Pigmented histiocyte accumulations: These appear in one third of the lesions. The accumulations vary from a few histiocytes to hundreds. Granulations similar to the ones in the epithelial cells (lipofuchsin granules) are found in the histiocyte cytoplasm.

Physiopathology of Brown patches is assumed to be the following: obstruction of one or more ductuli efferentes, causing dilatation of their proximal segments—associated or not with spermatocele or sperm granuloma—; the passage of histiocytes into the ductuli; and phagocytosis of the progressively degraded spermatozoa. The material within the proximal segments is then phagocytized by the epithelial cells of the ductuli efferentes, followed by the passage of pigmented material into the interstitium, which produces an inflammatory reaction (Fig. 19–5).

Vasectomy

Male sterilization through vasectomy has spread widely, not only in developing Asian and Eastern European countries, but also in the Western world. With relative frequency, pathologists receive vas deferens samples corroborating vasectomy or tissue samples from inflammatory lesions secondary to vasectomy.

Arvis (1976)—who has revised complications that are secondary to vasectomy—has found precocious, secondary, and late complications.

Precocious Complications

Among the precocious complications of vasectomy the following have been mentioned:

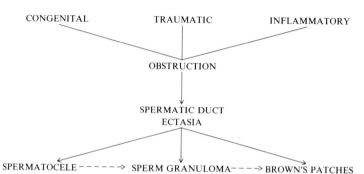

FIGURE 19–5. *Lesions secondary to epididymal obstruction. The continuous lines show normal development of lesions. The dotted lines show a possible evolution.*

1. Vagal reactions, including heart failure (rare).
2. Inability in finding vas deferens (0.1 percent of the cases). This figure includes those cases in which the vas deferens is congenitally absent, and those in which the spermatic cord is voluminous and/or is associated to varicocele or hernia, which make it difficult to find the vas deferens.
3. Haematoma. Between 0 and 18.2 percent of the cases.
4. Infection. A local reaction with transitory edema is normally produced, but scar infection (6 percent of the cases), abscess at ligature level (3 percent) and scrotal abscess (3 to 5 percent) have also been observed.
5. Epididymitis and vas deferens inflammation (0.2 to 6.1 percent of the cases). These patients require the proper antibiotic and antiinflammatory treatment.
6. Scrotal pain that may or may not be associated with inflammatory processes.

Secondary Complications

Secondary complications can appear during the first weeks. They show the following profiles:

1. Deferento-cutaneal fistula (less than 1 percent of patients). This may appear between three and eleven weeks after vasectomy. This can be caused by elimination of ligature material, necrosis, or an infection in the proximal portion of the vas deferens.
2. Defectuous cicatrization (0.2 to 1 percent), with skin retraction and subcutaneous tissue adherences.
3. Various degrees of hydrocele formation.
4. Sperm granuloma. This is the most common, although frequently undiagnosed, complication. It develops in 15 to 50 percent of the vasectomized patients and occurs between 3 weeks and eight months after the vasectomy. It is asymptomatic in half of patients and painful in the other half. On exploration it is shown to be a small 2 to 4 cm diameter tumor in the proximal portion of the vas deferens. It is usually caused by an insufficient ligature, which may or may not be associated with infection. Sperm granuloma formation is four times more frequent with vas deferens ligature than with vas deferens fulguration.

Late Complications

These are characterized by the persistence or reappearance of spermatozoa in the ejaculate. Spermatozoon survival in the spermatic ducts depends on the environment created within the epididymis and vas deferens. Human spermatozoa rarely survive over 15 days in the vas deferens and those that do lose their motility (which is necessary for fertilization) during the third week (Bedford and Zelikovsky, 1979). The reappearance of motile spermatozoa after three weeks suggests renewed vas deferens permeability (Freund and Couture, 1983). This is not rare and is observed in vasa deferentia that have been ligated. Factors favoring spontaneous reanastomosis are: haematoma; tissue necrosis; and sperm granuloma.

Another late complication is the presence of antisperm antibodies. These antibodies are present in 2 percent of fertile men. Following vasectomy over half of the patients develop antisperm antibodies (Silber and co-authors, 1977). The mechanism that causes only some patients to develop these antibodies is unknown, although it may be related to reabsorption of spermatozoa or their degradation products. Long term studies (Hellema and others, 1979) show that autoantibody levels produced secondary to vasectomy tend to remain high in the following years, which influences the possible fertility of men undergoing vasovasostomy (Fuchs and Alexander, 1983). One year after the vasectomy, agglutinating antibodies were detected in 73 percent of the patients; sperm immobilizing antibodies in 42 percent; and anti-nuclear antibodies in 29 percent (Hellema and Rümke, 1978). The type of antibodies developed appears to be related to the technique used. While there is no difference between the percentages of patients who show sperm agglutinating antibodies and were vasectomized either by vas ligation or by fulguration, the percentage of patients developing sperm immobilizing antibodies is lower with fulguration (Alexander and Schmidt, 1977). There is also a relationship between the presence of spermatic granuloma and a higher frequency of sperm immobilizing antibodies.

The possibility that vasectomy may influence an increase in arteriosclerosis has been reported by Fahrenbach and others (1980). In a comparative study between vasectomized and non-vasectomized men, Petitti and co-authors (1983) have found that neither the incidence of acute myocardial infarction, other ischemic heart disease, nor that of all atherosclerotic disease was significantly different between the two groups.

The testicular lesions found in vasectomized men consist of: tubular lumen dilatation; hypospermatogenesis or incomplete maturation arrest; and immature germinal elements sloughing (Gupta and associates, 1975).

In regard to pathogenesis, the seminiferous epithelium lesions are believed to be more related to intratubular pressure atrophy than to a hormonal or immunologically mediated atrophy (Jenkins and others, 1979). Nevertheless, an immunological mechanism is strongly suggested in some experimental testicular lesions in animals. These lesions include: lymphocyte infiltrations; basement membrane thickening; and immune complex deposits on seminiferous tubule walls (Alexander and Anderson, 1979).

The testicular lesions are cured quickly if re-anastomosis is successful, but although it is possible for the majority of the operations to produce a normal number of spermatozoa in the ejaculate, their motility and viability are clearly diminished (Middleton and Urry, 1980).

In order to avoid an increase in pressure of the proximal spermatic ducts after vasectomy, vas deferens diversion to the urinary bladder (vasocystostomy) has been successfully carried out in rabbits (Hooker, 1980).

Although most papers refer to the state of seminiferous epithelium, there is now sufficient experimental evidence to suppose that Leydig cells are also affected (Aoki and Fawcett, 1978; Risbridger and others, 1981). The hyperplasia of Leydig cells is the principal alteration observed. However, it occurs only in the ipsilateral testis; this supports the hypothesis for the existence of important local factors in controlling Leydig cell function. If there is a mechanism by which damaged seminiferous epithelium would affect the Leydig cells, it remains unknown.

REFERENCES

1. Alexander NJ, Schmidt SS: Incidence of antisperm antibody levels and granulomas in men. Fertil Steril 28:655, 1977
2. Alexander NJ, Anderson DJ: Vasectomy: Consequences of autoimmunity to sperm antigens. Fertil Steril 32:253, 1979
3. Aoki A, Fawcett DW: Is there a local feedback from the semiferous tubules affecting activity of the Leydig cells? Biol Reprod 19:144, 1978
4. Arvis G: La vasectomie: ses aspects techniques, les consequences du blocage de l'excrétion déférentielle. Ann Urol 10:163, 1976
5. Bandhauer, K.: Untersuchungen über immu-

nobiologische Ursachen der männlichen Sterilität. Klin Med Wien 18:204, 1963
6. Bedford JM, Zelikovsky G: Viability of spermatozoa in the human ejaculate after vasectomy. Fertil Steril 32:460, 1979
7. Belker AM, Konnak JW, Sharlip ID, Thomas AJ: Intraoperative observations during vasovasostomy in 334 patients. J Urol 129:524, 1983
8. Chiari R, Drujan B: Spermatozelenoperation und Fertilität. Urologe 19:268, 1980
9. Dubin L, Amelar R: Etiologic factors in 1294 consecutive cases of male infertility. Fertil Steril 22:469, 1971
10. Fahrenbach HB, Alexander NJ, Senner JW, Fulgham DL, Coon LJ: Effect of vasectomy on the retinal vasculature of men. J Androl 1:299, 1980
11. Freund MJ, Couture M: The presence of spermatozoa in the semen of vasectomized men. J Androl 3:313, 1982
12. Friberg J, Fritjofsson Å: Inguinal herniorrhaphy and sperm-agglutinating antibodies in infertile men. Arch Androl 2:317, 1979
13. Fuchs EF, Alexander NJ: Immunologic considerations before and after vasovasostomy. Fertil Steril 40:497, 1983
14. Glassy FJ, Mostofi FK: Spermatic granulomas of the epididymis. Am J Clin Pathol 26:1303, 1956
15. Gupta AS, Kothari LK, Dhruva A, Bapna R: Surgical sterilization by vasectomy and its effect on the structure and function of the testis in man. Brit J Surg 62:59, 1975
16. Hellema HW, Rümke P: Sperm autoantibodies as a consequence of vasectomy. I: Till one year post-operation. Clin Exp Immunol 31:18, 1978
17. Hellema HW, Samuel T, Rümke P: Sperm autoantibodies as a consequence of vasectomy II: Long-term follow-up studies. Clin Exp Immunol 38:31, 1979
18. Hendry WF, Knight RK, Whitfield HN, Stansfeld AG, Pryse-Davies J, Ryder TA, Pavia D, Bateman JR, Clarke SW: Obstructive azoospermia: respiratory function tests, electron microscopy and the results of surgery. Brit J Urol 50:598, 1978
19. Hooker RH: Changes in the testes and epididymides of rabbits following long term vasectomy or vasocystostomy: Correlation with results of vasovasostomy. Biol Reprod 22:297, 1980
20. Jenkins IL, Mui VY, Blacklock NJ, Turk JL, Hanley HG: Consequences of vasectomy: an immunological and histological study related to subsequent fertility. Brit J Urol 51:406, 1979
21. Kennedy SW, Heidger PM: Fine structure of the spermatic granuloma of the rat vas deferens following vasectomy. Anat Rec 198:461, 1980
22. Makler A, Geresh I: An attempt to explain occurrence of patent reproductive tract in azoospermic males with tubular spermatogenesis. Int J Fertil 24:246, 1979
23. Makler A, Hampel N: Tubular atrophy due to congenital occlusion of vasa efferentia in azoospermic male. Int J Fertil 20:253, 1975
24. Middleton RG, Urry RL: Vasovasostomy and semen quality. J Urol 123:518, 1980
25. Mitchinson MJ, Sherman KP, Stainer-Smith AM: Brown patches in the epididymis. J Pathol 115:57, 1975
26. Molnar J von, Bacsi E, Rappai G: Ueber Samenzellen aus Spermatozelen. Dermat Monatsch 164:35, 1978
27. Petitti DB, Klein R, Kipp H, Friedman GD: Vasectomy and the incidence of hospitalized illness. J Urol 129:760, 1983
28. Phadke AM: Spermiophage cells in man. Fertil Steril 26:760, 1975
29. Povysil C: Spermatic granulomas of ischaemic origin in the rat epididymis. Invest Urol 15:219, 1976
30. Risbridger GP, Kerr JB, Peake RA, Kretser DM de: An assessment of Leydig cell function after bilateral or unilateral efferent duct ligation: Further evidence for local control of Leydig cell function. Endocrinology 109:1234, 1981
31. Rovinescu I, Reid RG: The granulomatous lesions of the testicle and epididymis. Urol Int 21:564, 1966
32. Schmidt SS, Morris RR: Spermatic granuloma: the complication of vasectomy. Fertil Steril 24:941, 1973
33. Schmidt SS, Brüschke EE: Anatomical sizes of the human vas deferens after vasectomy. Fertil Steril 27:271, 1976
34. Silber SJ, Galle J, Friend D: Microscopic vasovasostomy and spermatogenesis. J Urol 117:299, 1977
35. Silber SS, Rodríguez-Rigau LJ: Quantitative analysis of testicle biopsy: determination of partial obstruction and prediction of sperm count after surgery for obstruction. Fertil Steril 36:480, 1981
36. Tamayo JL, Ruffolo FH: Spermatic cord tumor. Mesonephric hamartoma of the vas deferens. Arch Surg 94:430, 1967
37. Warner JJ, Kirchner FK, Wong SW, Dao AH: Vasitis nodosa presenting as a mass of the spermatic cord. J Urol 129:380, 1983
38. White RD, Paulson DF: Obstruction of the male reproductive tract. J Urol 118:266, 1977
39. Wong T, Straus FH: Testicular biopsy in the study of male infertility. II: Posttesticular causes of infertility. Arch Pathol 95:160, 1973
40. Young D: Surgical treatment of male infertility. J Reprod Fert 23:541, 1970

20

LESIONS OF THE TUNICA VAGINALIS

The tunica vaginalis is not only the site of congenital lesions (see chapter 6), but is also the site of acquired disorders that can be either inflammatory, reactive, or neoplastic in origin.

Hydrocele

Hydroceles are an accumulation of fluid within the layers of the testicular tunica vaginalis, the processus vaginalis along the spermatic cord, or both. Hydroceles are more frequent in the testicular tunica vaginalis than in the spermatic cord. Testicular tunica vaginalis fluid is formed primarily by the visceral layer of the tunica albuginea and hydroceles occur when the parietal layer of the tunica vaginalis loses its capacity to reabsorb the fluid. The following types of hydroceles can be observed:

1. Congenital: characterized by an accumulation of liquid within the tunica vaginalis and the processus vaginalis, due to an embryologic defect which results in the occlusion or obliteration of the structure.
2. Infantile: differentiated from the former only in that the processus vaginalis is closed at the external inguinal ring level.
3. Hernial: there is an accumulation of liquid within the hernial sac; it can be associated with either congenital or infantile types.
4. Cystic: it adopts the form of a cyst due to the persistence of a segment of the vaginalis process.
5. Spermatic: produced by the rupture of a spermatocele inside the tunica vaginalis.
6. Scrotal-abdominal hydrocele or "L´ hydrocele en bissac" (Dupuytren, 1834): a variety of "high" infantile hydrocele with processus vaginalis obliteration at the level of the internal inguinal ring at the bottom of the superior sac that extend towards the abdominal cavity (Brothers and Feldtman, 1981).

Hydroceles occur with a frequency that can be estimated as one percent of all patients in a general hospital. The incidence is higher in tropical countries. The affectation is most frequent in newborns and in adults after thirty years of age. The right side is affected slightly more often than the left and in 10 to 15 percent of the cases, the hydrocele is bilateral.

On an etiological basis, hydroceles can be classified as idiopathic and secondary, although it is accepted that most of the idiopathic hydroceles are secondary to asymptomatic trauma or infection.

Grossly, a noninfected hydrocele is characterized by a clear liquid, containing six to ten percent solids (proteins, salts, cholesterol). In children the wall of the hydrocele is: thick; swollen; formed by connective tissue; and can either lack, or show a decrease in, the subserosal lymphatic vessels. In these cases, it is thought that the fluid accumulation is due to the absence of efferent lymphatic draining channels (Nemetschek-Gansler and others, 1976) (Fig. 20–1A).

Secondary hydrocele can be observed in most of the processes that affect the testes and epididymides: specific or nonspecific epididymitis (for example, gonorrhea, tuberculosis); parasite infections such as filariasis and in most cases of or-

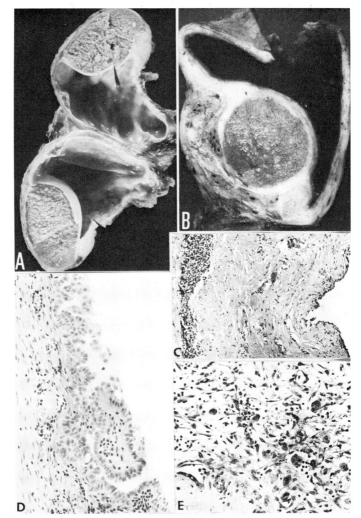

FIGURE 20–1. *A, Idiopathic hydrocele. In spite of the marked dilatation of the vaginalis cavity, the testicular parenchyma hardly presents any alteration. B, Hydrocele secondary to tuberculous epididymitis. Both the albuginea and the parietal layer of the tunica vaginalis are greatly engrossed. The testis presents focal atrophy. C, Vaginalis showing a dense banded infiltrate, formed by lymphocytes and plasma cells. H&E (x60). D and E, mesothelial hyperplasia. D, Papillar pattern of hyperplasia of mesothelial cells in a hydrocele of long evolution. H&E (x125). E, Mesothelial cells forming small solid clumps or glandular structures within the vaginalis wall together with inflammatory infiltrates. H&E (x100).*

chitis including syphilitic and idiopathic granulomatous orchitis (Fig. 20–1B).

Histologically, in the acute stage a fibrous exudate predominates, which may eventually become organized, and result in a moderate thickening of the tunica vaginalis. Later, both the testis and the tunica vaginalis are covered by a thick fibrous layer lacking in cells with practically no inflammatory infiltrate. At other times adherences can form, in which case the tunica vaginalis would appear partly or completely septate (Fig. 20–1C and 20–2A).

The surgical techniques used to treat hydrocele have recently been reviewed by Rodríguez and associates (1981).

MESOTHELIAL HYPERPLASIA

In response to various irritative stimuli, the vaginalis serosa reacts the same way as do the pleura, pericardium, or peritoneal lining of the hernial sacs, that is, by undergoing mesothelial cell hyperplasia (Rosai and Dehner, 1975) (Fig. 20–1D and E).

The most frequent cause is an infected hydrocele. Cellular proliferation can adopt two forms: papillary and infiltrating. In the first case, the epithelium lining the connective tissue papilla becomes polystratified. At the base of these papillas an intense inflammatory infiltrate can be seen. In the second type, which

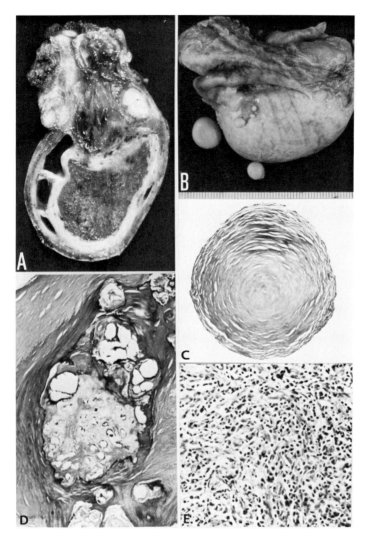

FIGURE 20–2. *A*, Transverse section of the testis and epididymis. At the epididymal level various nodules of caseous necrosis can be seen. Septi between the albuginea and the parietal layer of the tunica vaginalis are evident. *B, C* and *D*, Nodular periorchitis. *B*, Multiple nodules free within the tunica vaginalis or attached to the testis, seen in the autopsy of a 56 year old patient. *C*, Concentric laminar structure, poor in cells, of one of the nodular formations from the former case. H&E (x20). *D*, Calcification foci in the hyalinized stroma in a nodular periorchitis. H&E (x25). *E*, Fibrous pseudotumor of the testicular tunica. The section was obtained from a nodule with a diameter of 3.5 cm., which shows a pleomorphic infiltrate that varies from one area to another, in which plasma cells, lymphocytes, and fibroblasts predominate. H&E (x125).

shows an infiltrating growth pattern, various elements can be recognized in the inflamed connective tissue of the tunica vaginalis: isolated mesothelial cells; epithelial cords; and glandular formations, for example. In this case, the differential diagnosis must be made with a mesothelioma or the metastasis of an adenocarcinoma. In some cases, epidermoid metaplasia has been observed.

PERIORCHITIS

Diffuse thickening of the testicular tunica vaginalis is a frequent finding in hematoceles or hydroceles that undergo trauma or inflammation (Honoré, 1978). In other cases, the process is not diffuse but nodular and perfectly well delimitated. Two thirds of these lesions affect the testicular tunics, ten percent affect the epididymis and the remainder are located on the spermatic cord.

From a pathological point of view two entities can be distinguished: nodular periorchitis and fibrous pseudotumor. The first entity mainly affects the testis and epididymis, whereas the second is mostly located in the spermatic cord. Histological transitional forms exist. These processes have repeatedly been described as fibromas.

Nodular Periorchitis

It is a process similar to that of hypertrophic chronic serositis that appears in the other serosas. It can be recognized by the presence of nodular thickening at any level of the tunica vaginalis, usually accidentally discovered either in autopsies or in surgery for some other testicular lesion. It can be found at any time between the third and sixth decades. Half of the patients have a hydrocele and in approximately one third there is evidence of a previous epididymo-orchitis or trauma.

A gross observation shows multiple nodules. Their size varies from 0.5 to various cm; they can be free, sessile, or pedunculated. They have a hard consistency, and are located on the testis or the parietal tunica vaginalis. Cross-sectioning shows the nodules to have a whitish color with either yellowish, calcified, or ossified areas. Histologically, most of the free nodules show a laminar and concentric structure. They are formed by intensely collagenized and poorly cellular connective tissue. In some of the sessile or pedunculated nodules, the cellularity is more abundant (sometimes chronic), nonspecific, inflammatory infiltrates can also be seen. In addition to these lesions, the tunica vaginalis usually demonstrates numerous small thickened areas that probably represent initial stages. The base of these lesions appear similar to those of the previous ones, except that its surface is covered with a layer of fibrin. The cause of this fibrinous exudate is, in most cases, unknown (Lewis and Pierce, 1962) (Fig. 20–2**B**, **C**, and **D**).

Fibrous Pseudotumor (Chronic Proliferative Periorchitis)

This condition consists of hypertrophic inflammatory lesions located, in order of decreasing frequency, in the following areas: spermatic cord; the epididymis; and the testicular tunicas (Mostofi and Price, 1973). Viewed grossly, they are poorly delimited tumors measuring various centimeters in diameter. Histologically, most of these lesions present inflammatory foci with abundant lymphocytes, plasma cells, histiocytes, and even eosinophilic leukocytes, together with a variable degree of fibrous proliferation. The resulting histologic picture is similar to that of a fibroxantoma, lipogranuloma, or sclerosing angioma (Strom, 1977) (Figs. 20–2**E** and 20–3**A**).

IDIOPATHIC FIBROMATOSIS

Idiopathic fibromatosis is a process of obscure cause that usually affects the retroperitoneum, causing bilateral stenosis of the ureters, or the mediastinum, or both regions at once, although continuity between the two regions has not been established.

Patients with retroperitoneal fibromatosis can also display pituitary fibrosis. Two forms of male genital system involvement have been observed in the development of the retroperitoneal fibrosis. The first is a diffuse form that affects the scrotum. The second form is testicular parenchymal involvement. In both forms the tissue that develops intra- or extratesticularly is fibrous and contains few inflammatory cells and abundant macrophages with foamy cytoplasm (Grossman and others, 1980).

MECONIUM VAGINALITIS

Meconium granuloma of the tunica vaginalis is secondary to meconium peritonitis. The cause of either one or the other is the perforation of the gastrointestinal tract during fetal life. The tunica vaginalis involvement may be the only clinical manifestation of the cystic fibrosis if the intestinal perforation resolved spontaneously.

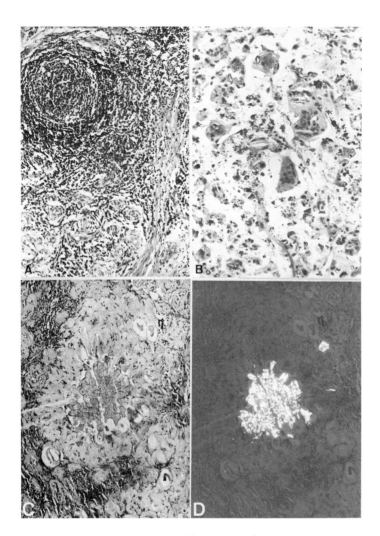

FIGURE 20–3. *A, Fibrous pseudotumor.* Fibrous proliferation with intense vascular neoformation and lymphatic nodules. H&E (x60). *B, Meconium granuloma.* Multinuclear foreign body giant cells, in whose interior can be seen laminar formations and bile pigments. H&E (x125). *C and D, Talc granuloma. C,* Tunica vaginalis with inflammatory infiltrates showing mostly lymphocytes around a polyhedrically structured material. H&E (x60). *D,* The same preparation observed with a polarized light microscope shows typical talc crystals (x60).

The tunica vaginalis is affected by the penetration of meconium through the processus vaginalis at some time between the sixth month of intrauterine life, when the processus vaginalis is formed, and at birth, when the process is occluded.

Meconium, when it reaches the peritoneal or vaginal serosa, causes sterile chemical peritonitis. Grossly, yellowish nodules can be seen on the tunica vaginalis. Histologically, a foreign body inflammatory reaction is found, with macrophages full of bile pigments and dystrophic calcification that can be detected radiologically (Fig. 20–3B).

The presence of scrotal calcification associated to a bilateral hydrocele should orient the diagnosis toward meconium granuloma of the tunica vaginalis.

The study of aspirated scrotal fluid can help in the diagnosis if meconium components can be confirmed (bile, lipids, mucin, salts, sloughed epithelial cells) (Heydenrych and Marcus, 1976).

GLOVE-POWDER GRANULOMA

It is characterized by inflammatory reactions of the foreign body type, similar to those observed in the peritoneum. The reactions can be produced either by the persistence of a processus vaginalis during abdominal surgery or directly by surgical procedures on the scrotal content. The materials most frequently found are licopodium, talc, and starch. Knowledge of a previous surgical intervention facilitates the diagnosis. The differential diagnosis includes tuberculosis, syphilis, sarcoidosis, and sperm granuloma.

In talc granulomas, polarization of the tissue reveals the pathognomonic doubly refractile crystals in the cytoplasm of the giant cells. In starch granulomas, the material is PAS positive and birefringent, showing a maltese cross-image under polarization (Healey and McDonald, 1977) (Fig. 20–3C and D).

TRAUMATIC TESTICULAR RUPTURE

This is a lesion found with increasing frequency. It is secondary to severe trauma to the scrotal region (Loup, 1979). In the four patients that we studied, the lesion was bilateral. The tunica albuginea was opened through which the testicular parenchyma, as well as large blood clots, could be seen. Bilateral orchiectomy was performed on all the patients (Fig. 20–4A). Although testicular ultrasound (Albert, 1980) and radionuclide imaging of the testis (Friedman and others, 1981) are useful for diagnostic purposes, they are

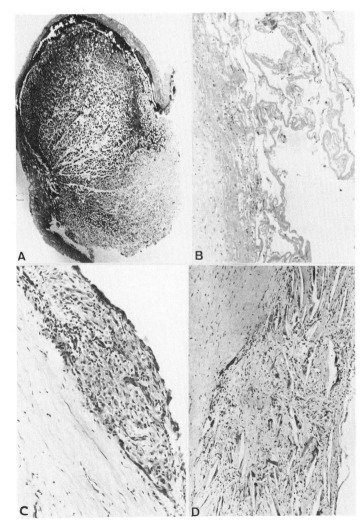

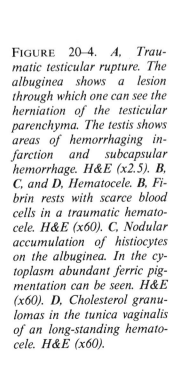

FIGURE 20–4. *A*, Traumatic testicular rupture. The albuginea shows a lesion through which one can see the herniation of the testicular parenchyma. The testis shows areas of hemorrhaging infarction and subcapsular hemorrhage. H&E (x2.5). *B, C,* and *D*, Hematocele. *B*, Fibrin rests with scarce blood cells in a traumatic hematocele. H&E (x60). *C*, Nodular accumulation of histiocytes on the albuginea. In the cytoplasm abundant ferric pigmentation can be seen. H&E (x60). *D*, Cholesterol granulomas in the tunica vaginalis of an long-standing hematocele. H&E (x60).

not generally performed. The only truly important procedure to increase the number of saved testicles in cases of blunt testicular trauma is early surgical exploration (Cass, 1983).

HEMATOCELE

Hematocele is the accumulation of blood within the vaginalis sac. It can be produced by a variety of causes. Some (traumas, spermatic cord- or testicular appendage torsion, or a subjacent tumor) are local. Other, less frequently, occurring hematoceles, are generalized and are associated with hematological alterations or to an increased tendency for the mucosa or serosa to bleed. The clinical presentation is that of a testicular tumor. In early studies, the tunica vaginalis appears to be full of blood clots or fresh blood and the surface of the tunica does not present any alterations. Later, the tunica may be full of spongy tissue the size of which can be many times that of the testis. This material is constituted mostly of fibrin (Fig. 20–4B, C, and D).

In long-standing hematoceles, the blood clots have organized into laminar structures that can appear calcified. The tunica is hard and irregular, and contains fibrous tissue showing macrophages, hemosiderin and calcified areas (Fig. 20–5).

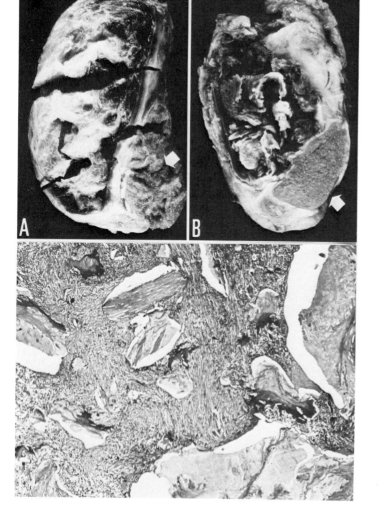

FIGURE 20–5. *A, Surgical specimen from an orchiectomy performed because testicular tumor was suspected. Most of the image shows a spongeous material within the vaginalis. The testis is pushed toward the periphery (arrow). B, Surgical specimen from an orchiectomy performed due to a probable teratoma. The tunica vaginalis contains numerous lamellar formations impregnated with calcium salts. The testis is pushed toward the periphery and compressed (arrow). C, Histological section of the tunica vaginalis seen in B. An organized hematoma with bony metaplasia and dystrophic calcification can be seen. H&E (x20).*

Mesothelioma of the Tunica Vaginalis

Tumors that originate in mesothelial cells may act in a benign manner (Herschman and Ross, 1974) and, infrequently, become locally aggressive and develop the potential to metastase (Johnson and coauthors, 1973; Fligiel and Kaneko, 1976). For many years, most of the malignant tumors affecting the tunica vaginalis were thought to be secondary. Thanks to the studies of Foster and Ackerman (1960) it is now known that mesotheliomas can present variable histological patterns including epithelial, fibrous, or mixed, and that these histological varieties are related to tumor location. The pleural mesotheliomas are predominantly fibrous, whereas those of the peritoneum and tunica vaginalis are mostly epithelial.

Malignant mesotheliomas of the tunica vaginalis are rare and are seen more often in older men. Clinically they appear with hydroceles. The tumor can be solid or cystic; the color can be white or yellowish; and the consistency is friable (Ackerman and Rosai, 1974).

Histologically, the tumors can present a papillary, tubulo-alveolar, solid, or sarcomatous pattern. The most frequent is a combination of the first two patterns. Numerous mitoses and atypias can be seen. In some cases, psammoma bodies

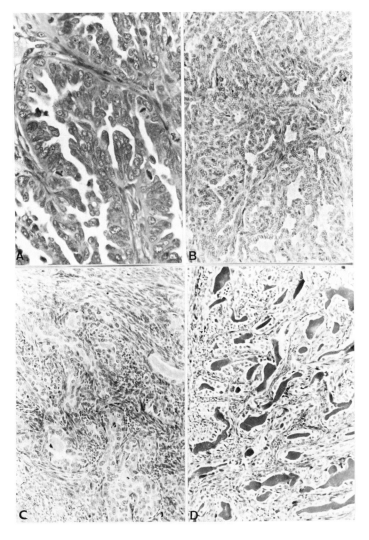

FIGURE 20–6. *Mesothelioma of the tunica vaginalis. A, Papillar pattern of a mesothelioma in the tunica vaginalis of a 46-year-old male. The mitotic index is high. Some mitoses present atypias. H&E (x250). B, Disposition of the mesothelial cells forming clefts and small glands. The mitotic index is low. H&E (x125). C, Mesothelial cells in a glandular disposition, close to others showing a sarcomatous pattern. H&E (x125). D, Presence of abundant mucopolysaccharides in the glandular lumens. Alcian blue-PAS (x125).*

have been described in the papillary areas. The criteria for the differentiation between benign and malignant lesions are the same as those used in lesions of other locations (Fig. 20–6).

Before establishing the diagnosis of a mesothelioma, other processes must be discarded:

1. Reactive mesothelial hyperplasias. They are secondary to hydrocele or an underlaying inflammatory process. Histologically, they may present either a papillary or glandular pattern. The two patterns show a more or less abundant inflammatory infiltrate, which is not related to the possible necrotic areas.
2. Metastasis. In the mesotheliomas, continuity can be demonstrated to exist between the tumor and the mesothelial vaginalis lining. On the other hand, mesotheliomas produce sulfated acid mucopolysaccharides whereas, normally, adrenocarcinomas elaborate neutral mucosubstances.

The prognosis of the mesothelioma is benign when the pattern is papillary, but the same lesions often become aggressive when the pattern is complex. Occasional metastasis have been observed in the inguinal lymphatic nodes (Eimoto and Inoue, 1977).

OTHER TUNICA VAGINALIS TUMORS

Isolated cases of neurofibroma of the tunica albuginea (Levant and Chetlin, 1948), leiomyoma (Albert and Mininberg, 1972), and hemangioma of the tunica albuginea (Pfitzenmaier and others, 1975) with benign courses have been described.

REFERENCES

1. Ackerman LV, Rosai J: Surgical Pathology, Mosby. St. Louis, Missouri: Mosby, 1974, 5th ed, p. 200
2. Albert PS, Mininberg DT: Leiomyoma of the tunica albuginea. J Urol 107:869, 1972
3. Albert NE: Testicular ultrasound for trauma. J Urol 124:558, 1980
4. Brothers LR, Feldtman RW: Abdominoscrotal hydrocele: youngest case report and review of the literature. J Urol 126:847, 1981
5. Cass AS: Testicular trauma. J Urol 129:299, 1983
6. Dupuytren G: Lecoma orales de clinique chirurgicale. Paris: Balliere, 1834, 4:444
7. Eimoto T, Inohue I: Malignant fibrous mesothelioma of the tunica vaginalis. A histologic and ultrastructural study. Cancer 39:2059, 1977
8. Fligiel Z, Kaneko M: Malignant mesothelioma of the tunica vaginalis propria testis in a patient with asbestos exposure. A case report. Cancer 37:1478, 1976
9. Foster EA, Ackerman LV: Localized mesotheliomas of the pleura; the pathologic evaluation of 18 cases. Am J Clin Pathol 34:349, 1960
10. Friedman SG, Rose JG, Winston MA: Ultrasound and nuclear medicine evaluation in acute testicular trauma. J Urol 125:748, 1981
11. Grossman A, Gibson J, Stansfeld G, Besser GM: Pituitary and testicular fibrosis in association with retroperitoneal fibrosis. Clin Endocr 12:371, 1980
12. Healey GB, McDonald DF: Talc granuloma presenting as a testicular mass. J Urol 118:122, 1977
13. Herschman BR, Ross MM: Papillary cystadenoma within testis. Am J Clin Pathol 61:724, 1974
14. Heydenrych JJ, Marcus PB: Meconium granulomas of the tunica vaginalis. J Urol 115:596, 1976
15. Honoré LH: Nonspecific peritesticular fibrosis manifested as testicular enlargement. Clinicopathological study of nine cases. Arch Surg 113:814, 1978
16. Johnson DE, Fuerst DE, Gallagher HS: Mesothelioma of the tunica vaginalis. South Med J 66:1295, 1973
17. Levant B, Chetlin MA: Neurofibroma of tunica albuginea testis. J Urol 59:1187, 1948

18. Lewis HY, Pierce JM: Multiple fibromas of the tunica vaginalis. J Urol 87:142, 1962
19. Loup J: Rupture traumatique du testicule. Ann Urol 13:231, 1979
20. Mostofi FK, Price EB: Tumors of the male genital system. In Atlas of tumor pathology. Washington D.C.: Armed Forces Institute of Pathology, 1973, Vol. 8
21. Nemetschek-Gansler H, Meinel A, Daum R: Die Wand der primären Hydrozele des Kindes. Licht- und elektronenmikroskopische Befunde. Virchows Archiv A Path Anat and Histol 371:373, 1976
22. Pfitzenmaier NW, Wurster K, Kjelle-Schweigler M: Hemangioma of the tunica albuginea testis. Urol Int 30:237, 1975
23. Rodríguez WC, Rodríguez DD, Fortuño, RF: The operative treatment of hydrocele: A comparison of 4 basic techniques. J Urol 125:804, 1981
24. Rosai J, Dehner LP: Nodular mesothelial hyperplasia in hernia sacs—a benign reactive condition simulating a neoplastic process. Cancer 35:165, 1975
25. Strom GW: Pseudotumor of testicular tunic. J Urol 118:340, 1977

21

TESTICULAR TUMORS

Testicular tumors are relatively rare: 2.88 per 10^5 per year occur in a selected 20- to 30-year-old population (U.S. Army). The frequency is 3.14 per 10^5 per year in 18- to 44-year-olds in the general United States population (Dixon and Moore, 1953). Similar percentages have been observed in Canada and Great Britain.

Testicular tumors represent little more than one percent of all tumors in men. However, they constitute one of the most interesting genito-urinary system tumor group because of their frequency in young men, their high degree of malignancy when untreated, and the great variety of histological patterns.

Ninety-three percent of testicular tumors originate in germinal cells. Seminoma, embryonal carcinoma, teratoma, yolk sac tumor, and choriocarcinoma are included in this group. Numerous observations emphasize the intratubular germinal cell origin of testicular tumors. The carcinoma *in situ* picture (Skakkebaek, 1972 and 1975) is well known in testicular biopsies of patients consulting for infertility, cryptorchid testes, or residual seminiferous parenchyma displaced by testicular tumors.

Three percent of testicular tumors are considered to be gonadal stromal tumors. Gonadal stromal cells are capable of differentiating into Sertoli cells as well as into Leydig cells. The ratio of Leydig cell tumors to Sertoli cell tumors is approximately three to one. Four percent of testicular tumors originate in nonspecialized stroma.

A small number of tumors (gonadoblastomas) are formed by germinal cells as well as by cells developed from gonadal stroma. They usually occur in dysgenetic gonads.

Primary Testicular Tumors

Germ Cell Tumors

Etiological Factors

The following factors are considered noteworthy in discussing testicular tumor etiology:
1. Genetic causes. The possibility that genetic factors play some role in the etiology of testicular cancer is supported by the ever more frequent descriptions of testicular cancer in several members of the same family. Since the first description by Champlin (1930) of testicular tumors in twins, these tumors have been observed in over 34 families and were found to occur as follows: in fathers and sons (Raghavan and co-authors, 1980; Kubelka and others, 1983); monozygotic twins (Levey and Grabstald, 1975); brothers who were not twins (Thomson and Sinclair, 1977); cousins (Shinohara and others, 1980); and so forth. Although the number of families already studied is insufficient, there are various factors that tend to repeat themselves: a higher incidence in twins (particularly in monozygotic ones); a slightly higher than average bilateral incidence; tumor presentation at the same age among family members; the phenomenon of tumor anticipation in offspring; and the appearance of progressively more malignant tumors in successive generations. A testicular cancer patients' probability for developing a second tumor is 500 times higher than the general population (Morris and others, 1976). A second primary

germ cell tumor occurs in 1 to 2.5 percent (Cockburn and co-authors, 1983; Bach and associated, 1983).

2. Cryptorchidism. Approximately 12 percent of all testicular neoplasms develop in undescended testes (Altman and Malament, 1967; Batata and others, 1976; Gehring and associates, 1974). This represents a malignancy risk in undescended testes that is 20 to 40 times higher than for scrotal testes (Campbell, 1942). It is not uncommon for a cryptorchid testis to be diagnosed as having an incipient malignant germinal tumor from material obtained by aspiration biopsy (Waxman, 1976) or biopsy (Dorman and others, 1979; Williams and Brendler, 1977) (Fig. 21-1A).

3. Dysgenetic testes. This cause is partly related to the anomalies observed in cryptorchid testes, but here the concept of dysgenesis is wider and refers to the presence of tubular dysgenesis (generally immature seminiferous tubules with an anomalous cell population) as well as to a testicular dysgenesis in which the anomaly is more serious and implies anomalous differentiation of a part of the primitive gonad. Gonadoblastomas frequently develop in these gonads.

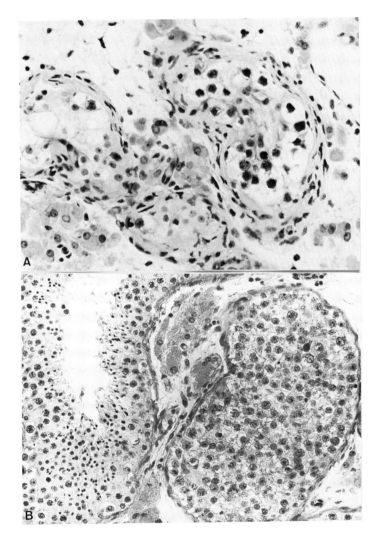

FIGURE 21-1. *A*, Undifferentiated intratubular germ cell tumor in a cryptorchid testis. The germ cells display marked polymorphism. H&E (x400). *B*, Comparison between normal seminiferous epithelium (left) and typical intratubular seminoma growth (right). H&E (x400).

4. Age. Not only is there a presentation age for each testicular tumor type, but the prognosis varies with the age. For example, infantile embryonal carcinoma (yolk sac tumor) and teratoma have a much more favorable prognosis in children than in adults (Exelby, 1980; Marshall and others, 1983). Teratoma, embryonal carcinoma, and choriocarcinoma occur in young adults. Classical seminoma appears in the 30 to 50 year-old age group and spermatocytic seminoma in men over 50 years of age.

Classification

Different germ cell tumor classifications have been suggested (Friedman and Moore, 1946; Mostofi, 1973; Pugh and Cameron, 1976). In order to unify different treatment guidelines, it is convenient to use the classification published in 1977 by the W.H.O. (Mostofi and Sobin, 1977). Table 21-1—based on Mostofi's 1980 classification—allows comparison between the different classifications.

This classification is based upon the histological picture of tumors only. Germ cell tumors are grouped under two large headings: tumors of one histological type (pure) and tumors of more than one histological type.

Tumors considered to be pure histological types are: seminoma; spermatocytic seminoma; embryonal carcinoma; yolk sac tumor; polyembryoma; choriocarcinoma; and teratoma (mature, immature, and with malignant transformation).

Tumors of more than one histological type are: embryonal carcinoma and teratoma (teratocarcinoma); choriocarcinoma associated to another tumor (specifying type); and other tumoral combinations (specifying type).

Histogenesis

The histogenesis of germ cell tumors has been the subject of enormous interest within the study of testicular cancer. The histogenesis of the extremely varied histological patterns of germ cell tumors is not only of academic interest, but has made possible the unification of the different germ cell tumor classifications.

The histogenetic theories can be summarized in two groups. The first is the theory of germ cell tumor double origin. Seminoma develops from germ cells. The other tumors that could be considered teratomas would develop from blastomeres that, by being displaced early in or during embryonary development, escape organizer influence. This hypothesis was principally supported by Willis (1967), and is shared by Collings and Pugh (1964) and Pugh and Cameron (1976).

The second theory is that of single origin. After demonstrating experimentally by Stevens (1967) and in experimental animals and humans by Pierce (1962), Pierce and Beals (1964), and Pierce and Abbell (1970) that teratomas can also develop from germ cells, all germ cell tumors should have a common origin. This point of view, presented by Ewing in 1942 and seconded by Friedman and Moore (1946) and Melicow (1955), has also been maintained by Teilum (1976) and Mostofi and Price (1973).

Pierce and Abbell's original idea considered embryonal carcinoma to be an omnipotent tumor. The germ cells would then give rise to two lines of tumoral development: seminoma and embryonal carcinoma. Embryonal carcinoma would be capable of differentiating into embryonal or extraembryonal tissues. Differentiation toward extraembryonal tissues would result in yolk sac tumors and choriocarcinomas; while embryonal differentiation would form teratomas.

An alternative theory has been considered by Mostofi (1973) who suggested that any germ cell tumor (seminoma, spermatic seminoma, embryonal carcinoma, teratoma, choriocarcinoma, and yolk sac tumor) can directly develop from germ

TABLE 21-1. *A Comparative Study of Different Germ-Cell Tumor Classifications (based on Mostofi, 1980)*

WHO	Friedman & Moore	Mostofi	Pugh & Cameron
-Tumors of only one histological type: •typical seminoma •spermatocytic seminoma •embryonal carcinoma	-Not used •seminoma •not included •embryonal carcinoma	-Tumors of only one histological type: •seminoma •spermatocytic seminoma •embryonal carcinoma adult type	-Not used •seminoma •spermatocytic seminoma •malignant teratoma undifferentiated (MTU includes yolk sac tumor in adults and some embryonal carcinomas and teratomas)
•yolk sac tumor (infantile embryonal carcinoma) •polyembryoma •pure choriocarcinoma •teratoma	•not included •not included •choriocarcinoma •teratoma	•infantile embryonal carcinoma •polyembryoma •pure choriocarcinoma •teratoma	•yolk sac tumor in children, MTU in adults •not included •not included •teratoma (includes WHO embryonal carcinoma, yolk sac tumor in adults, teratoma and choriocarcinoma)
+mature teratoma +immature teratoma +teratoma with malignant transformation	+teratoma +teratoma +teratocarcinoma	+mature teratoma +immature teratoma +teratoma with malignant areas excluding seminoma, embryonal carcinoma and choriocarcinoma	+teratoma, differentiated +teratoma, differentiated +malignant teratoma, intermediate (MTI)
-Tumors of more than one histological type: •embryonal carcinoma + teratoma (teratocarcinoma)	-Not used •teratocarcinoma (also including teratoma ± embryonal carcinoma ± seminoma ± choriocarcinoma	-Tumors of more than one histological type: •embryonal carcinoma + teratoma (teratocarcinoma)	-Not used •malignant teratoma intermediate (MTI) and some MTU
•choriocarcinoma and any other type •other combinations specify types	•teratocarcinoma •teratocarcinoma	•specify tumor types •specify tumor types	•malignant teratoma trophoblastic •malignant teratoma undifferentiated; malignant teratoma, intermediate; combined tumors for those with seminoma

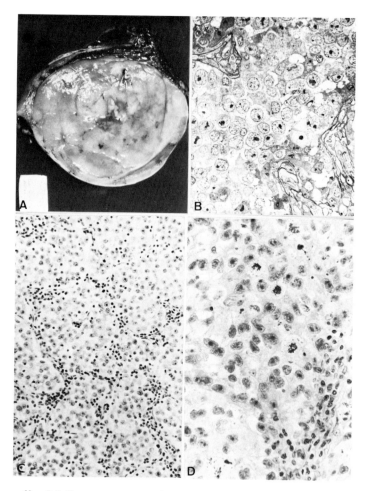

FIGURE 21-2. Seminoma. A, Tumor, with greyish appearance and necrotic central zones, that occupies most of the testicular parenchyma. B, Tumor cells displaying relative uniformity. The nucleolus is prominent and the cytoplasm is clear. One-micron-thick section of epon-embedded material. Toluidine blue (x450). C, Tumor cells grouped into small lobules, which are separated from each other by slender connective tissue septa in which numerous lymphocytes stand out. H&E (x60). D, Marked cellular polymorphism and abundant mitoses, characteristic of the anaplastic seminoma. H&E (x450).

cells. Malignant germ cells have been repeatedly observed within seminiferous tubules (Azzopardi and others, 1961; Skakkebaek, 1972 and 1975) and their development into classical and/or spermatocytic seminoma, embryonal carcinoma and syncytiotrophoblast cells, or yolk sac tumor has been illustrated (Teoh and associates, 1960; Mostofi, 1973). These malign intratubular cells can invade the tunica propria and develop into an infiltrating testicular tumor. Embryonal carcinoma would also be able to give rise to choriocarcinomas and yolk sac tumors as well as teratomas.

Histological Types

Seminoma. This is a germ cell tumor formed by polyhedric cells with clear cytoplasm, reminiscent of primordial germ cells and placed in a stroma with abundant lymphocytes.

This tumor has a low degree of malignancy and is very radiosensitive. Seminoma comprises 30 to 40 percent of all testicular tumors. They are more frequent in patients who: are from rural areas; are elderly (in the fourth and fifth decades of life) and have cryptorchid testes (Mostofi, 1973). They have also been described in prepubertal patients (Perry and Servandio, 1980) (Fig. 21-2).

Two different types of tumors must be considered under the name seminoma: typical seminoma and spermatocytic seminoma. Typical seminoma reflects the characteristic just described. Spermatocytic seminoma will be described later. Both tumor types manifest major clinical, macroscopic, histological, and evolutive differences that more than justify their consideration as two different types: classical or typical seminoma and spermatocytic seminoma.

Classical or Typical Seminoma. Clinically, the typical seminoma's most frequent symptom is a gradual increase in testicular size. This increase is painful in many cases. Other clinical symptoms, present only in isolated cases, are: gynecomastia and infertility. The right testis is affected more often than the left one (5/4). Gross observation shows that the testis is filled by an expansive mass that pushes the parenchyma into the form of a peripheral crescent. When sectioned, the tumor is lobulated, its consistency is soft, and it is brown or pink in color. Areas of necrosis and hemorrhage are frequent. Seminoma spreads to the epididymis and spermatic cord in eight percent of the cases (Fig. 21–2A).

Histologically, the tumor is formed by polyhedral big cells with clear cytoplasm. The nucleus is centrally located and round. The nuclear membrane has an irregular outline. The chromatin is granular and contains one or two nucleoli. Mitoses are scarce. Abundant glycogen granules are observed in the cytoplasm. The plasma membrane is well defined. This is an important criterion because it helps to distinguish seminoma from embryonal carcinoma, although this is not always possible (Fig. 21–2B). Ultrastructural studies of seminoma (Pierce, 1966; Holstein and Körner, 1974; Schulze and Holstein, 1977) have shown that, contrary to the information in earlier literature, the tumor is not made up of a uniform type of cell, but that at least three different tumoral cell types, probably corresponding to degrees of differentiation, can be recognized. These are:

1. Undifferentiated cells: These have few organelles, only a few mitochondria with electron lucent matrix, poorly developed Golgi complex and endoplasmic reticulum, and abundant ribosomes.
2. Intermediately differentiated cells: These are characterized by an increase of the Golgi complex and endoplasmic reticulum development, the presence of electrondense granular inclusions surrounded by a membrane, and variable quantities of glycogen granules.
3. Differentiated cells: In addition to the accentuated endoplasmic reticulum and Golgi complex development, there are numerous eosinophilic inclusions in the cytoplasm (reminiscent of proacrosomic granules) and numerous polymorphic mitochondria.

Isolated tumoral giant cells with several nuclei, syncytiotrophoblast cells, and foreign-body giant cells have been observed in some tumors (Fig. 21–3A and 21–4A).

The tumoral cells form nests or lobules separated by thin septa of stroma. The stroma may display three interesting features: lymphocytic infiltration (in the connective tissue septa, sometimes forming lymphatic nodules) is always present (100 percent of cases); granulomatous reaction in half of the cases; and fibrous reaction, which gives a scirrous appearance to some tumors (Fig. 21–2C). When the tumor shows necrosis, this can be of two types: simple, with nuclear pyknosis and cellular disintegration; or coagulation necrosis.

Most of the varieties of seminoma that have been observed histologically, such as intratubular seminoma, scirrous seminoma, and cribriform seminoma, have little influence on prognosis. In other cases, such as anaplastic seminoma and seminoma with trophoblastocarcinoma, their identification is justified due to the effect these conditions may have on prognosis.

Intratubular Seminoma. This results from tumoral cell growth within the se-

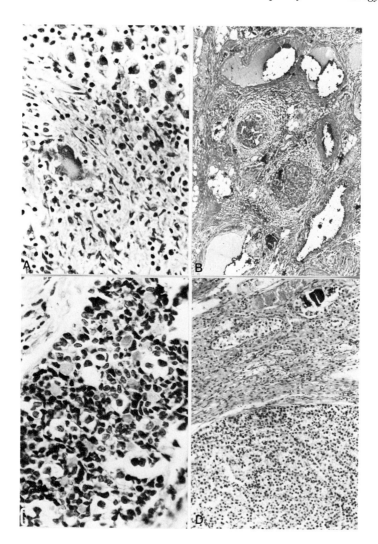

FIGURE 21–3. *A, Granulomatous pattern observed in seminoma. A giant cell surrounded by lymphocytes and tumoral cells. H&E (x125). B, Histological section of spermatic cord in which several vessels full of tumoral cells can be seen. The testicular tumor is an embryonal carcinoma. H&E (x25). C, Gonadoblastoma. A proliferation of atypical germ cells surrounded by Sertoli-granulosa cells. Several Call-Exner bodies are mixed among the cells. H&E (x125). D, Section from a testicular dysgenetic gonad in a 15-year-old pseudohermaphrodite. A developing seminoma beside tubular formations containing calcifications in their interior can be seen. H&E (x60).*

miniferous tubules. The resultant picture of seminiferous tubules containing only one type of cell contrasts sharply with the wealth of cytological detail in tubules with normal spermatogenesis. The intratubular growth is frequently observed in groups of seminiferous tubules in the testicular parenchyma located at the periphery of a classic seminoma. On other occasions the atypical germ cells intratubular growth has been an incidental finding in postpubescent excised cryptorchid testes and oligospermic patients' biopsies (Schütte and associates, 1981). Microinvasive seminoma has been suggested as the name for these cases of intratubular seminoma that begin to infiltrate the interstitium (von Eyben and co-authors, 1981) (Fig. 21–1**B**).

Scirrhous Seminoma. The stroma accompanying classical seminoma is generally scarce, thin, and populated with lymphocytes. However, in some tumors, the stroma may transform itself into an extremely collagenized fibrous matrix either after irradiation or spontaneously. The identification of tumor cells in these cases can be difficult. Some nests or strings of cells with a hyperchromatic nucleus and scarce, pale cytoplasm can barely be discerned. PAS and Best techniques are useful in diagnosis as allows the detection of

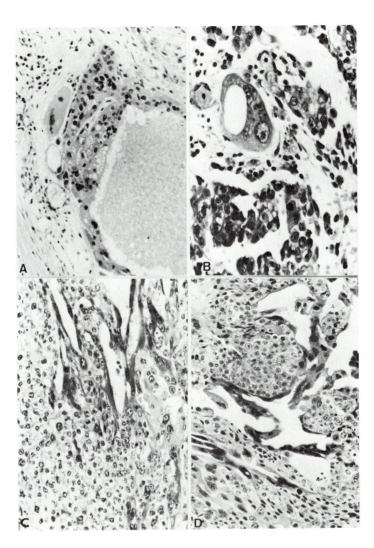

FIGURE 21-4. *A*, Syncytiotrophoblast cells observed in a seminoma with trophoblastocarcinoma. H&E (x125). *B*, Syncytiotrophoblast cells seen in an embryonal carcinoma. H&E (x250). *C*, Choriocarcinoma. The cytotrophoblast cells stand out due to their relative uniformity and clear cytoplasm. The syncytiotrophoblast cells are grouped around the acicular clefts. H&E (x125). *D*, Villous cytotrophoblast projections covered by syncytiotrophoblast. H&E (x125).

small glycogen granules in the tumor cell cytoplasm.

Cribriform and Sclerosing Seminoma.
Damjanov and associates (1980) have described a form of seminoma without lymphocytic infiltrates in which the tumor cell nests are separated from each other by wide bands of an acellular collagenized stroma. The nested cells are laid in a cribriform or trabecular pattern. Although this patient had metastasis, he was well four years after orchidectomy. Chemotherapy was used as part of the postoperative treatment.

Anaplastic Seminoma. Ten percent of seminomas show marked anaplasia. Although the gross appearance is similar to classical seminoma, anaplastic seminoma cell nuclei are hyperchromatic, larger than those of classical seminoma, more vesiculous and with a larger number of mitoses (3 to 5 mitoses per high power field) (Fig. 21-2D). Lymphocytic infiltrates are less abundant. There is no granulomatous reaction. Ultrastructural studies reveal characteristic cells that are like those of classical or typical seminoma, pineal seminoma, thymic seminoma, and ovarian dysgerminoma (Janssen and Johnston, 1976). There is no unanimous opinion regarding the prognosis. According to Johnson and others (1975), the prognosis is like that of classical seminoma; while according to Maier and Sulak (1973), this form is more aggressive and has a mortality rate more elevated than that of other forms of seminoma.

Seminoma with Trophoblastocarcinoma.
This term, suggested by Friedman and Pearlman (1970), refers to those seminomas that contain giant cells that have syncytiotrophoblast morphological characteristic. These tumors can produce HCG (see section entitled testicular tumor markers). Thirteen percent of Dixon and Moore's (1952) seminoma series are seminomas with trophoblastocarcinoma, which have a 20 percent mortality rate after two years. This form of seminoma should be distinguished from classical seminoma because of its histological pattern and high aggressiveness (Fig. 21-4A).

Once seminoma has been diagnosed, many sections must be examined in order to ascertain the presence of any other germ cell tumor. Should their presence be confirmed, the prognosis for seminoma must be evaluated in relation to the accompanying tumor.

Spermatocytic Seminoma. This is a rare tumor, which represents approximately 4.4 percent of all seminomas. It was distinguished from classical seminoma by Masson in 1946, based on its particular, clinical, histological, and macroscopic characteristic.

Clinically speaking this is a tumor of older men. Over 50 percent of the patients are over 50 years of age when diagnosed (Rosai and associates, 1969 a; Walter, 1980), and their average age is 65. The tumor grows slowly and, many times, is asymptomatic when compared with classical seminoma, which is frequently painful. This tumor has never been observed originating outside the gonad. In ten percent of the cases are bilateral whereas classical seminomas are bilateral in two percent of cases (Talerman, 1980 b). It is not more common in cryptorchid testes nor is it more frequently associated with other germ cell tumors.

When cut, the tumor shows a yellowish or pale grey, soft, and friable surface, which is mucoid or gelatinous. There may be cystic degeneration, but areas of necrosis and hemorrhage are infrequent. These tumors are well circumscribed and some appear to be encapsulated. The tumors tend to form nodules that can coalesce.

Histologically, the cells are irregularly grouped with hardly any connective septa. Mitoses are frequent. The cells are round and loosely distributed in the mucoid areas and polyhedral in the more solid areas. A characteristic is the great variety of cell sizes, giving rise to the classification into three cell types:

1. Medium-size cells (15 to 20 microns). They are the most abundant. They differ from classical seminoma cells in that their nucleus is spherical, hyperchromatic, and the cytoplasm is less abundant, has little glycogen and imprecise limits.
2. Giant cells (50 to 150 microns). These are uni- or multinucleated. The nuclei are oval or indented, and the cytoplasm is heavily eosinophilic and lacks glycogen granules.
3. Small cells (6 to 8 microns). These are similar to lymphocytes, but their cytoplasm may be acidophilic. They are considered to be degenerative cells.

An interesting cytological detail that defines the tumor is the chromatin distribution in most of the giant cells, which is similar to the spiremes formed in the meiotic prophase of the primary spermatocytes. These tumors show no lymphocytic infiltrate nor granulomatous stromal reaction. An intratubular growth of the tumor is frequently found in areas far away from the tumor.

Ultrastructural observations (Rosai and associates, 1969 b; Walter, 1980) confirm Masson's studies (1946) and reaffirm the suitability of the term "seminoma espermatocytaire," which he proposed. The form of the nucleolus and the chromatin configuration, similar to that of the leptotenic spermatocyte, are important nuclear characteristics. Intercellular bridges, a well-developed Golgi complex with proacrosomic granules and basal bodies with initiate flagellar structures are the outstanding cytoplasmic characteristics. These ultrastructural characteristics also favor Masson's hypothesis (1946) that spermatocytic seminoma is a spermatogonium-derived tumor capable of producing abortive spermatozoa. Intercellular bridges are typical of types A and B spermatogonium, spermatocytes, and spermatids (Bloom and Fawcett, 1975), and are a constant finding in spermatocytic seminoma that has not been observed in typical seminoma (Pierce, 1966) nor anaplastic seminoma (Janssen and Johnston, 1976). The high degree of cellular cohesion obtained by the intercellular bridges probably affects the tumor's histological behavior. The tumor cells are practically incapable of invading the tunica albuginea or the epididymis, and nearly incapable of metastasizing (Schoborg and others, 1980). See Table 21-2 for differential diagnosis between spermatocytic and classical seminoma.

Testicular tumor markers (alpha-fetoprotein, AFP, and HCG subunit beta) are negative. Radical orchidectomy is considered the best treatment.

Embryonal Carcinoma. This is a germinal cell tumor in which the cells display an embryonal epithelial and anaplastic appearance. They group forming: acini; tubules; papillae; and solid growths.

Twenty percent of testicular germinal cell tumors are embryonal carcinomas. It appears in adults only and is minimally radiosensitive. It appears clinically in the third decade, and a third of patients already have metastases by the time they consult a physician (Friedman and Moore, 1946; Mostofi and Price, 1973).

Seen grossly, this is one of the smallest tumors. When diagnosed, the tunica albuginea may have already been destroyed and, in 10 to 20 percent of the cases, the epididymis and spermatic cord are infiltrated. When cut, contrary to seminoma, the surface is a variagated mosaic of grey-white areas that are granular, soft, or solid and which alternate with hemorrhagic and necrotic areas (Figs. 21-5**A** and 21-3**B**).

Under the microscope, the cells forming the tumor vary in size and shape. Their appearance is epithelial and they lack precise cytoplasmic limits. The cytoplasm can be vacuolated or amphophilic. The nucleus is very irregular and has one or more nucleoli. Mitoses are frequent. Giant cells and syncytiotrophoblast-like cells are also seen. The cells can group into solid structures, acini, tubules, or papillae. The stroma varies from scarce to abundant and it may be loose, sarcomatous or hyalinized (Fig. 21-5**B** and **C**).

Embryonal carcinoma is very like the cells of the recently implanted embryo before these begin to show any kind of cellular differentiation and is, therefore, considered to be a tumor with the capacity of developing into other germ cell tumors.

Some embryonal carcinomas can show extraembryonic differentiation toward either yolk sac or trophoblast. In the first case, the embryonal carcinoma is accompanied by yolk sac tumor and in the second by syncytiotrophoblast cells. The extension of yolk sac tumor within the embryonal carcinoma tumor is extremely variable, ranging from microscopic foci to almost the entire tumor. There are high AFP serum levels in these cases. The negative effect of the presence of yolk sac tumor on prognosis, which is markedly worsened, has been known for several years (Talerman, 1975).

When the tumor differentiates toward a trophoblast, syncytial cells can be abundant (Fig. 21-4**B**). Serial measurements of HCG in these patients' serum is

TABLE 21-2. *Typical and Spermatocytic Seminoma. Differential Diagnosis Table (modification of Talerman).*

	Spermatocytic Seminoma	Typical Seminoma
Incidence	3.5 to 7.5 percent (1.7 to 12 percent)	92.5 to 96.5 percent (88 to 98.3 percent)
Presentation age	over 40 years of age	between 25 and 50 years of age
Localization	only testes	testis, ovary, mediastinum, retroperitoneum, pineal region
Bilateral incidence	10 percent	2 percent
Undescended testis incidence	no known reported cases	8.5 percent
Association with other tumors	none	25 percent
Gross appearance	grey to yellowish, solid, soft gelatinous, mucoid	yellow to pink, solid, firm, trabecular pattern
Histological details:		
tumor cell nucleus	round, dark, large, large variation in size and shape	ovoid, vesicular, little variation in size and chromatin distribution
tumor cell cytoplasm	dense, scarce, acidophilic, scarce or lacking in glycogen	clear or slightly granular, abudant, glycogen rich
edema	present, frequently give rise to pseudoglandular or microcystic pattern	absent
stroma	scarce and delicate	prominent, often abundant, fibrosis
lymphocytes	absent	present, may be abundant
granulomas	absent	present, may be abundant
Growth pattern	intrabular growth more often than interstitial	interstitial growth more often than intratubular
Metastasis	rare	frequent
Radiosensibility	very radiosensitive	very radiosensitive
Prognosis	Excellent, better than typical seminoma	very good with the proper treatment

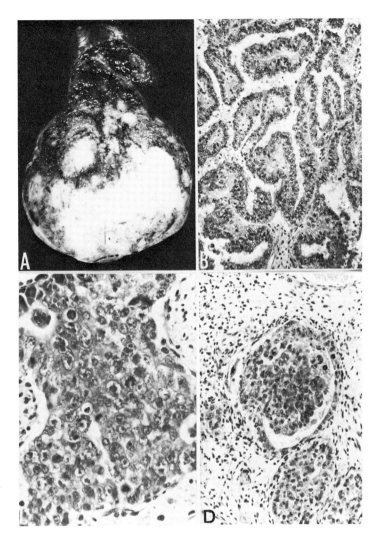

FIGURE 21-5. *Embryonal carcinoma. A,* Most of the testis has been replaced by a whitish tumor, layed out in different-sized nodules. *B,* Papillar pattern of embryonal carcinoma. H&E (x125). *C,* Solid tumoral cell arrangement. There is intense anisocytosis and frequent atypical mitoses. H&E (x250). *D,* Tumoral cell arrangement on the inside of a cavity lined by cubic cells; a characteristic of polyembryoma groupings. H&E (x125).

of interest in determining the prognosis (see testicular tumor markers in this chapter).

Yolk Sac Tumor. This term is used to refer to tumors that mostly occur during infancy and, in the past, were known as: orchioblastoma; testicular clear cell adenocarcinoma; infantile embryonal carcinoma; or endodermal sinus tumor (Pierce and co-authors, 1970). The name "yolk sac" tumor comes from Teilum's histogenetic hypothesis (1976), postulating these tumors differentiate toward extraembryonic structures and, preferentially, toward the yolk sac. This tumor has been described in the ovary, vagina, sacro-coccygeal region, mediastinum, and pineal region (Teilum, 1976).

It is the most common infant tumor, and constitutes 60 percent of infantile testicular tumors, frequently appearing in boys under 42 months of age. It appears as a fast-growing testicular mass that tends toward spontaneous arrest. It may also be observed in adults, in which case it is usually not alone, but associated to some other nonseminomatous tumor. Forty-four percent of embryonal carcinomas have areas of yolk sac tumor (Talerman, 1980 c).

Viewed grossly, the testis has a

smooth, elastic surface. When cut, it is mucoid and cystic, and has yellowish areas. The tumor usually does not disrupt the tunica albuginea nor infiltrate the spermatic cord (Fig. 21–6A).

Microscopically, the tumor is made up of cells with pale or vacuolated cytoplasm that form different patterns. Sometimes different-sized cysts are formed; other times they group into solid nests in which glandular lumens or ductal formations can be detected. Variable quantities of glycogen and lipids are detected in the cytoplasmic vacuoles (Fig. 21–6B and C). The tumor's stroma is loose, immature, or edematous.

A characteristic architectural pattern are glomeruloid or Shiller-Duval bodies. These are formed by a connective axis that has one or several capillaries, covered by the visceral and parietal layers with an epithelial appearance. The tumor may contain some teratoid elements.

Numerous spherical, hyaline globules with different sizes can be seen in the epithelial cell cytoplasm and in the stroma (Fig. 21–6D). These globules contain a diastase-resistant, PAS positive material in which AFP and alfa$_1$ antitrypsin, human yolk sac synthesized substances, have been identified (Gitlin and Perricelli, 1970).

Comparative ultrastructural studies between endodermic sinus tumors and the human yolk sac (Nogales-Fernández and associates, 1977) have supplied data that support their similarity. These authors have emphasized the presence of material,

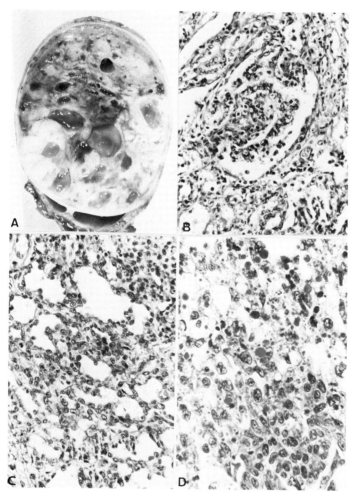

FIGURE 21–6. *Yolk sac tumor. A*, The cystic and mucoid appearance, characteristic of a yolk sac tumor section, is seen in this two-year-old boy. *B*, Glomeruloid body, formed by ·a central part which is reminiscent of a capillary tuft, and a flattened cell capsule. H&E (x100). *C*, Glandular formations coated by cells with a prominent nucleus and scarce cytoplasm. H&E (x100). *D*, Differently-sized PAS-positive inclusions in the cytoplasm of tumoral cells. H&E (x250).

like the basal lamina, forming both intra- and extra cellular aggregates. This material probably corresponds to the cytoplasmic eosinophilic inclusions or the extracellular eosinophilic globules. The cell nucleus has deep grooves with a nucleolonema like those in seminoma cells, and their cytoplasm has abundant mitochondria, free ribosomes, glycogen granules, and microfilaments. When these cells surround a glandular or cystic space numerous microvilli on the apical face and junctional complexes between the cells appear.

The prognosis for patient's with yolk sac tumor is not good. The 65 percent survival rate reported by Jeffs (1973) probably corresponds to tumors that have not yet spread.

Polyembryoma. Polyembryoma designates embryonal carcinomas that have a large number of embryoid bodies (Evans, 1957). The embryoid bodies measure less than 1 millimeter and may be for example, spherical, globular, or cylindrical. They are formed by a disc, a cavity, and a tubular structure. They are surrounded by an immature connective stroma, that may have syncytio- or cytotrophoblast cells, which recalls the appearance of a two- or three-week-old embryo (Fig. 21-5D).

As these embryoid bodies may be present in many teratomas and embryonal carcinomas, the term polyembryoma is used only when there is an elevated number of embryoid bodies. Polyembryoma is considered to be an embryonal carcinoma, which is initiating teratoid differentiation.

Choriocarcinoma. This tumor is formed by syncytiotrophoblast and cytotrophoblast. The pure tumor is rare (0.3 percent of all testicular tumors according to Mostofi and Price (1973)). It is most frequently associated with other testicular tumors such as embryonal carcinoma and teratoma (Bär and Hedinger, 1976). A testicular choriocarcinoma diagnosis should be limited to an isolated choriocarcinoma presentation, that is pure choriocarcinoma. It is more frequent in the second and third decades of life. Many times the first symptom is the appearance of metastases.

Viewed grossly, the testicular size is normal or it has a small nodule. The tumor has a hemorrhagic appearance. Histologically, the tumor has two basic cell types: syncytiotrophoblast cells—multi-nucleated cells with hyperchromatic nuclei and eosinophilic vacuolated cytoplasm; and cytotrophoblast cells—medium-sized polyhedric cells with precise cytoplasm limits (Fig. 21-4C and D).

The syncytiotrophoblast cells usually form a peripheral crown around the cytotrophoblast cells. Syncytiotrophoblast cells synthesizes HCG which can be detected with immunohistochemical methods. The measurement of HCG subunit beta in serum allows tumoral development to be followed.

A small percentage of patients that die from testicular choriocarcinoma metastasis show no testicular tumor. The seriated study of these patients' testes on occasion reveals irregular scars or basophilic, hematoxylinophilic, deposits. It is admitted that the primary tumor has spontaneously regressed (called a "burned-out" tumor). Ultrasound has been successfully utilized to detect a focus of a burned-out testicular tumor (Shawker and co-workers, 1983).

Teratoma. This is a complex tumor, formed by elements derived from more than one blastodermal leaf that reach different maturative and organizational stages. It can appear at any age, but more frequently occurs during the first three decades.

An increase in testicular size is observed macroscopically. When cut, cysts of different sizes and forms with gelatinous and mucous content are notable. Any necrotic or hemorrhagic zones should be carefully studied since they usually correspond to immature zones (Fig. 21-7).

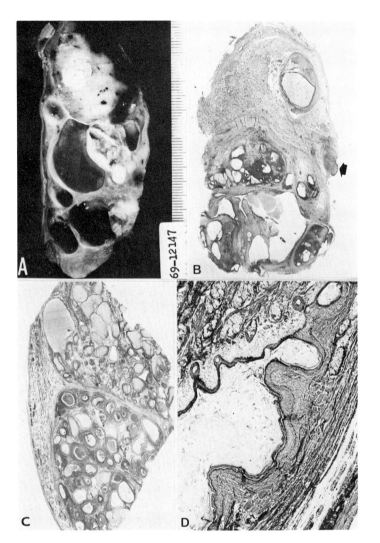

FIGURE 21–7. Teratoma. A, Cystic testicular tumor. The cyst content varies from a clear liquid to masses of keratin. B, Complete histological section of a testis showing numerous cavities corresponding to a well-differentiated teratoma with a small seminoma nodule (arrow). H&E (x1.5). C, Organoid teratoma from a 2-year-old boy. Only a small part of the testicular parenchyma, compressed below the tunica albuginea, is recognizable. H&E (x10). D, Dermoid cyst. Cystic formation lined by keratinized polystratified epithelium with skin appendages in its surroundings. H&E (x25).

Histologically, the following tissues are found:

1. Ectodermal derivatives such as epidermoid epithelium (with or without keratinization) and nervous tissue.
2. Endodermal derivatives such as gastrointestinal tract, respiratory tract and mucous glands.
3. Mesodermal derivatives such as bone, cartilage and muscle.

The term organoid teratoma is used when an abortive organ is formed in tumor areas: neural tissue (choroid plexus), gastrointestinal (intestine, pancreas, liver), respiratory (trachea), eye, etc.

From a histological point of view, teratomas can be classified as:

Immature Teratoma. This term was suggested by Mostofi and Price in 1973, and refers to tumors of varying differentiation ranging between embryonal carcinoma and mature teratoma, excluding either extreme. These represent from 20 to 30 percent of all testicular tumors. They are usually formed by primitive neuroectoderm, endoderm, mesoderm, or tissues with incomplete maturation in the form of cartilage, bone, mucous glands, transitional or cubic epidermoid epithelium, and smooth or skeletal muscle (Fig. 21–8).

Mature Teratoma. These are 5 to 10 percent of all testicular tumors. Histologi-

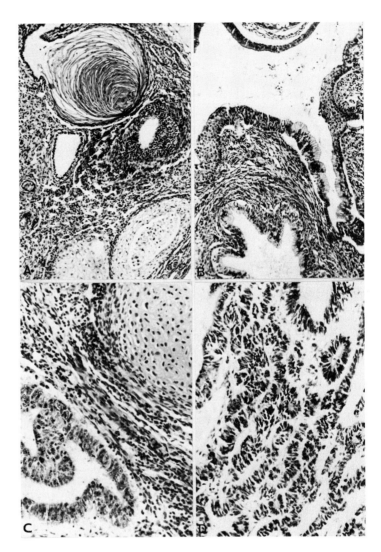

FIGURE 21–8. *Immature teratoma. A*, Cystic formations, lined by different types of epithelium, separated by immature nervous tissue. H&E (x60). *B*, Cystic formation in which mucous-secreting, respiratory and non-keratinized stratified epithelium can be recognized. H&E (x60). *C*, Nodule of immature cartilage, associated to atypical glandular structures and a rhabdomyoblastic stroma. H&E (x125). *D*, Immature nervous tissue observed in the wall of a testicular cystic teratoma. The numerous neuroblast rosettes and cords stand out. H&E (x125).

cally, these tumors show tissues derived from the differentiated, well-defined germ layers, which may be organoids.

A high percentage of mature and markedly differentiated teratomas (20 percent according to Brodner and associates (1980)) contain enteroendocrine cells (enterochromaffin cells, somatostatin, glucagon, pancreatic polypeptides secreting cells) which are detectable with immunohistochemical techniques. This is in agreement which the high percentage of teratomas containing intestinal musosa.

Teratomas appearing in boys under 12 years of age are usually mature and organoid and have an extremely benign course (Brown, 1976). Even in those cases in which the tumor contains undifferentiated areas, these do not metastasize at these ages, and the prognosis is excellent. In patients over 12 years of age, and even if the tumor is mature, it can metastasize, and, does do so in 29 percent of the patients. The metastases appear in the retroperitoneal lymph nodes. The prognosis for adults with mature teratoma is very good when radical orchidectomy and retroperitoneal lymphadenectomy are performed, and the cure rates—95 percent at five years—approach those of seminoma.

Testicular *dermoid cyst* is rare. It is considered to be a form of mature teratoma. The cysts are formed by epidermal and dermal elements with hair follicles and sebaceous glands. Like the ovarian dermoid cyst, testicular dermoid cysts may have bone, cartilage and even teeth. Thyroid gland tissue is rare in men, but pancreatic tissue can be occasionally observed. Mostofi and Price (1973) observed no cases with metastasis (Fig. 21–7**D**).

An *Epidermoid cyst* in the testis is rare and has been considered in Chapter 6, one-hundred-fifty cases have been described in the literature, most of them reviewed by Shah and others (1981). Clinical and histogenetic reasons justify their inclusion among testicular tumors. They appear clinically as testicular tumors and are so treated. Their histogenesis is under discussion (see Chapter 6). Most authors consider them to be derivatives of a germ layer or the unilateral development of a teratoma (Price and Mostofi, 1969; Nagel and Polley, 1955; Samuel and Tweedale, 1961).

When diagnosing an epidermoid cyst it is necessary to keep in mind Price and Mostofi's (1969) strict diagnostic criteria. These are: a localized lesion in the testicular parenchyma, the cyst content is keratin; the cyst wall is composed of a fibrous tissue lined partially or completely by squamous epithelium, an absence of teratomatous elements or skin appendages like sebaceous glands or hair follicles, and a lack of fibrosis in the neighboring testicular parenchyma. The last two criteria distinguish epidermoid cysts from teratoma (a potentially malignant lesion). A lack of scars or zones of focal fibrosis in the parenchyma are important in order to discard a "burnt out" malignant germ-cell tumor.

Testicular Carcinoid. This is a rare tumor appearing in 0.23 percent of all testicular tumors. It appers in middle-aged or old patients. Clinically it follows the same course as other testicular tumors: an increase in testicular size, which may be painful, and tender. It is not accompanied by a carcinoid syndrome. Like other testicular tumors, the left side is preferentially affected.

Histologically, the tumor is composed of cells that form nests, cords or gland-like structures. Like most digestive system carcinoids, the cells are characteristically uniform. The nucleus is spherical, with abundant chromatin clumps and one nucleolus. The cytoplasm is acidophilic and granular. The larger tumors can have necrosis of hemorrhagic foci. Cellular polymorphism may be evident in some cases with the appearance of giant cells and bizarre cells. Masson-Fontana's technique reveals argentaffin granules primarily in cells that are on the edge of the nests. Electron microscopic examination reveals granules which are characteristic of enteroendocrine secretion: electron-dense, polymorphic 50 to 350 nm granules, that occasionally have a peripheral halo, and are surrounded by membrane. The tumors can have a markedly hyalinized fibrous stroma.

The tumor normally appears alone, but it can be accompanied by teratomatous elements.

Two histogenetic hypotheses explaining carcinoid development in the testis have been suggested. Since there are no enteroendocrine cells in the testis (Brodner and associates, 1980), carcinoids may either be the result of the differentiation of teratoma elements (teratomas with intestinal epithelium have a large number of enteroendocrine cells); or be the product of a unilateral teratoma development, given the omnipotential capacity of germ cells. Since most carcinoids do not associate with teratomas, the second hypothesis for carcinoid origin is the most satisfactory.

Testicular carcinoid evolution is benign although there has been some cases reported with metastases and carcinoid syndrome (Berdjis and Mostofi, 1977).

Tumors with More Than One Histological Type. The W.H.O. classification distinguishes the following types:

1. Embryonal carcinoma and teratoma.
2. Choriocarcinoma and any other type (specifying type).
3. Other combinations (specifying types).

Forty percent of testicular tumors show more than one histological pattern; for this reason the pathologist should study multiple sections of testicular tumors before establishing a diagnosis. Although all combinations have been described, embryonal carcinoma with mature or immature teratoma, also known as teratocarcinoma is the most frequent association; and represents about 24 percent of all testicular tumors.

Choriocarcinoma associated with any other type of tumor has been separately considered, due to the serious prognosis of this combination (twenty percent survival after 5 years). Other frequent combinations are teratoma, embryonal carcinoma and seminoma; embryonal carcinoma and seminoma.

Germinal Cell Tumor Metastasis

Many germ cell tumors initially are disseminated through the lymphatic system and may continue their spread by vascular dissemination. The primary drainage for the right testis tumors is to the interaortic-caval, precaval, preaortic, paracaval, right common iliac, and right external iliac lymph nodes; they then drain to the para-aortic, left common iliac and right external iliac lymph nodes (Ray and others, 1974). The primary drainage for the left testis tumors is to the para-aortic, preaortic, left common iliac and left external iliac lymph nodes (Fig. 21–9). Inguinal lymph nodes in patients with a previous history of herniorrhaphy, orchidopexy, or other inguinal surgery, usually have a higher frequency mestastasis (Crawford and co-authors, 1983). Crossed metastases are infrequent (Zattoni and others, 1983). They occasionally affect

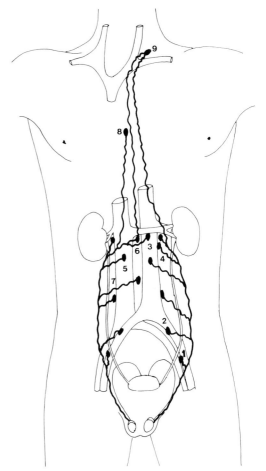

FIGURE 21–9. *Lymph nodes involved in testicular tumor spread. 1, External iliac nodes. 2, Common iliac nodes. 3, Preaortic nodes. 4, Paraaortic nodes. 5, Precaval nodes. 6, Interaortacaval nodes. 7, Paracaval nodes. 8, Mediastinic nodes. 9, Supraclavicular nodes.*

mediastinal and supraclavicular lymph nodes. Choriocarcinomas habitually spread through the blood stream.

Seminoma metastases, found at autopsy, affect, in descending order of frequency, the para-aortic and aortic lymph nodes, liver, lungs, left kidney, left adrenal gland, peritoneum, pancreas, pleura, right adrenal gland, and right kidney.

Classical (typical) and anaplastic seminoma metastasize as seminoma in 65 percent of the cases, embryonal carcinoma in 26 percent, and teratoma in 4 percent. Spermatocytic seminoma very rarely produces metastases (0.5 percent).

Embryonal carcinoma metastasizes to the following organs, in descending order of frequency: para-aortic and iliac lymph nodes, lung, liver, pleura, bones, and gastrointestinal tract. Histological examination of embryonal carcinoma metastases show 96 percent to be embryonal carcinoma, 8 percent to be teratoma and 5 percent to be choriocarcinoma.

Yolk sac tumor remains localized within the testis for a long time, but once metastases begin, they spread widely by vascular dissemination. It preferentially invades the lungs, liver and peritoneum. The three-year survival rate is 64 percent. The prognosis is improved in infants under two years of age and in first stages of tumoral development.

Teratomas metastasize to the preaortic and iliac lymph nodes, liver, lungs, bones, trunk, pleura and intestine, in order of descending frequency. The histological pattern of metastases is teratoma and embryonal carcinoma (63 percent), and choriocarcinoma (25 percent).

Choriocarcinomas metastasize through the vascular system as well as the lymphatic system, although the former is more common. There are metastases to the lungs and the para-aortic and iliac lymph nodes in 100 percent of cases; with less frequency, hepatic, intestinal, splenic, adrenal and cerebral metastases occur. The metastases are in the form of choriocarcinoma in all organs.

A tendency toward tumor maturation in the metastases is observed when the histological patterns of the primary testicular tumor and their metastases are compared. Eight percent of testicular tumors diagnosed as embryonal carcinoma, and about 50 percent of those diagnosed as pure teratoma or teratoma and embryonal carcinoma, display metastases of pure teratoma or teratoma with other tumoral elements (Dixon and Moore, 1952). In 1980, Mostofi suggested three factors that may play a role in tumor maturation: the omnipotential germ cell capacity; the microenvironment where they develop; and the influence of organizers.

Germ cell capacity for differentiation into different somatic tissues has been experimentally shown in isolated embryonal carcinoma cells (Martin, 1975; Kleinsmith and Pierce, 1964).

The place in which tumor cells develop may condition tumoral structure. Using embryonal carcinoma and teratoma cells from tumors in rats produced by transplanting genital ridge cells from the same species, Stevens (1967) observed that the cells developed into mature or immature teratoma when placed in the testis; abundant embryoid bodies when implanted intraperitoneally; and teratoma when they were placed subcutaneously. It is well known that in man metastases are preferentially mature teratoma in the retroperitoneum, lung and mediastinum; while areas of choriocarcinoma are seen in the liver, lungs, kidneys and brain.

The effect of organizers on testicular tumors is less understood, but it is well known that factors such as age, radiation, or chemotherapy can affect tumor maturation. This maturation is not only not produced in other cases, but some well differentiated tumor forms can evolve toward teratocarcinoma when they metastasize. Metastases which persist after adequate treatment with chemotherapy probably require biopsy (Carr and others, 1981) for a proper cellular characterization.

Testicular Tumor Markers

The development of specific radioimmunoassay methods (Vaitukaitis, 1972; Javadpour and Chen, 1981) and immunohistochemical techniques (Kurman and co-authors, 1977) that detect certain substances produced by tumor cells has made possible their identification in the patient's serum as well as in the tumor cells. These proteins or "markers," which are easily detectable in plasma, are extremely useful in ascertaining tumor stage, enabling the prediction of clinical metastases and following response to therapy.

The proteins most frequently synthesized by tumoral cells are: alpha-fetoprotein (AFP) and human chorionic gonadotropin (HCG). Both marker levels should be measure simultaneously.

AFP is the most abundant protein in the human fetus. It is synthesized in the yolk sac, liver, and gastrointestinal tract of many species. At the end of the first year, AFP levels decline below 16ng/ml (Waldmann and McIntire, 1974). Before considering its value in detecting testicular tumors, it is necessary to mention different clinical conditions that have high AFP values. For instance, elevated values can be found in patients with malignant tumors in the liver, pancreas, stomach, intestines, and extrahepatic biliary system; in patients with hepatic metastases; and they have also been observed in patients with ataxia-telangiectasia and thyrosinemia.

AFP levels are extremely high in all yolk sac tumors (Talerman and associates, 1980 a). AFP is present in tumors formed exclusively by the yolk sac as well as in tumors such as embryonal carcinoma or teratoma which show areas of yolk sac. Once the possibility of hepatic disease has been eliminated, slight AFP elevations are found in patients with pure embryonal carcinoma. The explanation for this discrete rise in AFP levels probably arises from the histogenetic dynamics of testicular tumors. Embryonal carcinoma is a generic term used to described tumors made up of cells, which, seen with a light microscope, are all similar; but they have different evolutionary potentials. Most likely, some tumor cells from embryonal carcinomas have developed an extraembryonic differentiation toward yolk sac structures.

HCG is synthesized by syncytiotrophoblastic cells in the placenta. This glycoprotein of approximately 45,000 daltons is made of two different subunits: alpha and beta. The alpha subunit amino acid sequence is basically identical to that of luteinizing hormone, however, beta subunit displays large amino acid sequence differences which gives it specificity. The normal serum level for the HCG beta subunit is 1 ng/ml. Patients with choriocarcinoma (100 percent of them), patients with seminoma (7.7 percent) and patients with embryonal carcinoma (60 percent) display extremely elevated HCG beta subunit levels. HCG can also be elevated in nontesticular carcinoma, such as neoplasms of the stomach, lung, pancreas, liver, and breast (Fukutani and others, 1983).

The importance of the AFP and HCG markers in the evaluation of tumor stages has been emphasized by Javadpour (1980). The margin of error in the evaluation of tumor stages drops to an acceptable level (between 5 and 14 percent) with these techniques. The persistence of high serum marker levels after orchiectomy invariably reflects that the tumor is developed to a Stage II or III. The persistence of high levels after lymphadenectomy indicates Stage III disease. Even though lymphadenectomy is negative, if marker determinations continue to be elevated, the patient has a Stage III tumor.

Serial AFP and HCG determinations allow the clinical course of patients with testicular tumors to be followed. The elevation of one or both markers after orchiectomy precedes clinical development of metastases, which must be suspected when the patient has not developed an intercurrent hepatic disease or other tumor.

HCG may be elevated in some seminomas. The presence of a discrete HCG elevation in 7.7 percent of seminomas can be attributed to different factors: the syncytiotrophoblast cells, present in some seminomas, can produce HCG, as Heyderman and Neville (1976) have shown using immunoperoxidase techniques;

Friedman and Pearlman (1970) have reported a "giant cell" seminoma variant (seminoma with trophoblastocarcinoma) which is more aggressive and radioresistant. It is also possible for the tumor to contain microscopic foci of embryonal carcinoma and/or choriocarcinoma which emphasizes the necessity for a careful histological examination of these tumors because of the possible implication of what may be found regarding prognosis and treatment.

If the AFP marker is observed in a seminoma, embryonal carcinoma with or without teratoma accompanies the seminoma, and this will alter the course of therapy to be followed. The moderate rise in AFP observed in patients with pure seminoma and hepatic metastasis may be secondary to the hepatic parenchymal regenerative changes, which, in turn, are caused by metastases (Javadpour, 1980).

Germinal Cell Tumor Treatment

The prognosis for testicular tumors is based on two basic facts: the histologic type of the tumor and the degree of extension at the moment of diagnosis. The following classification into three stages is very useful in evaluating the clinical stage:

— Stage I: The tumor is limited to the testis without invasion of the capsule or spermatic cord.
— Stage II A: Microscopic tumor which affects up to six well-encapsulated lymph nodes.
— Stage II B: A clearly-bordered macroscopic tumor or a microscopic tumor which infiltrates a lymph node capsule and extends to the retroperitoneal fat.
— Stage II C: Voluminous tumor infiltrating a large quantity of retroperitoneal fat; it can be completely resected.
— Stage II D: Voluminous tumor infiltrating a large quantity of retroperitoneal fat; it cannot be totally surgically removed.
— Stage III: Tumor with metastasis outside the retroperitoneum.

Once the histological type of tumor has been established, and after a detailed study of multiple sections from the orchiectomy specimen, the stage of the tumoral development must be considered in order to establish therapeutic guide-lines. The pathologist, who has stated whether the tunica albuginea, the epididymis or the spermatic cord are infiltrated, supplies some additional data.

Various procedures are useful for truly ascertaining if the tumor is Stage I or if it has already spread. These included chest x-rays, tomograms in cases of any suspicious lesion, bipedal lymphangiography, measurement of AFP and subunit beta HCG levels. Computerized tomography and ultrasoundgraphy may also be useful in some cases (Marincek and co-workers, 1983). In order to perform a complete evaluation of the patient with non-seminomatous testicular tumor, retroperitoneal lymphadenectomy should be performed.

It is important to remember that, as in any other oncological field, teamwork between the urological surgeon, pathologist, radiologist, radiotherapist and oncologist is necessary.

The treatment for seminoma is radiotherapy immediately after surgery. The guide lines for typical as well as anaplastic seminoma are similar, according to the opinion of most authors. The areas to be treated and the doses used have been reviewed by Slawson (1978) and Caldwell and others (1980).

Lymphography is negative in 70% of seminomas (Calman and associates, 1979) and the proportion of patients with microscopic metastasis, although unknown, should be very low. Some authors add no other treatment to orchidectomy (Ytredal and Bradfield, 1972) for those cases with negative lymphograms (Stage I), while others recommend using 2500 rad over 2.5 weeks to the inguinal and para-aortic regions (Maier and coworkers, 1968).

In Stage II tumors, irradiation should include lymph nodes of the mediatinum and supraclavicular regions as well as the inguinal and abdominal lymph nodes (Lee and Pérez, 1974; Doornbos and others, 1975; Quivey and associates, 1977) Radiation therapy above the diaphragm in patients with Stage II A testicular tumors may be unnecessary (Sause, 1983). Cure rates in Stage I and II—considered together—are 90 percent after 2 to 5 years.

All patients who present initially with either Stage III tumors or bulky Stage II should be treated with multiple drug chemotherapy including cis-platinum. If this regimen is not completely effective, the residual tumor should be irradiated or removed surgically (Wajsman and co-authors, 1983). Survival rates reach 80 to 90 percent after 2 years.

The treatment for nonseminomatous tumors includes radical orchidectomy, retroperitoneal lymph node dissection, and for most patients, chemotherapy. The prognosis, negative up until a few years ago, now approaches the cure rate for seminoma (Einhorn and Williams, 1980). Eighty-five to ninety percent of Stage I non-seminomatous tumors are cured simply with orchidectomy and retroperitoneal lymph node dissection. Approximately 60 percent of non-seminomatous tumors are in Stage I or II at the moment of diagnosis. The therapeutic guide-lines most commonly followed are:

—Stage I: Chemotherapy, theoretically, need not be used. A strict monthly control, during the first year and every two months during the second year, consisting in chest X-rays and tumor marker determinations has been proposed. The early detection of metastases and the use of adequate chemotherapy provide over a 90 percent cure rate. This treatment, though questionable, avoids requiring indiscriminate chemotherapy for all Stage I tumors that would only benefit 10 to 15 percent of patients (Bredael and others, 1983).

—Stage II: It has been demonstrated in many series that the dissection of the retroperitoneal lymph nodes, while necessary for the evaluation of the stage of tumoral development, is not completely effective. Between 40 percent and 50 percent of patients with retroperitoneal lymph node dissections develop recurrent disease. These occasionally occur in distant lymph nodes and at other times in the lung. Most recurrences occur during the first year, so that they may be caused by micrometastases which were already present at the time of lymphadenectomy. Using chemotherapy, containing vinblastine, actinomycin D, bleomycin, and chlorambucil, 84 percent of the patients are free of disease (Vugrin and others, 1981 b). When Stage II tumors are broken down into the aforementioned substages, the results show a three-year survival rate of 100 percent in Stage II A, 66 percent in Stage II B, and 45 percent in Stage II C.

The adverse prognosis for patients with large tumors that could not be removed or with extra-nodal masses must be attributed, at least in part, to the possibility that they were really Stage III tumors.

—Stage III: In patients with advanced testicular carcinoma treatment protocols have utilized more aggressive drugs. Following the Vugrin and associates (1981 a), cisplatinum is combined with the drugs used for Stage II disease. In general, when abdominal involvement is advanced, the prognosis is worse (29 percent), compared to that when the involvement is preferentially thoracic (67 percent). Not all tumors behave the same way to chemotherapy. Embryonal carcinomas have the best prognosis (Wittes and others, 1976). Pure choriocarcinoma is an extremely aggressive tumor, responding poorly to chemotherapy, and has a short period of survival (Vugrin and co-authors, 1979). The results obtained with either radiotherapy or surgery, exclusively, have been reviewed by Babaian and Johnson (1980).

Some tumors spontaneously experience involution and the tumor is reduced to a scar near the rete testis ("burned-out" testicular tumor). At times these scars are so small that they may not be noticed. Most contain hyalinized seminiferous tubules, macrophages with hemosiderin, plasma cells, and hematoxylinophilic bodies. Some have teratoid elements or foci of seminoma.

When an extra-gonadal germ cell tumor (seminoma, embryonal carcinoma, teratoma, or choriocarcinoma) present clinically, these scars must be carefully looked for, since these tumors can be no more than the metastasis from a "burnt-out" testicular tumor (Azzopardi and Hoffbrand, 1965; Munro and others, 1983; Powell and co-authors, 1983).

Specialized Gonadal Stroma Tumors

If we consider that Leydig, Sertoli, granulosal and thecal cells derive from the gonadal stroma, the following oncological possibilities exist: Leydig cell tumors, Sertoli cell tumors, granulosal cell tumors, combined tumors and undifferentiated gonadal stroma tumors (Crump, 1983). Although all these possibilities may occur in practice, given their low frequency and similar prognosis only two groups shall be considered: Leydig cell tumors and Sertoli cell tumors.

Leydig Cell Tumor

Leydig cell tumors represent between 1.6 and 3 percent of all testicular tumors (Mostofi and Price, 1973; Pugh, 1976). These tumors are more frequent in adults than in children. Two thirds of these tumors develop in postpubertal patients. Presentation ranges from 2 to 82 years of age, with a childhood frequency peak between 1 and 5 years of age, and in adults between 25 and 35 years of age (35 percent of the cases). Nine percent of the cases have cryptorchid antecedents. In 18.5 percent of the cases, the tumor develops in the contralateral testis (Lubetzki and associates, 1980).

Leydig cell tumors present as a variable endocrine condition which is generally a precocious puberty and genital enlargement in children and feminization or lack of symptoms in the adult. During infancy, an androgens increase a clinical picture of genital enlargement with diverse manifestations occurs: an increase in penis size, the appearance of body-hair on the scrotum, acne, voice change, an increase in muscular development, erections, epiphyseal closure, and dwarfism (Gracia and others, 1980). Some 50 prepubertal Leydig cell tumors have been reported.

Thirty percent of adult patients display endocrinological symptoms. The most frequent clinical findings are: gynecomastia, decrease of sexual libido, and contralateral testicular atrophy. An increase in estrogen, progesterone, and prolactin levels has been repeatedly observed (Caldamone and associates, 1979; Pérez and others, 1980).

Gross examination generally shows the tumor to be unilateral. Of 151 tumors reviewed by Hugues and Caron (1976), 73 (48.3 percent) were located in the right testis, and 61 (40.4 percent) in the left one; 7 (4.6 percent) were bilateral and 3 (2 percent) were paratesticular. The tumor is formed by one or several well defined yellowish parenchymal nodules (Fig. 21–10A and 21–11A) (Nistal and others, 1974; Shimp and associates, 1977).

Different cell types can be observed histologically. The following predominate: medium-sized cells with eosinophilic cytoplasm (Figs. 21–10B and 21–11B), and large uni-, bi-, or multinucleated cells.

The cells form variable histological patterns: sheet, fascicles, and nests. The stroma may be scarce, fibrous, mixoid or calcified. The surrounding parenchyma may show atrophy due to nonfunctioning tumor compression, precocious seminiferous tubule maturation in boys with virilizing tumors and maturation arrest, hypospermatogenesis or an absence of germ cells in estrogen-producing tumors. An interesting diagnostic detail is the presence of Reinke's crystals in Leydig cell tumors, but these are present in less than half of the tumors.

With the electron microscope the functional tumors display cells which closely recall normal Leydig cells. These tumor cells contain abundant smooth endoplasmic reticulum, which at times forms concentric nonfenestrated cisternae, nu-

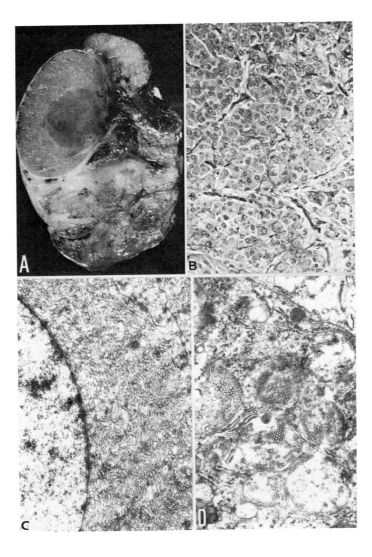

FIGURE 21–10. *Functioning Leydig cell tumor. A, Well-defined, one cm nodular formation located in the testicular mediastinum of a 5-year-old boy. B, Solid uniform proliferation of eosinophilic cells with ample cytoplasm. H&E (x125). C, Smooth endoplasmic reticulum hyperplasia observed in a tumoral Leydig cell. (x25,000). D, Clump of mitochondria with tubular cristae in tumoral Leydig cells. (x25,000).*

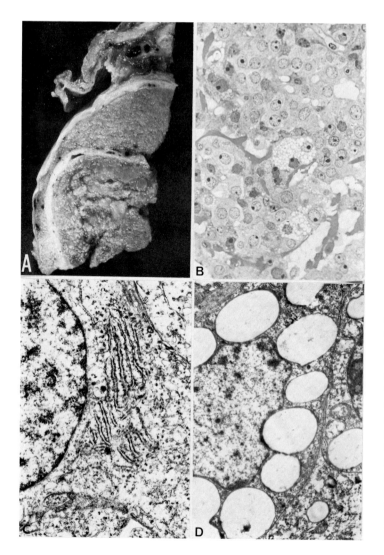

FIGURE 21–11. *Nonfunctioning Leydig cell tumor* **A**, *Testicular section showing part of a well-encapsulated tumor.* **B**, *Solid proliferation pattern of tumoral cells among which some cells loaded with lipids stand out. One-micron section of eppon-embedded material. Toluidine blue (x250).* **C**, *Leydig cell from the above tumor in which abundant free ribosomes and rough endoplasmic reticulum cisternae are seen (x25,000).* **D**, *Leydig cell with numerous lipid droplets forming a perinuclear crown (x8000).*

merous mitochondria displaying tubular cristae, lysosomes, and lipid droplets. They are differentiated from normal Leydig cells but their bizarre multiple nucleoli, the numerous foldings of the nuclear envelope and the low number of paracrystalline inclusions, Reinke's crystals and lipofuchsin pigment granules (Sohval and others, 1977) (Figs. 21–10C and **D**; and 21–11C and **D**). There are no ultrastructural differences between feminizing and virilizing tumors (Sohval and others, 1982). Non-functional tumors have less smooth endoplasmic reticulum development. Cytologically, their cells are less differentiated.

Between 10 and 14 percent of Leydig cell tumors are malignant (Lockhardt and others, 1976; Ober and co-authors, 1976; Shemiakin, 1971; Davis and associates, 1980; Sworn and Buchanan, 1981), and metastases may appear 10 years after orchiectomy. The malignant Leydig cell tumors usually occur at an older age than benign ones (an average age of 60 years). In these cases, cellular polymorphism, atypical mitoses, the absence of lipofuchsin granules in the cytoplasm, and the presence of tumor embolisms in the lymphatic vessels suggest a malignant behavior (Gharpure, 1950). It is difficult to establish a prognosis based on histology in many cases, and the only sure criteria for malignancy are the presence of metastasis (Klippel and others, 1979). There are no known cases of malignant Leydig cell tumors occurring during infancy.

Malignant Leydig cell tumors behave biochemically like adrenal corticoid carcinomas (Lipsett and associates, 1966). These tumors have low 3-β-hydroxysteroid activity, produce large quantities of dehydroepiandrosterone sulphate, and patients develop high levels of 17-urinary ketosteroid as well as elevated testosterone levels, which are almost exclusively due to peripherical dehydroepiandrosterone conversion to testosterone.

Given the similarity between malignant Leydig cell tumor and adrenal carcinoma, which is perhaps explicable by the very close embryological origin of the Leydig cells and the adrenal cortex, along with the deficient Leydig cell tumor response to irradiation and polychemotherapy, adrenolytic agent (O,P'-DDD) (mitotane or 1,1-dichloro-2(o-chlorophenyl)-2-(p-chlorophenyl) ethane) treatment has been attempted with limited success (Azer and Braunstein, 1981).

Leydig cell tumor differential diagnosis basically includes two conditions:
1. Leydig cell hyperplasia. In certain cases, the hyperplasia may be so intense as to suggest a Leydig cell tumor. The diffuse testicular involvement and conservation of the tubular architecture, even though the seminiferous tubules may be atrophied, are criteria for hyperplasia.
2. The second condition is the presence of an intratesticular adrenal choristoma. Radial cellular orientation, the presence of several cell layers, and a characteristic cytology can be recognized in adrenal choristoma. The cells have a thin nuclear membrane and a vesiculous nucleus with scarce dense chromatin. The Leydig cell nuclear membrane is thick and several prominent nucleoli are outstanding. Based only on the cellular morphology it is sometimes not possible to distinguish between adrenal cortical tissue and Leydig cell tumors (Galian and others, 1971). This is not surprising when one recalls that the embryologic origin of gonadal stroma and the adrenal cortex is mesodermal and that both glands are intimately related during embryologic development. The frequency of adrenal rests along the spermatic cord, epididymis and testis is so high that nearly 30 percent of newborns possess them.

In the adrenogenital syndrome, both testes frequently increase in size due to the presence of adrenal choristomas. For many years it has been postulated that steroid treatment diminished testicular size and confirmed the adrenal origin of the disease. Although this is true in many cases, there are others in which is does not occur (Newell and associates, 1977). On the other hand, testicular growth is not always bilateral in the adrenogenital syndrome.

Sertoli Cell Tumor

The Sertoli cell tumor derives from primitive gonadal stroma and it may be constituted by only Sertoli cells, only granulosa cells, only fusiform (thecal-like) cells, as well as by combination of the three cell-types. In addition, the tumor may or may not have Leydig cells.

The first case of Sertoli cell tumor was reported by Teilum in 1949, who called it "androblastoma," balancing the "arrhenoblastoma" described in 1930 by Meyer in the ovary. Both are known as gonadal stromal tumors, a term used by Mostofi and others (1959), in English speaking countries.

The Sertoli cell tumor is a rare tumor constituting between 0.4 percent (Dixon and Moore, 1952) and 1.2 percent (Pugh, 1976) of all testicular tumors. The number of cases published in the review by Kalis and Goulandris (1974) barely reached 70. New cases have recently been reported (Mantoudis and associates, 1979; Gabrilove and others, 1980).

Clinically it appears at all ages. A fifth of the reported cases have occurred during the first 10 years of life, a third between 20 and 39 years of age, and another fifth between 40 and 60 years of age (Mostofi and co-authors, 1959). The clinical presentation consists of a testicular tumor, which may or may not be painful, and in a third of the patients gynecomastia is present. The left testis is more frequently affected (about twice as often) than the right. The patients may or may not present feminization symptoms. Elevated androgen levels have been detected in some cases while high pregnanediol and estradiol levels have been found in others. The plasma levels of androgens, estrogens, gonadotropins and 17-ketosteroids are normal in some tumors.

Grossly, these tumors are well defined, encapsulated, and, when cut, are yellowish or greyish, and occasionally cystic. Three different cell-types can be observed in Sertoli cell tumors, although the three cell-types are not necessarily present in all tumors:

1. Polyhedric or columnar cells. These have a large, vesiculous nucleus, well defined nuclear membrane, abundant euchromatin and a small nucleolus. The cytoplasm may be ample and vacuolated with abundant lipid inclusions (Marshall and associates, 1977). These cells form tubular structures which are reminiscent of seminiferous tubules.
2. Cells similar to Leydig or luteal cells, with abundant eosinophilic cytoplasm. These cells form clumps or are isolated among other cell-types.
3. Spindle-shaped stromal cells. They have an elongated nucleus, eosinophilic cytoplasm. These cells frequently form bundles between the seminiferous tubules.

These different cell-types are considered to give rise to the three histological tumor types: epithelial tubular tumor; sarcomatous tumor; and mixed tumor type (Fig. 21-12). A recently described form of Sertoli cell tumor with distinctive clinical and pathologic features was designated as "large-cell calcifying Sertoli cell tumor". This appears usually in both testes and during the first two decades of life, associated with malformative stigmatas and marked endocrine alterations. The ample cytoplasm and the presence of intra-and extracellular calcifications are characteristic features (Proppe and Scully, 1980; Proppe and Dickersin, 1982).

Nearly 10 percent of Sertoli cell tumors develop metastasis (Morin and Loening, 1975). Poor prognostic criteria are marked anaplasia, a large amount of mitoses, and infiltration of the tunica albuginea or spermatic cord. Retroperitoneal lymph node dissection is justified when macroscopic and microscopic tumor examination suggest malignancy. The value of radiotherapy and chemotherapy for controlling metastasis is under discussion.

Germ Cell and Gonadal Stroma Tumors (Gonadoblastoma)

These tumors characteristically possess intermingled germ cells and gonadal stromal cells. The gonadal stromal cells are similar to the granulosa or Sertoli cells, but cells recalling Leydig or luteal cells are also frequently found.

The term gonadoblastoma was introduced by Scully (1953) to describe these tumors that frequently originate in dysgenetic gonads. Scully's report (1970) on tumors from 74 patients has supplied most

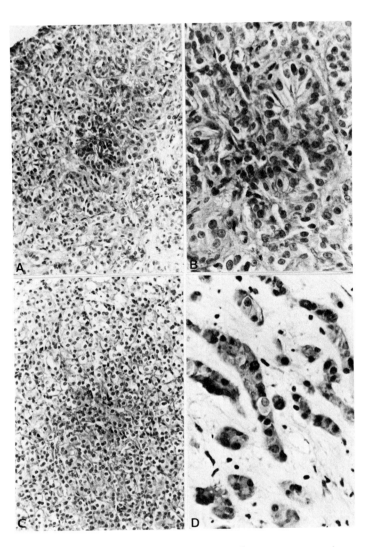

FIGURE 21-12. Sertoli cell tumor. A, Group of tumoral cells forming rosetoid structures. H&E (x125). B, Cylindrical cells grouped into tubular structures. H&E (x250). C, Cellular sheet formed by numerous cells with scarce connective tissue support. H&E (x125). D, Large cord-like tumoral cell proliferation in loose stroma, characteristic of large-cell calcifying Sertoli cell tumor. H&E (x250).

of the clinical, hormonal, and genetic data that are known.

The age of presentation varies from one to seventy-three years of age. Clinically, 25 of these patients displayed a female phenotype, 35 displayed female phenotype with signs of virilization, and 13 patients displayed a male phenotype. The gonad containing the tumor was a streak gonad in 22 cases, a testis in 18, and in 61 cases was unknown. The tumor was bilateral in a third of the cases. In half of the cases where the tumor was in a streak gonad, the opposite gonad was also a streak gonad and nearly always contained a second gonadoblastoma. In 9 of the 16 cases where the tumor was in a testis, the opposite gonad was streak, and in 3 patients this streak gonad contained a second gonadoblastoma. In the 5 cases where both gonads were testes, 4 had gonadoblastomas in only one testis and one was a bilateral gonadoblastoma.

The karyotype study carried out on 30 patients showed that the karyotype of 26 patients was 46,XY or 45,X/46,XY; one patient had the 45,X karyotype; and the remaining patient's karyotype showed mosaicism.

Grossly, the tumor size varied from a few centimeters to being a histological finding only (the tumor was only discovered during the histological study in one-fourth of the patients) (Fig. 21–13). The larger tumors were greyish. Most of the tumors showed granular calcifications; some tumors were almost completely calcified. Histologically the tumor displays a nodular structure, which is constituted by different cell types (Fig. 21–3C and **D**):

1. Germ cells: These are large cells with abundant clear cytoplasm, a vesiculated nucleus and large nucleolus.
2. Small cells similar to Sertoli or granulosa cells, with irregular hyperchromatic nucleus and scarce cytoplasm. They are arranged either on the periphery of the tumoral nests, around germ cells, or surrounding hyaline bodies.
3. Cells similar to Leydig or luteal cells, which have a more ample cytoplasm, that are polygonal and located in the stroma, constituted by the above mentioned cell-types, surrounding the tumor nests.

Ultrastructural studies have enabled the identification of interesting details of the tumor. Gonadoblastoma germ cells are morphologically similar to those in the human testis, fetal ovary, seminoma and dysgerminoma. The Sertoli- or granulosa-

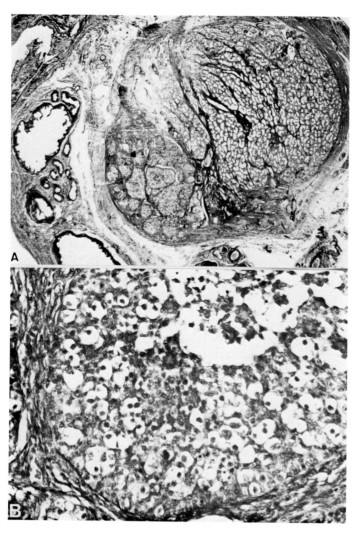

FIGURE 21–13. *Gonadoblastoma. A, Middle section from the gonad of a patient with Sohval's syndrome. A lobulate nodular structure is seen at the testicular periphery. H&E (x10). B, Each of the tumoral lobules is composed by the proliferation of small-sized cells around germ cells which stand out due to their clear cytoplasm. H&E (x150).*

like cells have irregular nuclei with abundant foldings, heterochromatin clumps preferentially attached to the nuclear envelope, a prominent nucleolus, abundant mitochondria, moderate endoplasmic reticulum development, and isolated lysosomes. These characteristics are similar to those of the normal ovarian granulosa cells or normal testicular Sertoli cells.

The hyaline bodies, which under the light microscope are reminiscent of Call-Exner bodies, are formed by laminar structures like those forming the basal lamina. This feature, along with the tumor nests being surrounded by a thick, multilaminar basal lamina as well as the presence of Charcot-Böttcher's crystals, lead Ishida and co-authors (1976) to suggest that the granulosa or Sertoli-like cells are really Sertoli cells.

The stromal cells located between the nodules are similar to Leydig and luteal cells, and are not present in all cases. Ultrastructurally they display nearly all the characteristic organelles of steroid-secreting cells: very abundant smooth endoplasmic reticulum, lipid droplets, mitochondria with tubular cristae; however, they lack Reinke's crystals. Even so, given the large number of electron dense cytoplasmic inclusions observed in these cells, Ishida and co-authors (1976) are inclined to feel these cells are more probably Leydig cells rather than luteal cells.

Ultrastructural findings suggest many gonadoblastomas originate in the dysgenetic testes of genetically male patients. The gonadoblastoma should be considered as an *in situ* carcinoma. Seminoma foci undistinguishable from typical seminoma are found in 50 percent of the gonadoblastoma. Teratoma, embryonal carcinoma, or yolk sac tumor were seen in either the contralateral or the same gonad in eight of Scully's (1970) 74 patients. Gallager and Lewis (1973) have reported a study of choriocarcinoma in a patient who previously had been diagnosed as having gonadoblastoma. Although some tumors have metastasized and caused death, in no case was the metastasis a gonadoblastoma.

The treatment for gonadoblastoma consists not only in its removal, but in extirpating both gonads. This same practice is followed in patients with gonadal dysgenesis.

Nonspecialized Gonadal Stroma Tumors

Testicular angiomas, leiomyomas and neurofibromas are considered to be nonspecialized gonadal stromal tumors. Leukemic infiltrations and testicular lymphomas are also included under the same heading. Osseous (Yoneda and others, 1979) and adipose (Honoré, 1979) metaplasia stand out among the pseudotumoral lesions that have been observed. All these gonadal stromal tumors have followed a benign course.

Testicular Angiomas

These are exceptional tumors that can adopt different histological patterns. Cavernous angioma (Morehead and Thomas, 1944) display the characteristic dilated blood vessels with thickened wall. Hemagioendothelioma is a tumor that has been frequently observed in extra testicular locations. Some cases of testicular hemangio-endothelioma have been reported in adults as well as children (Stein, 1975; D'Esposito and associates, 1976). This tumor is constituted by a proliferation of endothelial cells, forming two or three layers located between the vascular lumen and the basement membrane. This formation is easily demonstrated using silver impregnation techniques for reticulum fibers. The reported tumors showed no signs of anaplasia and were considered to be benign. Testicular capillary hemangioma (Nistal and co-authors, 1982) differs from hemangioendothelioma in the uniformity of the vascular lumen, the small size of the vessels, and the presence of only one endothelial cell layer lining the vascular lumen (Fig. 21–14A). Masson's vegetant endothelioma, which has also been described in the testis (Cricco and Buck, 1980), is considered secondary to the organization and canalization of a thrombosed blood vessel.

Testicular Fibromas

These are listed on the American series of nongerminal tumors (Dixon and Moore, 1953) and only incidentally in the British series (Collins and Pugh, 1964). Its existence is controversial.

Testicular Leiomyomas

A primary testicular leiomyoma was described by Honoré and Sullivan (1970) in a 65-year-old patient. The authors suggest that it may have originated from peritubular myofibroblasts.

Testicular Neurofibromas

A intratesticular neurofibroma has been described by Livolsi and Schiff (1977) in a 23-year-old patient.

Leukemic Infiltration

In the course of leukemia, the testes can undergo infiltration by tumoral cells. The testes may be converted into a res-

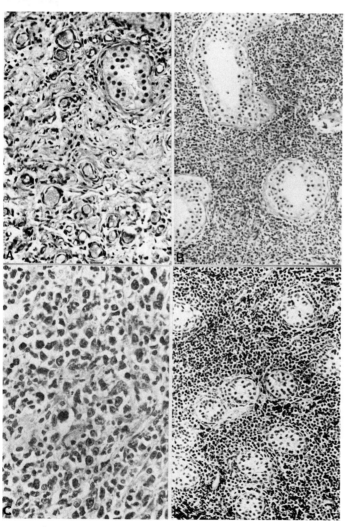

FIGURE 21–14. *A, Testicular angioma showing the proliferation of small blood vessels in an intensely collagenized stroma. H&E (x125). B, Primary testicular lymphoma. Tumoral cells infiltrate the intertubular space isolating the seminiferous tubules. H&E (x60). C, Marked polymorphism in a light malignant primary testicular lymphoma. H&E (x250). D, Leukemic infiltration in the testis of a 3-year-old boy. H&E (x60).*

ervoir of tumoral cells during the course of a leukemia, and may—months or years after the clinical cure of the disease—give rise to secondary disseminations. Not less than 16 to 22 percent of the clinically cured patients show recurrence that begins in the testes. The mechanism by which the testis provides a special environment for the tumoral cells is unknown. Bilateral testicular irradiation of 2500 rad is recommended for these patients (Sullivan and others, 1980) (Fig. 21-14**D**).

Testicular Lymphoma

When the pathologist diagnoses lymphoma on a surgical specimen corresponding to a testis, he is faced with three possibilities with different prognoses. First, it may be a terminal testicular leukemia or lymphoma infiltration. Second, the lymphoma seen in the testis may be the initial manifestation of a lymphoma that had been hidden until that moment and that may have developed in the paraaortic, pelvic, or other lymph nodes. Third, the tumor may be a primary testicular tumor.

The literature questions the existence of primary testicular lymphoma (Melicow, 1955; Tanenbaum and associates, 1972). Nevertheless, it must be admitted that it is a present-day reality. There are patients who, with no other treatment but orchidectomy (occasionally associated with regional lymph node irradiation), live free of disease for over 60 months (Eckert and Smith, 1963; Gowing, 1976; Wooley and co-authors, 1976).

Nevertheless, the criteria for testicular lymphoma diagnosis are not the same in the different previously reported papers. They are as follows: a testicular mass as the first sign of lymphoma (Wooley and others, 1976); an increase in testicular size as the first and principal symptom when previous or synchronous lymphoma affectation is absent (Talerman, 1977); patients in whom the lymphoma appeared to have originated primarily in the testis, although some had clinical supraclavicular, abdominal, pelvic or inguinal lymph node involvement (Jackson and Montessori, 1980); or somewhat stricter criteria like those of Paladugu and associates (1980) which demand: (1) that the testis be the site of the principal tumor mass; (2) that there be no clinical evidence of lymph node involvement at the time of diagnosis; (3) that the diagnosis be histologically confirmed before initiating treatment; and (4) that the minimum survival time be at least six months.

The frequency of primary testicular lymphoma is difficult to establish given the different criteria used in its diagnosis. A review of our material suggests that it constituted approximately 3.2 percent of primary testicular tumors.

The age of presentation varies between eight and seventy-eight years of age, but the average age is 64. In patients over fifty, 25 to 50 percent of the testicular tumors have a lymphoreticular lineage. Primary testicular lymphomas show no preference for either testis, and no higher frequency has been registered in cryptorchid or ectopic testes, or those with inflammatory or traumatic antecedents. Testicular lymphoma is frequently bilateral (21 percent of the cases). It is synchronous in 4 percent of the cases and metachronous in 17 percent, which makes it the tumor which most commonly affects both testes.

Grossly, primary testicular lymphomas produce a symetrical increase in testicular size. When cut they are greyish, soft, and have a certain tendency towards forming nodules. The testicular parenchyma gradually disappears, and can either not be recognizable, or else be reduced to a small peripherical crescent. The epididymis is affected in over half the cases.

Microscopically the tumor cells form thick cords or a sheet separating the seminiferous tubules and causing the seminiferous epithelium to atrophy (Fig. 21-14**B** and **C**). The most preserved tubules only contain Sertoli cells and a few spermatogonia. Most of the tubules are hyalinized. Unlike other primary tumors, necrotic or hemorrhagic zones are usually not identified. Blood vessels are frequently infiltrated. Reticular fibers are abundant and tend to form concentric rings around the most preserved tubules and between the tumor cells.

It is difficult to ascertain cytologically which class of lymphoma primarily affects the testis. There are several reasons for this: lymphoma classification criteria are still not definitive and it is difficult to apply them to lymphomas outside the lymph nodes; the low incidence of testicular lymphoma; and the necessity for the use of immunohistochemical techniques when one desires to definitively classify some cases.

Our cases, as well as the previously reported cases, are all diffuse forms with no testicular nodular lymphomas being recognized. In a study by Jackson and Montessori (1980) on 16 testicular lymphomas (that originally had been considered to be histiocytic in Rappaport's (1966) classification, and were reclassified following Lukes and Collins's (1974) criteria), six of the original cases could be included within the lymphoma group known as large cleaved cell, five in the large noncleaved cell, and the other five in the large noncleaved cell probably of the immunoblastic sarcoma subtype. One of our cases was, in its day, considered to be a reticulosarcoma, and turned out to be an immunoblast sarcoma. Other authors report similar experiences. Talerman (1977) also arrived at the conclusion that one third of testicular lymphomas have a plasmacytoid differentiation. Only isolated cases of testicular plasmocytoma have been reported (Soumerai and others, 1980).

Once a testicular lymphoma has been diagnosed, a lymphangiogram or preferentially, a laparotomy should be performed to determine the tumor stage. Lymphangiography frequently has false negatives (three patients with negative lymphangiograms, according to Paladugu and co-authors (1980) criteria had metastases in the lymph nodes). The results of liver, para-aortic lymph nodes, spleen, mesenteric lymph nodes, and bone marrow biopsy studies show a high degree of metastases. For these authors, only two out of nine cases turned out to be negative. This reflects even more the difficulty of defining whether the lymphoma is part of a disseminating primary testicular lymphoma and when the testicular involvement is only part of a "hidden" lymphoma. An extremely restrictive criteria would certainly exclude some primary testicular lymphomas.

The high frequency of metastases indicate the poor prognosis of many testicular lymphomas. Only 14.5 percent of the patients have a localized illness or have survived 5 years. An attempt has been made to correlate the cytological picture of the tumor with its evolution, and the bad prognosis of immunoblastic sarcomas, closely followed by large noncleaved cell lymphomas, when compared to the relatively good prognosis of large cleaved lymphomas has been corroborated. Tendencies toward nodularity and sclerosis are thought to be signs of a good prognosis (Talerman, 1977).

The spread patterns followed by testicular lymphomas are the same as those followed by primary testicular tumors. Metastases appear, in this order of frequency, in: lymphatic, iliac, para-aortic, mediastinic and supraclavicular lymph nodes, in 86 percent of the autopsies performed. The same frequency is found in pulmonary involvement; which clearly contrasts with the frequency of pulmonary involvement for testicular germ cell tumors. The key to this large number of pulmonary metastases may be the high proportion of tumor involvement of testicular intraparenchymal veins. The kidney, liver, and brain are also affected in this order, but always in more than 50 percent of cases.

A differential diagnosis is classically raised between primary testicular lymphoma and seminoma, embryonal carcinoma, and idiopathic granulomatous orchitis. Classical or typical seminoma is the tumor most frequently confused with lymphoma (Gowing, 1976). Seminoma cells are larger than those of lymphoma, their cytoplasm is clearer and the nucleus contains one or two large nucleoli; the cellular outline is more distinct. Abundant glycogen is observed with the Best's carmin stain. Silver impregnation techniques show few reticular fibers condensing in sclerosed zones or around the seminiferous tubules, while in lymphomas, reticular fibers surround each cell and form concentric rings around the seminiferous tubules (Melicow, 1955). The lymphocytes present in most seminomas are mature and are placed along the connective tissue septa separating the tumor cell masses. Typically seminomas usually appear in young adults. Embryonal carcinoma is characterized by the epithelial appearance of the tumor cells, and tubular, papillary, or glandular structures are observed.

The inflammatory infiltrate found in idiopathic granulomatous orchitis affects the seminiferous tubule walls until they are destroyed. The infiltrates are focal in the early stages and polymorphic, including histiocytary cells, macrophages, plasma cells, lymphocytes and eosinophilic leukocytes, in the more advanced stages. Instead of the tubular atrophy observed in lymphomas, the seminiferous tubules contain macrophages in the idiopathic granulomatous orchitis. This typical cellular polymorphism in idiopathic granulomatous orchitis suggests a differential diagnosis more with Hodgkin lymphoma rather than with non-Hodgkin lymphomas. However, it must be said that well-documented primary testicular Hodgkin lymphomas are unknown.

Even though the tumor is Stage I (localized exclusively in the testis), orchidectomy followed by combined chemotherapy is the most advisable treatment for testicular lymphomas. Central nervous system prophylaxis with intrathecal metrotrexate, cytosine arabinosides, or cranial irradiation are strongly suggested in Stage II and III tumors.

Secondary Testicular Tumors

Secondary testicular tumors are rare, except for testicular involvement occurring in the course of leukemia and lymphomas. In order of frequency: bronchial carcinoma, prostate adenocarcinoma, and even more infrequently, renal adenocarcinoma, melanomas, and tumors of the gastrointestinal tract, pancreas, adrenal cortex, retina, urinary bladder, ureter, biliary duct system, salivary glands, penis, contralateral testis and appendix can metastasize in the testis (Pienkos and Jablokow, 1972; Werth and co-authors, 1982). Price and Mostofi (1957) have observed several cases in which the metastases simulated a primary testicular tumor.

Intratesticular Spermatic Duct Tumors

The most frequent tumor of the intratesticular duct system is the *rete testis adenocarcinoma*. This tumor is preferentially cystic; its growth compresses and atrophies the testicular parenchyma. It appears in adults during the fifth and sixth decades of life (Whitehead and associates, 1972; Turner and Williamson, 1973).

Histologically this tumor is constituted by a cubic or columnar epithelium consisting of cells with elongated, pale nucleus and scarce cytoplasm. The epithelial lining frequently forms papillas and the number of mitoses and atypias is usually low. The stroma supporting the tumor tends to display marked collagenization (Fig. 21-15).

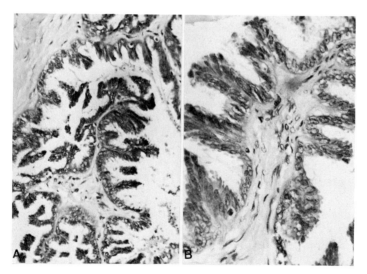

FIGURE 21–15. *Rete testis adenocarcinoma. A, Cellular proliferation adopting papillar pattern over highly hyalinized stroma. H&E (x60). B, Tumor papilla constituted by a central axis of connective tissue and an external coat of cylindrical cells with vesiculous nucleus that are occasionally ciliated. H&E x125).*

Before diagnosing rete testis adenocarcinoma, the possibility of adenocarcinoma metastasis from other sites, mesothelioma or rete testis infiltration by seminoma cells should be considered.

The criteria for differential diagnosis between rete testis adenocarcinoma and other testicular tumors include: preferential involvement of testicular mediastinum, absence of direct extension through the tunica albuginea, demonstration of transition from the tumor cells to the normal rete testis cells, lack of histological or hormonal evidence for teratoma, and absence of any other primary tumor.

In some cases radiotherapy or chemotherapy have been associated with orchiectomy when recurrence or metastasis developed (Gisser and others, 1977). Metastases develop in lymph nodes, lungs, skin, liver and bones, in order of decreasing frequency. Most patients die within the first year after diagnosis.

REFERENCES

1. Altman BL, Malament M: Carcinoma of the testis following orchidopexy. J Urol 97:498, 1967
2. Azer PC, Braunstein GD: Malignant Leydig cell tumor: objective tumor response to O,P'-DDD. Cancer 47:1251, 1981
3. Azzopardi JG, Mostofi FK, Theiss EA: Lesions of testes observed in certain patients with widespread choriocarcinoma and related tumors. Am J Pathol 38:207, 1961
4. Azzopardi JG, Hoffbrand AV: Retrogression in testicular seminoma with viable metastasis. J Clin Pathol 18:135, 1965
5. Babaian RJ, Johnson DE: Management of stages I and II nonseminomatous germ cell tumors of the testis. Cancer 45:1775, 1980
6. Bach DW, Weissbach L, Hartlapp JH: Bilateral testicular tumor. J Urol 129:989, 1983
7. Bär W, Hedinger C: Comparison of histologic types of primary testicular germ cell tumors-consequences for the WHO and the British nomenclatures Virchows Arch. A Path Anat and Histol 370:41, 1976
8. Batata MA, Whitmore WF, Hilaris BS, Tokita N, Grabstald H: Cancer of the undescended or maldescended testis. Am J Roentgenol 126:302, 1976
9. Berdjis CC, Mostofi FK: Carcinoid tumors of the testis. J Urol 118:777, 1977
10. Bloom W, Fawcett DW: A textbook of histology. Philadelphia-London-Toronto: W.B. Saunders Co., 1975, 10th ed
11. Bredael JJ, Vugrin D, Whitmore WF: Recurrences in surgical stage I nonseminomatous germ cell tumors of the testis. J Urol 130:476, 1983
12. Brodner CG, Grube D, Helmstaedter V, Kreienbrink ME, Wurster K, Forssmann

WG: Endocrine GEP-cells in primary testicular teratoma. Virchows Arch A Path Anat and Histol 388:251, 1980
13. Brown NJ: In Pugh R.C. (ed) Pathology of the testis Oxford, England: Blackwell Scientific Publications, 1976
14. Caldamone AA, Altebarmakian V, Frank IN, Linke Ch A: Leydig cell tumor of testis. Urology 14:39, 1979
15. Caldwell WL, Kademian MT, Frias Z, Davis TE: The management of testicular seminomas. Cancer 45:1768, 1980
16. Calman FM, Peckham MJ, Hendry WF: The pattern of spread and treatment of metastasis in testicular seminoma. Brit J Urol 51:154, 1979
17. Campbell HE: Incidence of malignant growth of the undescended testicle. Arch Surg 44:353, 1942
18. Carr BI, Gilchrist KW, Carbone PP: The variable transformation in metastases from testicular germ cell tumors: the need for selective biopsy. J Urol 126:52, 1981
19. Champlin HW: Similar tumors of testis occurring in identical twins. JAMA 95:96, 1930
20. Cockburn AG, Vugrin D, Batata M, Hajdu S, Whitmore WF: Second primary germ cell tumors in patients with seminoma of the testis. J Urol 130:357, 1983
21. Collins DH, Pugh RC: The Pathology of testicular tumors. London: E.S. Livingstone Ltd., 1964
22. Crawford ED, Cain DR, Black WC, Borden TA: Inguinal lymph node metastases following a torek orchiopexy. Urology 21:300, 1983
23. Cricco CF, Buck AS: Hemangioendothelioma of testis. Second reported case. J Urol 123:131, 1980
24. Crump WD: Juvenile granulosa cell (sex cord-stromal) tumor of fetal testis. J Urol 129:1057, 1983
25. Damjanov I, Niejadlik DC, Jeffrey V, Rabuffo V, Donadio JA: Cribiform and sclerosing seminoma devoid of lymphoid infiltrates. Arch Pathol Lab Med 104:527, 1980
26. Davis S, Dimartino NA, Schneider G: 17-β-hydroxysteroid dehydrogenase deficiency in malignant interstitial cell carcinoma of the testis. J Clin Endocrinol Metab 51:1293, 1980
27. D'Esposito RF, Ferraro LR, Wogalter H: Hemangioma of the testis in an infant. J Urol 116:677, 1976
28. Dixon FJ, Moore RA: Testicular tumors; a clinicopathological study. Cancer 6:427, 1953
29. Dixon FJ, Moore RA: Tumors of the male sex organs. In Atlas of Tumor Pathology. Washington D.C.: Armed Forces Institute of Pathology, 1952, sec. 8, fasc. 31b and 32, p. 120
30. Doornbos JF, Hussey DH, Johnson DE: Radiotherapy for pure seminoma of the testis. Radiology 116:401, 1975
31. Dorman S, Trainer TD, Lefke D, Leadbetter G: Incipient germ cell tumor in a cryptorchid testis. Cancer 44:1357, 1979
32. Eckert H, Smith JP: Malignant lymphoma of the testis. Brit Med J 2:891, 1963
33. Einhorn LH, Williams SD: Chemotherapy of disseminated testicular cancer. A random prospective study. Cancer 45:1339, 1980
34. Evans RW: Developmental stages of embryolike bodies in teratoma testis. J Clin Pathol 10:31, 1957
35. Ewing J: Neoplastic diseases. A treatise of tumors. Philadelphia-London: W.B. Saunders Co., 1942, 4th ed
36. Exelby PR: Testicular cancer in children. Cancer 45:1803, 1980
37. Friedman NB, Moore RA: Tumors of the testis: A report on 992 cases. Milit Surgeon 99:573, 1946
38. Friedman M, Pearlman AW: Seminoma with trophocarcinoma. Cancer 26:46, 1970
39. Fukutani K, Libby JM, Panko WB, Scardino PT: Human chorionic gonadoptropin detected in urinary concentrates from patients with malignant tumors of the testis, prostate, bladder, ureter and kidney. J Urol 129:74, 1983
40. Gabrilove JL, Freiberg EK, Leiter E, Nicolis GL: Feminizing and non-feminizing Sertoli cell tumors. J Urol 124:757, 1980
41. Galian PH, Ganter P, Galian G, Delesque M, Dadoune JP, Abelanet R: Etude anatomopathologique, ultrastructurale et histoenzymologique de deux cas d'inclusions corticosurreniennes intra-testiculaires. Virchows Arch A Path Anat and Histol 354:239, 1971
42. Gallager HS, Lewis RP: Sequential gonadoblastoma and choriocarcinoma. Obstet Gynecol 41:123, 1973
43. Gehring GG, Rodríguez FR, Woodhead DM: Malignant degeneration of cryptorchid testes following orchiopexy. J Urol 112:354, 1974
44. Gharpure VV: A case of malignant interstitial-cell tumor of the testis in man. J Pathol Bacteriol 62:113, 1950
45. Gisser SD, Nayak S, Kaneko M, Tchertkoff V: Adenocarcinoma of the rete testis: A review of the literature and presentation of a case with associated asbestosis. Hum Pathol 8:219, 1977
46. Gitlin D, Perricelli A: Synthesis of serum albumin, prealbumin, α-foetoprotein, α_1-antitrypsin and transferrin by the human yolk sac. Nature 288:995, 1970
47. Gowing NF: Malignant lymphoma of the tes-

tis. In Pugh RC (ed) Pathology of the testis. London: Blackwell Scientific Publications, 1976 p. 334
48. Gracia R, Nistal M, Gallego ME, Lledó G, Oliver A, Utrilla J, Gancedo P: Tumor de células de Leydig con pseudopubertad precoz. An Esp Pediat 13:593, 1980
49. Heyderman E, Neville AM: Syncytiotrophoblasts in malignant testicular tumours. Lancet 2:103, 1976
50. Holstein AF, Körner F: Light and electron microscopical analysis of cell types in human seminoma. Virchows Arch A Path Anat and Histol 363:97, 1974
51. Honoré LH, Sullivan LD: Intratesticular leiomyoma: a case report with discussion of differential diagnosis and histogenesis. J Urol 114:631, 1975
52. Honoré LH: Fatty metaplasia in a postpubertal undescended testis: A case report. J Urol 122:841, 1979
53. Hugues FC, Caron M: Les tumeurs leydigiennes Etude generale a propos d'une observation. Sem Hop Paris 52:1157, 1976
54. Ishida T, Tagatz GE, Okagaki T: Gonadoblastoma. Ultrastructural evidence for testicular origin. Cancer 37:1770, 1976
55. Jackson SM, Montessori GA: Malignant lymphoma of the testis: Review of 17 cases in British Columbia with survival related to pathological subclassification. J Urol 123:881, 1980
56. Janssen M, Johnston WH: Anaplastic seminoma of the testis. Ultrastructural analysis of 3 cases. Cancer 41:538, 1976
57. Javadpour N: The role of biologic tumor markers in testicular cancer. Cancer 45:1755, 1980
58. Javadpour N, Chen H: Improved human chorionic gonadotropin detection with carboxyl-terminal radioimmunoassay of the beta subunit on concentrated 24-hour urine in patients with testicular cancer. J Urol 126:176, 1981
59. Jeffs RD: Management of embryonal adenocarcinoma of the testis in childhood: an analysis of 164 cases. "Cancer in childhood." Proceedings of the 17th Clinical Conference of the Ontario Cancer Research Foundation. Golden JO (ed) New York: Plenum Press, 1973, p. 68
60. Johnson DE, Gómez JJ, Ayala AG: Anaplastic seminoma. J Urol 114:80, 1975
61. Kalis EG, Goulandris ND: Androblastoma-Sertoli cell tumour. J Urol 112:618, 1974
62. Kleinsmith LJ, Pierce BG: Multipotentiality of single embryonal carcinoma cells. Cancer Res 24:1544, 1964
63. Klippel RF, Jonas U, Hohenfellner R, Walther D: Interstitial tumor of testis: a delicate problem. Urology 14:79, 1979
64. Kubelka J, Sarkar NN, Belitsky P: Familial occurrence of testicular neoplasia: case report of testicular seminoma in father and son. J Urol 130:140, 1983
65. Kurman RJ, Scardino PT, McIntire KR, Waldmann TA, Javadpour N: Cellular localization of alpha-fetoprotein and human chorionic gonadotropin in germ cell tumors of the testis using an indirect immunoperoxidase technique. A new approach to classification utilizing tumor markers. Cancer 40:2136, 1977
66. Lee F, Pérez CA: Radiation therapy in the management of testicular tumors. J Urol 111:201, 1974
67. Levey S, Grabstald H: Synchronous testicular tumors in identical twins. Urology 6:754, 1975
68. Lipsett MB, Sarfaty GA, Wilson H, Bardin GW, Fishman LM: Metabolism of testosterone and related steroids in metastatic interstitial cell coriocarcinoma of the testis. J Clin Invest 45:1700, 1966
69. Livolsi VA, Schiff M: Myxoid neurofibroma of the testis. J Urol 118:341, 1977
70. Lockhardt JL, Dalton DL, Vellmor RT, Glenn FP: Nonfunctioning interstitial cell carcinoma of the testis. Urology 8:392, 1976
71. Lubetzki J, Guillausseau PJ, Galian A, Guillausseau Cl, Piel-Desruisseaux JL, Cedard L, Wassef M, Mosse A, Evard D: Tumeur testiculaire à cellules de Leydig chez l'adulte: Un cas avec études clinique, biologique, anatomo-pathologique (optique ultrastructurale). Ann Med Interne 1311:157, 1980
72. Lukes RJ, Collins RD: Immunologic characterization of human malignant lymphomas. Cancer 34:1488, 1974
73. Maier JG, Mittemeyer BT, Sulak MH: Treatment and prognosis in seminoma of the testis. J Urol 90:72, 1968
74. Maier JG, Sulak MH: Radiation therapy in malignant testis tumors. Part II: Carcinoma Cancer 32:1217, 1973
75. Mantoudis SM, Apostolidis NS, Legakis NC, Philippakis MG: Sertoli cell tumour of the testis. Brit J Urol 51:412, 1979
76. Marincek B, Brutschin P, Triller J, Fuchs WA: Lymphography and computed tomography in staging nonseminomatous testicular cancer: limited detection of early stage of metastatic disease. Urol Radiol 5:243, 1983
77. Marshall FF, Kerr WS, Kliman B, Scully RE: Sex cord-stromal (gonadal stromal) tumors of the testis: A report of 5 cases. J Urol 117:180, 1977
78. Marshall S, Lyon RP, Scott MP: a conserv-

ative approach to testicular tumors in children: 12 cases and their management. J Urol 129:350, 1983
79. Martin GR: Teratocarcinomas as a model system for the study of embryogenesis and neoplasia. Cell 5:229, 1975
80. Masson, P.: Etude sur le séminome. Rev Canad Biol 5:361, 1946
81. Melicow MM: Classification of tumors of testis: a clinical and pathological study based on 105 primary and 13 secondary cases in adults, and 3 primary and 4 secondary cases in children. J Urol 73:547, 1955
82. Meyer R: Tubuläre (testikuläre) und solide Formen des Andreioblastoma Ovarii und ihre Beziehung zur Vermännlichung. Beitr. Z Path Anat U Z Allg Path 84:485, 1930
83. Morehead RP, Thomas WC: Cavernous hemangioma of the testicle. J Urol 51:548, 1944
84. Morin LJ, Loening S: Malignant androblastoma (Sertoli cell tumor) of the testis. A case report with a review of the literature. J Urol 114:476, 1975
85. Morris SA, Vaughan ED, Constable WC: Problems in management of primary bilateral germ cell testicular tumors: report of 3 cases and review of literature. J Urol 115:566, 1976
86. Mostofi FK, Theiss EA, Ashley DJB: Tumors of specialized gonadal stroma in human male subjects. Cancer 12:944, 1959
87. Mostofi FK: Testicular tumors; epidemiologic, etiologic, and pathologic features. Cancer 32:1186, 1973
88. Mostofi FK, Price EB: Tumors of the male genital system. In Atlas of Tumor Pathology. Washington D.C.: Armed Forces Institute of Pathology, 1973, series 2, fasc. 8
89. Mostofi FK, Sobin LH: In International histological classification of tumors. n. 16. Geneva, Switzerland: World Health Organization, 1977
90. Mostofi FK: Pathology of germ cell tumor of testis. A progress report. Cancer 45:1735, 1980
91. Munro AJ, Dunca W, Webb JN: Extragonadal presentations of germ cell tumours. Brit J Urol 55:547, 1983
92. Nagel LR, Polley VB: Epidermoid cyst of the testis. J Urol 73:124, 1955
93. Newell, ME, Lippe BM, Ehrlich RM: Testes tumors associated with congenital adrenal hyperplasia: a continuing diagnostic and therapeutic dilemma. J. Urol 117:256, 1977
94. Nistal M, López-Rubio F, Figols J: Tumor de células de Leydig. Estudio ultraestructural. Arch Esp Urol 27:301, 1974
95. Nistal M, Paniagua R, Regadera J, Abaurrea MA: Testicular capillary hemangioma. Brit J Urol 54:433, 1982
96. Nogales-Fernández F, Silverberg SG, Bloustein PA: Yolk sac carcinoma (endodermal sinus tumor). Ultrastructure and histogenesis of gonadal and extragonadal tumors in comparison with normal human yolk sac. Cancer 39:1462, 1977
97. Ober WB, Kabakow B, Hecht H: Malignant interstitial cell tumor of the testes: a problem in endocrine oncology. Bull NY Acad Med 52:561, 1976
98. Paladugu RR, Bearman RM, Rappaport H: Malignant lymphoma with primary manifestation in the gonad. A clinicopathologic study of 38 patients. Cancer 45:561, 1980
99. Pérez C, Novoa J, Alcañiz J, Salto L, Barceló B: Leydig cell tumor of the testis with gynaecomastia and elevated estrogen, progesterone and prolactin levels: case report. Clin Endocrinol 13:409, 1980
100. Perry C, Servandio C: Seminoma in childhood. J Urol 124:932, 1980
101. Pienkos EJ, Joblokow VR: Secondary testicular tumors. Cancer 30:481, 1972
102. Pierce GB: The pathogenesis of testicular tumors. J Urol 88:573, 1962
103. Pierce GB, Beals TF: The ultrastructure of primordial germinal cells of the fetal testis and of embryonal carcinoma cells of mice. Cancer Res 24:1553, 1964
104. Pierce GB: Ultrastructure of human testicular tumors. Cancer 19:1963, 1966
105. Pierce GB, Bullock WK, Huntington RW: Yolk sac tumor of the testis. Cancer 25:644, 1970
106. Pierce GB, Abell MA: Embryonal carcinoma of the testis. Pathology annual, Sommers Sheldon C, (series ed) New York: Appleton-Century-Crofts, 1970, p. 27.
107. Powell S, Hendry WF, Peckham MJ: Occult germ-cell testicular tumours. Brit J Urol 55:440, 1983
108. Price EB, Mostofi FK: Secondary carcinoma of the testis. Cancer 10:592, 1957
109. Price EB, Mostofi FK: Epidermoid cyst of the testis: a clinical and pathological analysis of 69 cases from the Testicular Tumor Registry. J Urol 102:708, 1969
110. Proppe KH, Dickersin, GR: Large-cell calcifying Sertoli cell tumor of the testis: light microscopic and ultrastructural study. Hum Pathol 13:1109, 1982
111. Proppe KH, Scully RE: Large cell calcifying Sertoli cell tumor of the testis: a report of ten cases and a review of two cases from the literature. Am J Clin Pathol 74:607, 1980
112. Pugh RC, Cameron KM: Teratoma. In Pugh RC (ed) Pathology of the testis. Oxford-London-Edinburgh-Melbourne: Blackwell Scientific Publications, 1976

113. Pugh RC: Pathology of the testis, Pugh RC (ed). Oxford-London-Edinburgh-Melbourne: Blackwell Scientific Publications, 1976
114. Quivey JM, Fu KK, Herzog KA, Weiss JM, Phillips TL: Malignant tumors of the testis: analysis of treatment, results and sites and causes of failure. Cancer 39:1247, 1977
115. Raghavan D, Jelihovsky T, Fox RM: Father-son testicular malignancy. Does genetic anticipation occur? Cancer 45:1005, 1980
116. Rappaport H: Tumors of the hematopoietic system. In Atlas of Tumor Pathology, Washington D.C.: Armed Forces Institute of Pathology, 1966, sec. 3, fasc. 8
117. Ray B, Hajou SI, Whitmore WF: Distribution of retroperitoneal lymph node metastases in testicular tumors. Cancer 33:340, 1974
118. Rosai J, Silber I, Khodadoust K: Spermatocytic seminoma. 1. Clinicopathologic study of six cases and review of the literature. Cancer 24:92, 1969a
119. Rosai J, Khodadoust K, Silber I: Spermatocytic seminoma. 2. Ultrastructural study. Cancer 24:103, 1969b
120. Samuel A, Tweedale DN: Epidermoid cyst of the testicle: report of a case and review of the literature. J Urol 85:311, 1961
121. Sause WT: Testicular seminoma—analysis of radiation therapy for Stage II disease. J Urol 130:702, 1983
122. Schoborg TW, Whittaker J, Lewis CW: Metastatic spermatocytic seminoma. J Urol 124:739, 1980
123. Schütte B, Holstein AF, Schulze C, Schirren C: Zur Problematik der Früherkennung eines Seminoms. Nachweis von Tumorzellen in der Biopsie aus den Hoden von 5 Patienten mit Oligozoospermie. Andrologia 13:521, 1981
124. Scully RE: Gonadoblastoma. A gonadal tumor related to the dysgerminoma (seminoma) and capable of sex hormone production. Cancer 6:455, 1953
125. Scully RE: Gonadoblastoma: A review of 74 cases. Cancer 25:1340, 1970
126. Shah KH, Maxted WC, Chun B: Epidermoid cysts of the testis: A report of three cases and an analysis of 141 cases from the world literature. Cancer 47:577, 1981
127. Shawker TH, Javadpour N, O'Leary T, Shapiro E, Krudy AG: Ultrasonographic detection of "burned-out" primary testicular germ cell tumors in clinically normal testes. J Ultrasound Med 2:477, 1983
128. Shemiakin OS: Leydig cell tumor with metastases in liver and spine. Arch Pathol 33:77, 1971
129. Shimp WS, Schultz AL, Hastings JR, Anderson WR: Leydig cell tumor of the testis with gynecomastia and elevated estrogen levels. Am J Clin Path 67:562, 1977
130. Shinohara M, Komatsu H, Kawamura T, Yokoyama M: Familial testicular teratoma in 2 children: familial report and review of the literature. J Urol 123:552, 1980
131. Shulze C, Holstein AF: On the histology of human seminoma. Development of the solid tumor from intratubular seminoma cells. Cancer 39:1090, 1977
132. Skakkebaek NE: Possible carcinoma-in-situ of the testis. Lancet 2:516, 1972
133. Skakkebaek NE: Atypical germ cell in the adjacent "normal" tissue of testicular tumors. Acta Path Microbiol Scand Sct A, 83 A, 127, 1975
134. Slawson RG: Radiation therapy for germinal tumors of the testes. Cancer 42:2216, 1978
135. Sohval AR, Churg J, Gabrilove JL: Ultrastructure of feminizing testicular Leydig cell tumors. Ultrastructural Pathology 3:335, 1982
136. Sohval AR, Chung J, Suzuki Y, Katz N, Gabrilove JL: Effects of a feminizing testicular Leydig cell tumour on nontumorous testicular tissue: an ultrastructural study. Clin Endocrin 6:127, 1977
137. Soumerai S, Gleason EA: Asynchronous plasmacytoma of the stomach and testis. Cancer 45:396, 1980
138. Stein JJ: Hemangioendothelioma of the testis. J Urol 113:201, 1975
139. Stevens LC: Origin of testicular teratomas from primordial germ cells in mice. J Natl Cancer Inst 38:549, 1967
140. Sullivan MP, Pérez CA, Herson J, Silva-Sousa M, Land V, Dyment PG, Chan R, Ayala RG: Radiotherapy (2500 rad) for testicular leukemia: local control and subsequent clinical events: a Southwest oncology group study. Cancer 46:508, 1980
141. Sworn MJ, Buchanan R: Malignant interstitial cell tumor of the testis. Hum Pathol 12:72, 1981
142. Talerman A: The incidence of yolk sac tumor (endodermal sinus tumor) elements in germ cell tumors of the testis in adults. Cancer 36:211, 1975
143. Talerman A: Primary malignant lymphoma of the testis. J Urol 118:783, 1977
144. Talerman A, Haije WG, Baggerman L: Serum alphafetoprotein (AFP) in patients with germ cell tumors of the gonads and extragonadal sites: correlation between endodermal sinus (yolk sac) tumor and raised serum AFP. Cancer 46:380, 1980a
145. Talerman A: Spermatocytic seminoma. Clinicopathological study of 22 cases. Cancer 45:2169, 1980b

146. Talerman A: Endodermal sinus (yolk sac) tumor elements in testicular germ-cell tumors in adults: comparison of prospective and retrospective studies. Cancer 46:1213, 1980c
147. Tanenbaum B, Sandford RS, Elquezabal A, Klinger ME: Testicular tumor: presenting sign of lymphoma. Cancer 29:1223, 1972
148. Teilum G: Estrogen-producing Sertoli cell tumors (androblastoma tubulare lipoides) of human testis and ovary; homologous ovarian and testicular tumors. III. J Clin Endocrinol 9:301, 1949
149. Teilum G: Special tumours of the ovary and testis. Comparative pathology and histological identification. Copenhagen: Munksgaard 1976, 2nd ed, p. 31
150. Teoh TB, Steward JK, Willis RA: The distinctive adenocarcinoma of the infant testis: an account of 15 cases. J Pathol Bacteriol 80:147, 1960
151. Thomson WO, Sinclair DM: Familial teratoma of testes. Brit J Urol 49:322, 1977
152. Turner RW, Williamson J: Andenocarcinoma of the rete testis. J Urol 109:850, 1973
153. Vaitukaitis JL, Braunstein GD, Ross GT: A radioimmunoassay which specifically measures human chorionic gonadotropin in the presence of human luteinizing hormone. Am J Obstet Gynecol 113:751, 1972
154. Von Eyben FE, Mikulowski P, Busch C: Microinvasive germ cell tumors of the testis. J Urol 126:842, 1981
155. Vugrin D, Cvitkovic E, Cheng E, Grabstald H, Golbey RB: Chemotherapy of testicular carcinoma with VAB IV. Proc Amer Soc Clin Oncol 20:338, 1979
156. Vugrin D, Cvitkovic E, Whitmore WF, Cheng E, Golbey, RB: VAB-4 combination chemotherapy in the treatment of metastatic testis tumors. Cancer 47:833, 1981a
157. Vugrin D, Whitmore WF, Cvitkovic E, Grabstald H, Sogani P, Barzell W, Golbey RD: Adjuvant chemotherapy combination of vinblastine, actinomycin D, bleomycin, and chlorambucil following retroperitoneal lymph node dissection for stage II testis tumor. Cancer 47:840, 1981b
158. Wajsman Z, Beckley SA, Pontes JE: Changing concepts in the treatment of advanced seminomatous tumors. J Urol 129:303, 1983
159. Waldmann TA, McIntire KR: The use of radioimmunassay for alphafetoprotein in the diagnosis of malignancy. Cancer 34:1510, 1974
160. Walter P: Séminome spermatocytaire. Etude de 8 observations et revue de la littérature. Virchows Arch A Path Anat and Histol 386:175, 1980
161. Waxman M: Malignant germ cell tumor insitu in a cryptorchid testis. Cancer 38:1452, 1976
162. Werth V, Yu G, Marshall FF: Nonlymphomatous metastatic tumor to the testis. J Urol 127, 142, 1982
163. Whitehead ED, Valensi QJ, Brown JS: Adenocarcinoma of the rete testis. J Urol 107:992, 1972
164. Williams TR, Brendler H: Carcinoma in situ of the ectopic testis. J Urol 117:610, 1977
165. Willis RA: Pathology of tumors, New York: Appleton-Century-Crofts 1967, 4th ed
166. Wittes RE, Yagoda A, Silvay O: Chemotherapy of germ cell tumors of the testis. I. Induction of remission with vinblastine, actinomycin D and bleomycin. Cancer 37:637, 1976
167. Wooley PV, Osborne CK, Levi JA, Wiernik PH, Canellos GP: Extranodal presentation of non-Hodgkin lymphoma in the testis. Cancer 38, 1026 (1976)
168. Yoneda F, Kagawa S, Kurokawa K: Dystrophic calcifying nodule with osteoid metaplasia of the testis. Brit J Urol 51:413, 1979
169. Ytredal DO, Bradfield JS: Seminoma of the testicle: prophylactic mediastinal irradiation versus periaortic and pelvic irradiation alone. Cancer 30:628, 1972
170. Zattoni F, Wajsman Z, Beckley SA, Lanteri V, Pontes JE: Treatment of sequential bilateral germ cell tumors of the testis following interval retroperitoneal lymph node dissection. J Urol 130:142 1983

22

TUMORS OF THE EPIDIDYMIS AND THE SPERMATIC CORD

TUMORS OF THE EPIDIDYMIS

Primary Tumors

The most frequent benign primary tumors of the epididymis are: adenomatoid tumor; leiomyoma; and papillary cystadenoma. In Beccia and associates' (1976) review of 341 tumors of the epididymis, 75 percent were benign and 25 percent were malignant. Of the 257 benign epididymal tumors, 73 percent (188) were adenomatoid tumors (55 percent of all epididymal tumors, benign and malignant); 11 percent were leiomyomas; 9 percent were papillary cystadenomas; and the remaining 7 percent included angioma, lipoma, dermoid cyst, fibroma, hamartoma, teratoma, cholesteatoma, and so forth. The most frequent malignant primary tumors in the epididymis are sarcomas.

Adenomatoid Tumor

This is the most frequent tumor in the paratesticular structures and corresponds to 32 percent of all tumors in these structures. The term "adenomatoid" tumor was first used by Golden and Ash, in 1945, to emphasize the likely epithelial glandular origin of the tumor. This tumor is preferentially located in the epididymis, although it has also been described in the tunica vaginalis and the spermatic cord. It is not an exclusively male genital system tumor; cases have been reported in the uterus, fallopian tubes, and ovaries (Jackson, 1958; Teel, 1958; Evans, 1943; Fajers, 1949; Akhtar and others, 1976). The most common presentation age is during the fourth and fifth decades of life. It is a slow-growing, asymptomatic tumor.

Macroscopically, these tumors are generally small and round, have a firm, elastic consistency and affect, in order of decreasing frequency: caput; cauda; and corpus epididymis. When cut they are whitish or greyish and fasciculated (Fig. 22–1).

Histologically, they are constituted by two structural types: epithelial cells and fibrous stroma. The epithelial cells from cords or glandular structures. They are cubic or flat cells with vacuolated cytoplasm. The stroma varies from loose to dense and sometimes contains numerous smooth muscular fibers, other times lymphoid tissue, and, in some cases, thick elastic fibers (Nistal and co-authors, 1978). Lymphocyte and monocyte migration into the glandular lumen from the stroma can be observed in most tumors.

The origin of these tumors have been the subject of discussion with several hypotheses being put forward: an endothelial origin suggested by the epithelial clefts; a mesonephric origin (Teilum, 1954); a Müllerian origin (Sundarasivarao, 1953); and a mesothelial origin (Masson et al., 1942). The last hypothesis has been completely confirmed with histochemical and electron microscope studies (MacKay and others, 1971; Ferenczy and associates, 1972). One of the most valuable histochemical findings was the elevated concentration of hyaluronic acid in the adenomatoid tumor, as well as in normal mesothelium (Castor and Naylor, 1969; Wagner and others, 1962), and in the mesotheliomas, in which the mesothelial origin is proven. Ultrastructurally, the cells lining the glandular spaces also show great similarity to those described by Hesseldahl and Larsen (1969) in the human

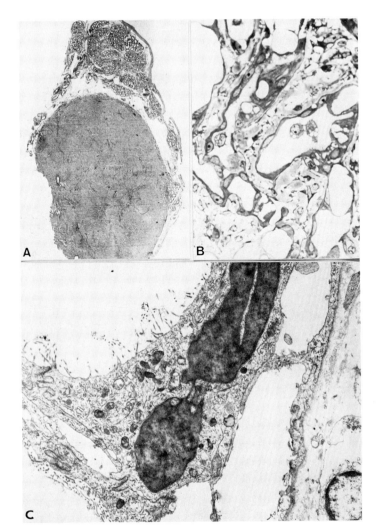

FIGURE 22–1. *Adenomatoid tumor of the epididymis. A, Nodular formation in the caput epididymis displacing the ductuli efferentes toward the periphery. H&E (x3). B, Glandular structures lined by cubical and flat cells containing numerous cytoplasmic vacuoles. One-micron section of epon-embedded material. Toluidine blue (x250). C, Epithelial cells from the glandular structures showing long, thin, apical microvilli as well as inter- and intracellular channels. (x7000).*

mesothelium. These cells possess irregular apical microvilli and sometimes cilia. Junctional complexes at the level of the apical face and twisting intercellular channels can be found between the cells.

The adenomatoid tumor is benign, even though the rete testis and the testicular parenchyma are infiltrated. This infiltration is observed in approximately 40 percent of tumors involving the caput epididymis.

Leiomyoma

This tumor appeared in a proportion of one to every nine adenomatoid tumors. It is bilateral in 15 percent of the patients and is frequently accompanied by hydrocele (5 percent of the cases). The age of maximum incidence is during the fifth decade (Longo and others, 1971). Its structure is similar to that of other leiomyomas located in other sites. The tumor is well delimited and constituted by bundles of smooth muscle cells that show no atypia (Fig. 22–2A).

Papillary Cystadenoma

This is a hamartomatous lesion located in the caput epididymis that is constituted by a papillary proliferation developing inside ectasic ductuli efferentes. In half of the cases the lesion is bilateral

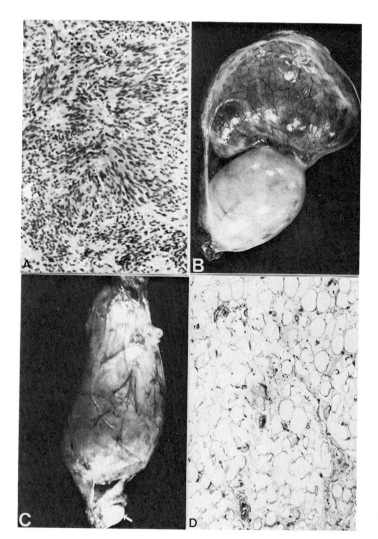

FIGURE 22–2. *A, Fusiform cells, with palisade-forming nuclei in a leiomyoma of the epididymis. H&E (x100). B, Cystadenoma of the epididymis. Cystic tumor in the epididymis derived from the ductuli efferentes in a 17-year-old male with V. Hippel Lindau's syndrome. C and D, Spermatic cord lipoma. C, Large (15 x 6 cm) tumor located in the inguinal duct. Arrow indicates testis. D, Adult adipose cells, separated by connective tissue septa. H&E (x60).*

(Fig. 22–2**B**). It is most frequently diagnosed during the second and third decades, and in addition to other symptoms, suggests the Hippel Lindau syndrome. The unilateral forms of epididymal cystadenoma are considered to be frustrated forms of this syndrome. Patients with bilateral cystadenomas and no other symptoms are probably carriers of an incomplete form of the disease. Papillary cystadenoma has been described as being associated with infertility in patients with severe oligospermia (Crisp and Roberts, 1975) or obstructive azoospermia (López de Santamaría and Bustos-Obregón, 1981).

Viewed grossly, it is a well encapsulated, 1.5 to 5 cm diameter cystic or solid formation that is located in the caput epididymis and can be present asymptomatically for several years. Histologically, it is composed of cysts derived from the ductuli efferentes. The epithelium is cuboid and the cells have vacuolated cytoplasm. Papillary formations grow in the interior of the cysts and can completely occupy them (Grant and Hoffman, 1963; Chan and co-authors, 1968). The cells lining the papillas are the same as the epithelial cells lining the cysts. Focal inflammatory infiltrates, small lipogranulomas, or areas similar to those of hemangioblastoma can be found in the stroma inside the papillas as well as in the capsular stroma (Price, 1971).

Sarcomas

The most frequent primary malignant tumors in the epididymis are sarcomas: fibrosarcoma (see spermatic cord), leiomyosarcoma and rhabdomyosarcoma (see spermatic cord). Sarcomas represent about 44 percent of all malignant tumors of the epididymis (Broth and others, 1968).

Primary leiomyosarcoma of the epididymis is a very rare tumor (only one case out of the 15 paratesticular leiomyosarcomas reported to the *British Testicular Tumor Panel* between 1958 and 1967), in comparison to the relatively high frequency with which it affects other structures of the male genital system such as the spermatic cord (Wallini and associates, 1975; Weitzner, 1967). Isolated cases have been described by Nistal and others (1976), Davides and co-authors (1975) and Farrell and Donnelly (1980).

The tumors highest incidence is at the end of the sixth decade. The macroscopic and microscopic characteristics vary from case to case. The tumors may be so small that they are only detected during surgery. One of the largest tumors was probably the one (over 22 cm in diameter) reported by Singh and Manhas in 1969. Externally, the majority do not have a capsule and they infiltrate the neighboring soft tissues. When cut, the surface is whitish and fasciculated. Hemorrhagic and necrotic areas are not common. Myxoid focal changes may be present. Histologically, the cells form bundles and, in many cases, show the characteristics of the smooth muscle cells (Fig. 22–3). Anysocytosis and anysokaryosis are notable and mitotic figures are frequent. Leiomyosarcoma differs from leiomyoma in the greater cellular polymorphism and the more numerous mitoses and atypias. Leiomyosarcoma preferentially spreads through the circulatory system as the primary leiomyosarcoma of the spermatic cord. Orchioepididymidectomy with high spermatic cord ligature and the local resectioning of neighboring structures, (which in some cases have been infiltrated) seems to be the more advisable treatment. One fourth of the patients show metastasis and recurrence.

Other Tumors

Fibromas (fibrous pseudotumors), some Brenner tumor; neuroectodermal tumor of infancy, and mucinous adenoid tumor cases have been observed in the epididymis.

Brenner Tumor. (Ross, 1968) show a structure like that of its ovarian homologue. It is located below the tunica albuginea, between the testis and the epididymis, and very close to the caput epididymis. Its prognosis is good. Its histogenetic origin is unknown (Goldman, 1970).

Neuroectodermal Tumor of Infancy. or melanotic hamartoma (retinal anlage tumor) (Zone, 1970) appears in the first months of life. The size barely surpasses two centimeters. Microscopically it is formed by two types of cells. One cell type is small, grouped into nests, and shows vesiculated nuclei with large nucleoli. The second cell type has larger cells with eosinophilic cytoplasm containing melanin pigment granulations in a remarkable amount. The stroma of the tumor is fibrous and frequently hyalinized. The mitotic index of tumor cells is low and the prognosis is very good.

Mucinous Adenoid Tumor. described by Mukerjee and associates (1976) is an epididymal tumor composed of epithelial cells, disposed in a tubular or trabecular pattern, and an abundant ground substance that is positive to mucopolysaccharide acid techniques and resistant to hyaluronidase. Since it does not produce

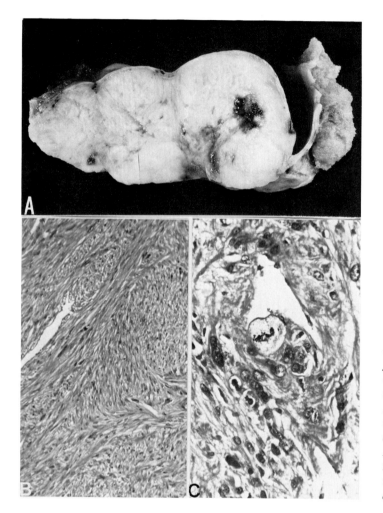

FIGURE 22–3. *Leiomyosarcoma of the epididymis.* **A**, *Voluminous tumor with a fasciculated appearance showing necrotic and hemorrhagic areas. The tumor has not infiltrated the testicular parenchyma, which is recognizable at the right of the picture.* **B**, *Fasciculated distribution of the muscle cells from the above tumor. H&E (x60).* **C**, *Marked cellular pleomorphism with atypical mitotic figures in the same leiomyosarcoma. H&E (x250).*

hyaluronic acid, this tumor cannot be included among classic mesotheliomas in a strict sense; however, until studies on new cases become available, it could be considered as an adenomatoid tumor or a mesothelioma with abundant mucin production. The reported cases displayed capsule invasion but no metastasis.

Secondary Tumors

Among the most frequent secondary tumors of the epididymis the following stand out: infiltration by an ipsilateral testicular tumor; contralateral testicular tumor; and metastasis and infiltration by spermatic cord sarcoma. Metastasis of carcinomas located in several parts of the body (in order of frequency: stomach; prostate; kidney; pancreas and colon) have been observed (Wachtel and Mehan, 1970; Puigvert and co-authors, 1978 Faysal and others, 1983).

TUMORS OF THE SPERMATIC CORD

Ninety percent of the scrotal extratesticular tumors affecting the epididymis, testicular tunica vaginalis, or spermatic cord are believed to originate from spermatic cord structures. Seventy percent of these tumors are benign and the other thirty percent are malignant. The most common benign tumor is lipoma. A great variety of sarcomas represent the malignant tumors (Sogani and associates, 1978). Except for rhabdomyosarcoma, which preferentially affects infants and children, the remaining sarcomas affect patients of advanced age.

Malignant tumors originate preferentially either in the inferior extreme of the spermatic cord or close to the testis. Tumor growth is preferentially intrascrotal. The clinical diagnosis includes: hernia; hydrocele; spermatocele; tuberculosis; syphilis; and tumors of the epididymis and testis. Most of the time, the diagnosis can only be made by the pathologist.

Benign Tumors

Lipoma

Lipoma is the most frequent spermatic cord benign tumor. It represents 66 percent of all benign tumors and nearly half (45 percent) of all spermatic cord tumors (El-Badawi and Al-Ghorab, 1965). It occurs mainly in the fourth and fifth decades. Prepubertal cases are infrequent (Kokotas and Papaharalambous, 1983). Lipoma, in contrast to what occurs with malignant tumors, is usually located in the inguinal canal. Its development is asymptomatic and more than a few cases have been discovered during autopsy. The surface of these tumors is lobulated and frequently they are not perfectly encapsulated. Many times, they are hypertrophic lobules of adipose tissue rather than true lipomas (Fig. 22–2C and D).

Other benign tumors and pseudotumoral lesions of the spermatic cord are:

1. *Dermoid cysts*: they are usually located in the inguinal portion of the spermatic cord.
2. *Lymphangiomas*: these can be located at any level of the spermatic cord.
3. Other tumors that have been described are leiomyomas, neurofibromas, and adrenal cortex heteropias.
4. The following are among the most frequent pseudotumoral lesions: spermatic cord lipogranulomas (Fig. 22–4B), fibromas or fibrous pseudotumors, usually present along the scrotal portion of the spermatic cord, and spermatic cord hematomas.

Spermatic Cord Hematoma

The causes for the spontaneous hemorrhages that occur in all organs and systems of the body can not always be ascertained. Other times manifestations of periarteritis nodosa, arteriovenous malformations, or hemorrhagic diathesis are

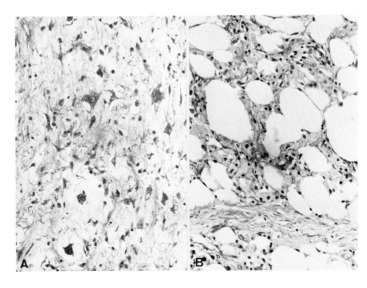

FIGURE 22–4. *A, Liposarcoma of the spermatic cord. Pleomorphic and multinucleated giant cells showing a vacuolated cytoplasm, in a myxoid stroma. H&E (x60). B, Lipogranuloma. Multinucleated giant cells with eosinophilic cytoplasm phagocyting neutral fats. H&E (x60).*

discovered. Spontaneous scrotal hemorrhage has been observed in patients with Henoch-Schönlein's syndrome with anticoagulant therapy after a trauma. A dozen cases of spontaneous idiopathic spermatic cord hematomas are listed in the literature. The typical symptoms develop in the following manner: a young man, after an intense exercise (without direct trauma to the abdominal or scrotal regions) suddenly feels a strong pain followed by swelling and the appearance of a mass within the scrotum (Lerman and Lerman, 1981). The rupture of the spermatic vein and/or one of its branches or the tearing of some of the cremasteric muscle fibers have been suggested as possible causes for this condition.

Malignant Tumors

Of 197 malignant spermatic cord tumors (reviewed by Beccia and others, 1976), 91 percent were sarcomas. Rhabdomyosarcomas, fibrosarcomas, leiomyosarcomas, liposarcomas, mesotheliomas, and more recently, malignant fibrous histiocytomas have been described.

Spermatic cord sarcomas are believed to derive from mesenchymal cells that are trapped inside the spermatic cord without undergoing any differentiation. Under certain circumstances, and for unknown reasons, they would be capable of giving rise to different tumor types by differentiating into fibrous connective, adipose, vascular, or muscular tissues, among others.

Rhabdomyosarcoma

This is the most frequent spermatic cord tumor and occurs primarily during the first decade of life. Viewed grossly, most of tumors appear as intrascrotal masses that reject the testis and epididymis. They are greyish with yellowish areas. Their consistency varies from firm to myxoid (Fig. 22–5).

Histologically, although the tumor can show different patterns that evoke the different stages of skeletal muscle development, several extremely characteristic cell types can be distinguished:

1. Cells with ample, eosinophilic cytoplasm and a peripheric nucleus.
2. Extremely elongated cells with eosinophilic cytoplasm.
3. Strap-like cells
4. Fusiform cells with cross striations.

Cellular polymorphism is very high in some cases.

Of the three histological rhabdomyosarcoma types—embryonal, alveolar, and pleomorphic—the most frequent pattern found in the spermatic cord of children is the embryonal type; nevertheless it is true that 15 percent of the cases show areas of alveolar rhabdomyosarcoma (Regadera and co-authors, 1982). The pleomorphic type is characteristic of adult patients (Kage and others, 1983).

The prognosis for rhabdomyosarcoma depends on various parameters: the clinical stage; patient's age; the localization; and the histological type. The most important of these parameters, and the one that best correlates with the evolution of a tumor, is the clinical stage. The prognosis is worse during the first year of life. Spermatic cord rhabdomyosarcomas are more malignant than those of the orbit, but less aggressive than those of the extraorbital neck and head. Regarding histological pattern, embryonal rhabdomyosarcomas have a more favorable prognosis than the pleomorphic and alveolar varieties. Rhabdomyosarcomas spread through the lymphatic system, preferently to the retroperitoneal lymph nodes (Exelby, 1980; Lawrence and associates, 1977; Malek and others, 1972; Trippitelli and co-authors, 1982).

Treatment of rhabdomyosarcomas of the spermatic cord include a combination of surgery, radiotherapy and chemotherapy. The surgery consists of radical orchiectomy and, if testicular biopsy has been performed, hemiscrotectomy and ipsilateral retroperitoneal and pelvic lymph node removal. Lymph node dissection allow the clinical stage evaluation and helps settle on an adjuvant therapy (Kaplan and co-authors, 1983). Patients with negative retroperitoneal node dissection receive only chemotherapy. The other patients are treated with radiation or chemotherapy. Doses of 3,500 to 4,000 rads are given over any area presenting tumor rests or any zone where positive lymph nodes have been removed. Chemotherapy includes combined cyclic treatment with combined drugs such as: vincristine; bleomycin; cyclophosphamide; adriamycin; actinomycin D; and methrotrexate, according to the guide lines that vary relatively little from one protocol to another (Razek and others, 1977; Rogers and co-authors, 1976; Chavimi and associates, 1975).

The prognosis for rhabdomyosarcoma, which was not good up until 20 years ago, has completely changed and the survival rate of some series is over 80 percent (Sago and Novicki, 1982).

Fibrosarcoma

Spermatic cord fibrosarcomas were reviewed in 1964 by Samellas, who found 21 cases. The number of published cases before Sogani and associates (1978) was 30. These tumors are found in adults, if we except the case of a six-year-old boy reported by Malek and others (1972). Tumor growth is slow and is formed by atypical fibroblasts that synthesize variable quantities of collagen. Fibrosarcomas are locally aggressive tumors that give rise to frequent recurrence, but they do not usually metastasize. Fibrosarcoma of the epididymis behaves in a similar manner.

Leiomyosarcoma

The first known case was reported by Patel and Charlier (1909). Kyle reviewed the literature in 1966 and found 21 cases, to which he added one of his own. New cases, making a total of 30, have been reported by different authors (Malek and others, 1972; Bissada and co-authors, 1976; Jenkins and Subbuswamy, 1972). Histologically, leiomyosarcoma of the spermatic cord is similar to that of the epididymis. Its origin may be in the spermatic vessel walls. These are locally aggressive tumors, prone to recurrence, and they occasionally spread. They spread preferentially by the circulatory system.

Liposarcoma

This is a rare tumor that represents approximately less than four percent of the malignant soft tissue tumors originating in the paratesticular structures (Johnson and associates, 1978). This tumor usually develops in elderly patients. Clinically the tumor can appear as either an increase in scrotal content or as a mass in an inguinal duct. The tumor growth is slow and progressive during up to ten years. Macroscopically it is lobulated, nonencapsulated, with a solid, soft consistency. When cut, the surface is greyish-white and brilliant. Microscopically, most tumors are well differentiated liposarcomas. They are constituted by lipoblasts with a voluminous nucleus and one or several cytoplasmic vacuoles. They are reminiscent of adult adipose tissue in some areas. The marked anysokaryosis, some mitoses, and presence of atypical giant cells are frequent findings. The presence of a "myxoid liposarcoma" pattern considerably helps the diagnosis. Spermatic cord liposarcomas show recurrence, however metastasis is rare (Senoh and others, 1978; Reyes, 1980) (Fig. 22-5A).

Malignant Fibrous Histiocytoma

This is an infrequent tumor that only recently has been described, which affects the spermatic cord (Sogani and co-authors, 1978; Williamson and associates,

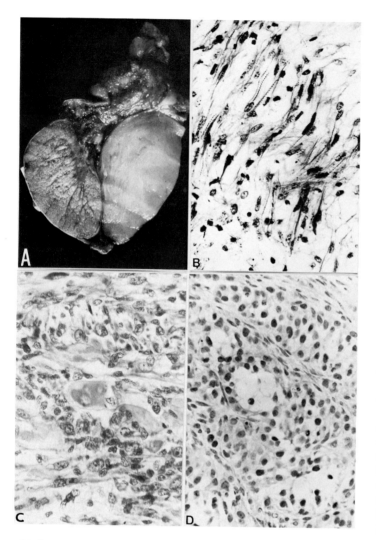

FIGURE 22–5. *Rhabdomyosarcoma of the spermatic cord. A,* Large tumor with a myxoid appearance in the initial segment of the spermatic cord, which rejects the testis. *B,* Rhabdomyoblast cell clump in which cross striation can be seen. P.T.H. (x250). *C,* Markedly pleomorphic tumoral cells. Cross striated multinucleated cells can be seen in the center of the picture. H&E (x250). *D,* Alveolar pattern observed in some areas of the rhabdomyosarcoma shown in A. H&E (x125).

1980). Of 200 malign fibrous histiocytomas collected by Weiss and Enzinger (1978), 68 percent affected extremities, 16 percent affected the abdomen and retroperitoneum, 9 percent affected the trunk, and 3 percent affected the head and neck. These authors expressly mentioned that they observed no case of malignant fibrous histiocytoma in the spermatic cord. Viewed grossly, these tumors are large, firm, greyish-white, nodular and adherent to neighboring structures.

Histologically, they consist of fusiform, fibroblastlike cells, with a voluminous nucleus, which form a storiform pattern mingled with histiocytary cells and an inflammatory infiltrate that varies in intensity from one zone to another. Multinucleate histiocytes with intensely vacuolated cytoplasm and notable atypias are easily recognizable in all cases.

The common treatment for adult spermatic cord sarcomas (fibrosarcomas, leiomyosarcomas, malignant fibrous histiocytomas, and liposarcomas) includes radical orchiectomy and ample local removal (Smailowitz and co-authors, 1983). This treatment seems to be effective only against small tumors that have a low histological level of malignancy. Para-aortic lymphadenectomy as the first part of a treatment followed by irradiation has been proposed in the tumors that are difficult to resect or have medium and high levels of malignancy (Blitzer and others, 1981; Sclama and co-workers, 1983). Chemotherapy, which is so effective in embryonal rhabdomyosarcoma in children, does not appear to be as effective in adults.

Other Tumors

Mesotheliomas (McDonald and others, 1983), as well as several myxomas that are difficult to classify with the present terminology, are other tumors that have been described as occurring in the spermatic cord. Eusebi and Massarelli (1971) have reported a case of pheochromocytoma of the spermatic cord and Krieger and co-authors (1980) have reported a neuroblastoma.

Even though malignant spermatic cord tumors are relatively frequent, other tumor spreading in the spermatic cord are exceptional (Anselmo and associates, 1979). However, metastases of colon, pancreas, prostate, parathyroid gland, and kidney carcinomas have been observed (Marković and others, 1983; Johansson and Lannes, 1983).

INFLAMMATORY PSEUDOTUMOR OF THE EPIDIDYMIS AND THE SPERMATIC CORD. FIBROUS PSEUDOTUMOR. FIBROMA.

Epididymis and spermatic cord pseudotumors are slow-growing reactive processes that eventually form variably-sized nodules. Although many have been described repeatedly as "fibromas" in the literature, we consider "fibrous pseudotumor," used by Mostofi and Price (1973), to be a term that is better adapted to the nature of this tumor.

Approximately two thirds of the fibrous pseudotumors are located in the testicular coverings, ten percent in the epididymis, and the remaining are located in the spermatic cord.

Seen grossly, this is a firm, well-limited lesion that is several centimeters in diameter. When cut, the color depends on the histological structure: whitish for cases with a predominance of fibrous tissue; with yellow areas for cases with inflammatory foci; and toasted brown if there is fat necrosis.

The histological pattern presented by most of these tumors is similar to that of the tunica albuginea pseudotumor, with inflammatory areas, lymphatic nodules, histiocytes, plasma cells, and a variable degree of necrosis. Fibroblast proliferation and the degree of collagenization in the lesion may, on occasion, be so intense as to justify a diagnosis of fibroma.

On other occasions, the histological pattern is that of a lipogranuloma. Besides the unspecific inflammatory infiltrate, in these cases, there are abundant empty spaces corresponding to lipid material that has been phagocytized by giant cells. This picture can be secondary to adipose tissue destruction (endogen lipids), to exogenous lipid, or silicon injections (Oertel and Johnson, 1977). In either case the prognosis is excellent.

REFERENCES

1. Akhtar M, Reyes F, Young I: Elastogenesis in adenomatoid tumor. Histochemical and ultrastructural observations. Cancer 37:338, 1976
2. Anselmo G, Rizzotti A, Gramegna V: A metastatic melanoma in the spermatic cord. Brit J Urol 51:416, 1979
3. Beccia DJ, Krane RJ, Olsson CA: Clinical management of non-testicular intrascrotal tumors. J Urol 116:476, 1976
4. Bissada NK, Finkbeiner AE, Redman JF: Paratesticular sarcomas: review of management. J Urol 116:198, 1976
5. Blitzer PH, Dosoretz DF, Proppe KH, Shipley

WV: Treatment of malignant tumors of the spermatic cord: A study of 10 cases and a review of the literature. J Urol 126:611, 1981
6. Broth G, Bullock WK, Morrow J: Epididymal tumors: 1 Report of 15 new cases including review of the literature. 2 Histochemical study of the so-called adenomatoid tumor. J Urol 100:530, 1968
7. Castor CW, Naylor B: Characteristics of normal and malignant human mesothelial cells studied in vitro. Lab Invest 20:437, 1969
8. Chan YH, Schinella RA, Draper JW: Papillary clear cell cystadenoma of the epididymis. J Urol 100:661, 1968
9. Chavimi F, Exelby PR, D'Angio GJ: Multidisciplinary treatment of embryonal rhabdomyosarcoma in children. Cancer 35:677, 1975
10. Crips JC, Roberts PF: A case of bilateral cystadenoma of the epididymis presenting as infertility. Brit J Urol 47:682, 1975
11. Davides KC, King LM, Paat F: Primary leiomyosarcoma of the epididymis. J Urol 114:642, 1975
12. El-Badawi AA, Al-Ghorab MM: Tumors of the spermatic cord: a review of the literature and a report of a case of lymphangioma. J Urol 94:445, 1965
13. Eusebi V, Massarelli G: Phaeochromocytoma of the spermatic cord: report of a case. J Path 105:283, 1971
14. Evans N: Mesotheliomas of the uterine and tubal serosa and the tunica vaginalis testis. Am J Pathol 19:461, 1943
15. Exelby PR: Testicular cancer in children. Cancer 45:1803, 1980
16. Fajers CM: Mesotheliomas of the genital tract: a report of 5 new cases and survey of the literature. Acta Path Microbiol Scand 26:1, 1949
17. Farrel MA, Donnelly BJ: Malignant smooth muscle tumors of the epididymis. J Urol 124:151, 1980
18. Faysal MH, Strefling A, Kosek J: Epididymal neoplasms: a case report and review. J Urol 129:843, 1983
19. Ferenczy A, Fenoglio J, Richart RM: Observations on benign mesothelioma of the genital tract (adenomatoid tumor). A comparative ultrastructural study. Cancer 30:244, 1972
20. Golden A, Ash J: Adenomatoid tumors of the genital tract. Am J Pathol 21:63, 1945
21. Goldman RL: A Brenner tumor of the testis. Cancer 26:853, 1970
22. Grant SM, Hoffman EF: Bilateral papillary adenomas of the epididymides. Arch Path 76:620, 1963
23. Hesseldahl H, Larsen JF: Ultrastructure of human yolk sac: endoderm, mesenchyme, tubules and mesothelium. Amer J Anat 126:315, 1969.
24. Jackson JR: The histogenesis of the "adenomatoid" tumor of the genital tract. Cancer 11:337, 1958
25. Jenkins DG, Subbuswamy SG: Leiomyosarcoma of the spermatic cord. A case report. Brit J Surg 59:408, 1972
26. Johansson JE, Lannes P: Metastases to the spermatic cord, epididymis and testicles from carcinoma of the prostate—five cases. Scand J Urol Nephrol 17:249, 1983
27. Johnson DE, Harris JD, Ayala AG: Liposarcoma of spermatic cord. Urology 11:190, 1978
28. Kage M, Kojiro M, Arakawa M, Nakamura Y, Kawada H: Paratesticular rhabdomyosarcoma. Acta Pathol Jpn 33:817, 1983
29. Kaplan WE, Firlit CF, Berger RM: Genitourinary rhabdomyosarcoma. J Urol 130:116, 1983
30. Kokotas NS, Papaharalambous ME: Lipoma of the spermatic cord in childhood. Brit J Urol 55:572, 1983
31. Krieger J, Chasko SB, Keuhnelian JG: Paratesticular neuroblastoma associated with subependymal giant cell astrocytoma. J Urol 124:736, 1980
32. Kyle VN: Leiomyosarcoma of the spermatic cord: a review of the literature and report of an additional case. J Urol 96:795, 1966
33. Lawrence W, Hays DM, Moon JE: Lymphatic metastasis with childhood rhabdomyosarcoma. Cancer 39:556, 1977
34. Lerman SH, Lerman PH: Spontaneous idiopathic hematoma of the spermatic cord: A report of 2 cases. J Urol 125:130, 1981
35. Longo VJ, McDonald JR, Thompson GJ: Primary neoplasms of epididymis; special reference to adenomatoid tumors. JAMA 147:937, 1971
36. López de Santa María J, Bustos-Obregón E: A case of bilateral cystadenoma of the epididymis causing obstructive azoospermia. Andrologia 13:548, 1981
37. MacKay B, Bennington JL, Skoglund RW: The adenomatoid tumor: fine structural evidence for a mesothelial origin. Cancer 27:109, 1971
38. Malek RS, Utz DC, Farrow GM: Malignant tumors of the spermatic cord. Cancer 29:1108, 1972
39. Marković B, Oprić M, Prica V, Colović V, Mandić R, Jeremić A: Metastasis to the funiculus spermaticus as the first sign of renal cell carcinoma. World J Surg 7:669, 1983
40. Masson P, Riopelle JL, Simard LC: Le mésothéliome béning de la sphère génital. Rev Can Biol 1:720, 1942

41. McDonald RE, Sago AL, Novicki DE, Bagnall JW: Paratesticular mesotheliomas. J Urol 130:360, 1983
42. Mostofi FK, Price EB: Tumors of the male genital system. In Atlas of tumor pathology (second series) Washington, D.C.: AFIP, 1973, 8:151
43. Mukerjee MG, Norris M, Strum DP, Mittemeyer BT, Borski AA: Mucinous adenoid tumor of the paratesticular tissue. J Urol 115:472, 1976
44. Nistal M, Cermeño de Giles F, Vázquez-Martul E, Velilla L: Leiomiosarcoma primario del epidídimo. Arch esp urol 29:109, 1976
45. Nistal M, Contreras F, Paniagua R: Adenomatoid tumor of the epididymis. Histochemical and ultrastructural study of two cases. Brit J Urol 50:121, 1978
46. Oertel YC, Johnson FB: Sclerosing lipogranuloma of male genitalia. Arch Pathol Lab Med 101:321, 1977
47. Patel M, Charlier A: Les tumeurs solides du cordon spermatique. Rev Chir 39:119, 1909
48. Price EB: Papillary cystadenoma of the epididymis. Arch Pathol 91:456, 1971
49. Puigvert A, Vázquez L, Santaularia JM: Metástasis en epidídimo de carcinoma de próstata. Arch esp urol 31:1, 1978
50. Razek AA, Pérez CA, Lee FA, Ragob AH, Askin F, Vietti T: Combined treatment modalities of rhabdomyosarcoma in children. Cancer 39:2415, 1977
51. Regadera JF, Nistal M, Vázquez-Estévez J, Rodríguez-Peralto JL: Rabdomiosarcomas genitourinarios infantiles: patología, clínica y evolución de 18 pacientes. Patología 15:131, 1982
52. Reyes CV: Spermatic cord liposarcoma. Urology 15:416, 1980
53. Rogers PC, Howards SS, Komp DM: Urogenital rhabdomyosarcoma in childhood. J Urol 115:738, 1976
54. Ross L: Paratesticular Brenner-like tumor. Cancer 21:722, 1968
55. Sago AL, Novicki DE: Rhabdomyosarcoma of spermatic cord. Urology 19:606, 1982
56. Samellas, W: Malignant neoplasms of spermatic cord. Liposarcoma. New York J Med 64:1213, 1964
57. Sclama AO, Berger BW, Cherry JM, Young JD: Malignant fibrous histiocytoma of the spermatic cord: the role of retroperitoneal lymphadenectomy in management. J Urol 130:577, 1983
58. Senoh K, Osada Y, Kawachi J: Spermatic cord liposarcoma. Brit J Urol 50:429, 1978
59. Singh A, Manhas DR: Leiomyosarcoma of the epididymis. J Surgery 31:293, 1969
60. Smailowitz Z, Kaneti J, Sober I, Krugliak L, Sacks M: Malignant fibrous histiocytoma of the spermatic cord. J Urol 130:150, 1983
61. Sogani PC, Grabstald H, Whitmore WC: Spermatic cord sarcoma in adults. J Urol 120:301, 1978
62. Sundarasivarao D: The Müllerian vestiges and benign epithelial tumours of epididymis. J Pathol Bacteriol 66:417, 1953
63. Teel P: Adenomatoid tumors of the genital tract: with special reference to the female. Amer J Obstet Gynecol 75:1347, 1958
64. Teilum G: Histogenesis and classification of mesonephric tumors of the female and male genital system and relationship to benign socalled adenomatoid tumors (mesotheliomas); comparative histological study. Acta Pathol Microbiol Scand 34:431, 1954
65. Trippitelli A, Rosi P, Selli C, Carini M, Turini D: Rhabdomyosarcoma of spermatid cord in adults. Urology 19:533, 1982
66. Wachtel TL, Mehan DJ: Metastatic tumors of the epididymis. J Urol 103:624, 1970
67. Wagner JC, Munday DE, Harrington JS: Histochemical demonstration of hyaluronic acid in pleural mesotheliomas. J Pathol Bacteriol 84:73, 1962
68. Wallini E, Popelier G, Renders G: Tumeurs paratesticulaires malignes. Discussion des problèmes de la dissémination des métastases et du traitement à propos de deux cas. Ann Urol 9:159, 1975
69. Weiss SW, Enzinger FM: Malignant fibrous histiocytoma: an analysis of 200 cases. Cancer 40:2010, 1978
70. Weitzner S: Leiomyosarcoma of the spermatic cord. Rocky Mtn Med J 64:73, 1967
71. Williamson JC, Johnson JD, Lamm DL, Tio F: Malignant fibrous histiocytoma of the spermatic cord. J Urol 123:785, 1980
72. Zone BM: Retinal anlage tumor of the epididymis: a case report. J Urol 103:106, 1970

INDEX

Acrocephalosyndactyly syndrome, 134
Adenomatoid tumor, 338–339
Adrenal cortical carcinoma, 184
Adrenal gland, 181–185
Adrenoleukodystrophy, 184–185
Adult testis, 26–51
   blood supply testis, 46–47
   germinal cells, 30
   Leydig cells, 42–46
   nerve supply, testis, 47–48
   seminiferous epithelium associations, 41
   seminiferous epithelium, cycle of, 41–42
   seminiferous tubules, 26–42
   Sertoli cells, 28–30
   spermatogenesis, 26, 32–36
   spermatogonia, 31–32
   spermiogenesis, 36–40
   spermatozoon, structure of, 40–42
   supporting structures, 26
   testicular interstitium, 42–48
   5-alpha reductase deficiency, 254–255
Alstrom-Edwards syndrome, 162–164
Antibiotics, 193
Arteriosclerosis, testicular lesions, 203–204
Arteritis, polyarteritis nodosa, 212–214
Ataxia and secondary hypogonadism, 174
Axoneme, 236–237

Basal cell nevus syndrome, 134
Beckwith-Wiedemann syndrome, 134
Bell Clapper elongation, 228
Biedmond syndrome, 175–176
Biotin deficiency, 197
Blastomycosis, 269–270
Borjeson syndrome, 176
Bowen's syndrome, 133
Brenner tumor, 341
Brown patches, epididymis, 283–284
Brucellosis, 270–271

Cadmium, 198
Calcium-poor diets, 198
Carpenter syndrome, 133, 175
Cerebrohepatorenal syndrome, 133
Choriocarcinoma, 311
Chromosome 4, short-arm delection syndrome, 133

Chromosome 21, long-arm delection syndrome, 134
Clorambucil, 193
Coccidiomycosis, 270
Cockayne's syndrome, 134
Colchicine, 193
Congenital adrenal hyperplasia, 181
Congenital anomalies, 72–93
   adenomatous hyperplasia, rete testis, 81
   adrenal cortex choristoma, 74–75
   anorchism, 87–89
   cartilaginous choristoma, 75
   choristoma and hamartoma, 74–79
   congenital testicular lymphangiectasis, 29
   cystic dysplasia, testis, 81–83
   cysts of testis and tunica albuginea, 77–78
   ectopic testicular parenchyma, 76–77
   ectopic testis, 90–92
   epidermoid cyst, 78–79
   epididymis, 83–87
   Giraldes organ, 74
   Haller's organ, 73
   Leydig-cell-only syndrome, 88
   paraganglia, 75–76
   Pedunculated hydatid of Morgagni, 72
   polyorchism, 89
   remnant embryonic structures, 72–74
   rete testis deficiency and ductuli efferentes connection, 80–81
   sessile hydatid of Morgagni, 72–73
   splenic choristoma, 75
   testes, number, size and location, 87–92
   testicular fusion, 89
   testicular hyperplasia, 90
   testicular hypoplasia, 89–90
   tubular development, 79–87
Congenital hemihypertrophy, 135
Contralateral testis, 202–203
Cornelia de lange's syndrome, 134
Cri-du-chat syndrome, 134
Cryptorchidism, 120–139, 299
   adult testes, 124
   bilateral maldescent, 125–128
   cancer, 130–131
   complications of, 129–131
   contralateral testis, 126
   dysgenetic testis, 121
   endocrinological syndromes, 133–135

Cryptorchidism (*continued*)
  epididymal anomalies, 129
  etiological factors, 120–121
  familial, 129
  genetic factors, 121
  histopathology, 122–128
  hormonal treatment, 132
  incidence, 120
  infertility, 130
  lesions and testis location, 126–127
  local anatomical anomalies, 121
  prepubertal testes, 122–123
  prognosis for differentiated histological testicular lesions, 127–128
  psychiatric problems, 131
  pubertal testes, 123
  testicular histological pattern after orchiopexy, 126
  testicular microlithiasis, 135–137
  testicular torsion, 131
  treatment, 131–133
  surgery, 132
  urological anomalies, 129
Cushing's syndrome, 184
Cyclophosphamide, 193
Cystic fibrosis, 186

del Castillo-Trabucco-de la Balze syndrome, 160–162
Dermoid cyst, 313–314, 343
Diabetes mellitus, 185–186
Diastrophic dwarfism, 134
Dibromo-chloro-propane (DBCP), 195
Diethylstilbestrol, 194
Down's syndrome, 159–160
Ductuli recti, 52
Dwarfism and secondary hypogonadism, 175
Dysgenetic testes, 299

Ectopic testis, 90–92
  femoral or crural, 91
  interstitial or superficial inguinal, 91
  pelvic, 91–92
  perineal, 91
  pubic-penile, 91
  transverse or crossed testicular ectopia, 91
Efferent ducts, 54–55
Embryonal carcinoma, 307–309
Endocrine gland disorders and testicular lesions, 178–189
  adrenal cortical carcinoma, 184
  adrenal gland, 181–185
  adrenoleukodystrophy, 184–185
  chronic liver diseases, 186–187
  congenital adrenal hyperplasia, 181
  Cushing's syndrome, 184
  cystic fibrosis, 186
  diabetes mellitus, 185–186
  feminizing adrenal hyperplasias, 182–183
  11-β hydroxylase deficiency, 182
  20-α-hydroxylase deficiency, 182–183
  21-hydroxylase deficiency, 182
  3-β-hydroxysteroid-dehydrogenase deficiency, 183
  hyperprolactinemia, 179–180
  hyperthyroidism, 180–181
  hypoprolactinemia, 179–180
  hypothyroidism, 181
  intrahepatic bile duct hypoplasia, 187
  kidney (chronic renal insufficiency), 187
  liver, 186–187
  nongenital affecting adrenal hyperplasias, 183
  pancreas, 185–186
  pituitary gland, 178–180
  pluriglandular insufficiency, 187–188
  postpubertal hypopituitarism, 178–179
  prepubertal hypopituitarism, 178
  thyroid gland, 180–181
  virilizing adrenal hyperplasias, 181–182
Epidermoid cyst, 314
Epididymal configuration, abnormalities, 84–87
  absence of, 85–86
  angulated, 84
  ductuli efferentes deficiency, 84–85
  ductus deferens, absence of, 87
  elongated epididymis, 84
  free epididymis, 84
  hyperplasia, 87
  hypoplasia, 86
  with mesorchium, 84
Epididymis, characteristics of, 52
  epididymal duct, 55–57
Epididymis, tumors of, 338–342
  adenomatoid tumor, 338–339
  Brenner tumor, 341
  leiomyoma, 339
  mucinous adenoid tumor, 341–342
  neuroectodermal tumor, infancy, 341
  papillary cystadenoma, 339–341
  primary tumors, 338–342
  sarcomas, 341
  secondary tumors, 342

Epididymis, see Spermatic ducts and epididymis
Epididymitis, 263-264
  acute, 263
  chronic non-specific, 264
Epididymo-orchitis, see Orchitis
Estrogens, 194-195

Fanconi's syndrome, 134
Feminizing adrenal hyperplasias, 182-183
Fibrosarcoma, 345
Folic acid, 197
Fraser's syndrome, 133
Fungi, 269-270

Genital duct formation, 2-3
Germ cell tumors, 298-320
  age factors, 300
  anaplastic seminoma, 305-306
  choriocarcinoma, 311
  classical or typical seminoma, 303
  classification, 300
  clinical staging, 318, 319-320
  cribriform and sclerosing seminoma, 305
  cryptorchidism, 299
  dermoid cyst, 313-314
  dysgenetic testes, 299
  embryonal carcinoma, 307-309
  epidermoid cysts, 314
  etiological factors, 298-300
  genetic causes, 298-299
  histogenesis, 300-302
  histological types, 302-315
  intratubular seminoma, 303-304
  metastasis, 315-316
  organoid teratoma, 312
  polyembryoma, 311
  scirrhous seminoma, 304-305
  seminoma, 302-303
  seminoma with trophoblastocarcinoma, 306
  spermatocytic seminoma, 306-307
  teratoma, 311-313
  testicular carcinoid, 314
  testicular treatment, 318-320
  testicular tumor markers, 316-318
  WHO classification, 314-315
  yolk sac tumor, 309-311
Gilbert-Dreyfus, Sebaoun and Belasich syndrome, 253
Glove-powder granuloma, 292-293
Goeminne's syndrome, 134
Gonadal dysgenesis, 241-242
Gonadoblastoma, 324-327

Hallerman-Streiff's syndrome, 134
Head abnormalities, spermatozoa, 227-232
  elongated head, 227-228
  irregular head, 230, 231
  macrocephalic head, 230
  microcephalic head, 229
  multinucleate spermatozoa, 232
  multiple head, 232
  multiple headed spermatozoa, 232
  round head, 229-230
  thin head, 228
  vacuolated head, 232
Hematocele, 294
Henoch-Schonlein's syndrome, 344
  purpura, 214
Histoplasma capsulatum, 270
Hormonal control, testicular function, see Testicular function, hormonal control
Hydrocele, 288-289
11-β-hydroxylase deficiency, 182
20-α-hydroxylase deficiency, 182-183
21-hydroxylase deficiency, 181-182
3-β-hydroxysteroid-dehydrogenase deficiency, 183
Hyperprolactinemia, 179-180
Hypertelorism-hypospadius, 134
Hypertension and vascular disorders, 204-205
Hyperthyroidism, 180-181
Hypogonadism, 145-164
  Alstrom-Edwards syndrome, 162-164
  autosomal chromosome aberrations, 159-160
  del Castillo-Trabucco-de la Balze syndrome (Sertoli-cell-only syndrome), 160-162
  classification of, 145-146
  Down's syndrome, 159-160
  false Klinefelter's syndrome, 152-153
  Klinefelter's syndrome, 146
    and malignant tumors, 153
  La Chapelle syndrome, 153-157
  myotonic dystrophy, 162
  Noonan's syndrome, 158-159
  prepubertal Klinefelter's syndrome, 153
  progressive muscular dystrophy, 162
  rudimentary testes syndrome, 164
  sex chromosome aberrations, 146-159
  Sohval-Soffer syndrome, 164
  true Klinefelter's syndrome, 146-151
  Weinstein's syndrome, 164
  Werner's syndrome, 162
  XYY syndrome, 157-158

Hypogonadotropic eunuchoidisms, 168
Hypogonadotropic hypogonadisms, 168
Hypopituitarism
  postpubertal, 178–179
  prepubertal, 178
Hypoprolactinemia, 179–180
Hypospermatogenesis, 103–105
Hypothyroidism, 181

Ichthyosis, 174
Idiopathic fibromatosis, 291
Idiopathic granulomatous orchitis, 271–272, 275
Idiopathic hypogonadotropic hypogonadism, 168–169
Idiopathic precocious puberty, 116
Immotile cilia syndrome, 237
Iodine deficiency, 198
Iron, 198
Isolated gonadotropin deficit, 168–169
Isosexual pseudoprecocious puberty, 116–118

Juvenile hypothyroidism, 115–116

Kidney (chronic renal insufficiency), 187
Klinefelter's syndrome, 146
  false, 152–153
  and malignant tumors, 153
  prepubertal, 153
  true, 146–151
Kraus-Ruppert syndrome, 174

LaChapelle syndrome, 153–157
Laurence-Moon-Rozabal-Bardet Biedl (LMB), 173–174
Lead, 198
Leiomyoma, 339
Leiomyosarcoma, 345
Lenz's micropthalmia syndrome, 134–135
Leopard's syndrome, 135
Leprosy, 268
Leukemic infiltration, 328–329
Leydig cell tumor, 320–323
Lipomas, 343
Liposarcoma, 345
Liver, 186–187
Lowe's syndrome, 133
Lubs, Vilar and Bergenstal syndrome, 253
Lymphangiomas, 343

Maestre de San Juan-Kallmann-de-Morsier syndrome, 169–171

Malakoplakia, 272–275
Male external genitalia, development of, 10–11
  schematic drawings, 5
Male genital tract, development, 1–13
  genital duct formation, 2–3
  male external genitalia, development of, 10–11
  male genital system, birth, 10
  spermatic ducts, development, 9–10
  testis, descent of, 11–12
  testis, development, 6–9
  undifferentiated external genitalia, 3–6
  undifferentiated gonad, evolution of, 1–2
Male pseudohermaphroditism, 245–259
  5-alpha reductase deficiency, 254–255
  17-alpha-hydroxylase deficiency, 248
  androgen synthesis defects, 246
  associated with other congenital anomalies, 259
  17.20 desmolase deficiency, 248
  dysgenetic male pseudohermaphroditism, 255–256
  Gilbert-Dreyfus, Sebaoun and Belasich syndrome, 253
  3-β-hydroxysteroid dehydrogenase deficiency, 248
  17-β-hydroxysteroid dehydrogenase deficiency, 248
  impaired metabolism of androgens by peripheral tissues, 248–252
  Lubs, Vilar and Bergenstal syndrome, 253
  mixed gonadal dysgenesis, 256–259
  Müllerian structure regression defect, 255
  persistent Müllerian duct syndrome, 257–259
  pregnenolone formation deficiency, 246–248
  Reifenstein syndrome, 253
  Rosewater, Gwinup and Hamwi syndrome, 253
  secondary to Leydig cell hypoplasia, 259
  type I incomplete male, 253
  type II incomplete male, 253–254
Malignant fibrous histiocytoma, 345–347
McCune-Albright syndrome, 115
Meckel's syndrome, 135
Meconium vaginalitis, 291–292
Mesothelial hyperplasia, 289–290
Mesothelioma, tunica vaginalis, 295–296
Middle piece abnormalities, 233–234
  bent middle piece, 233
  cytoplasmic droplets, 233

elongated middle piece, 233
short or absent middle piece, 233–234
Morphological abnormalities, *see* Specific abnormalities
Mucinous adenoid tumor, 341–342
Müllerian structure regression defect, 255
Myotonic dystrophy, 162

Neuroectodermal tumor, infancy, 341
Nongenital affecting adrenal hyperplasias, 183
Nonspecialized gonad stroma tumors, 327–331
   leukemic infiltration, 328–329
   testicular angiomas, 327–328
   testicular fibromas, 328
   testicular leiomyomas, 328
   testicular lymphoma, 329–331
   testicular neurofibromas, 328
Noonan's syndrome, 133, 158–159

Oculocerebrorenal syndrome, 133
Opitz's syndrome, 134
Orchitis, 265–275
   acute epididymo-orchitis, 265
   brucellosis, 270–271
   chronic epididymo-orchitis, 265–266
   coxackie B virus infection, 265
   fungi, 269–270
   granulomatous epididymo-orchitis, 266–275
   idiopathic granulomatous orchitis, 271–272, 275
   leprosy, 268
   malakoplakia, 272–275
   nonspecific chronic orchitis, 265–266
   parasites, 270
   syphilis, 268–269
   tuberculosis, 266–268
Osteochondritis, 135

Pancreas, 185–186
Pantothenic acid, 197
Papillary cystadenoma, 339–341
Parasites, 270
Pasqualini-Bure-McCullagh syndrome, 171–173
Periorchitis, 290–291
   fibrous pseudotumor, 291
   nodular periorchitis, 291
Persistent Müllerian duct syndrome, 257–259
Phosporus and manganese deficiency, 198
Phylariasis, 270

Physical-chemical agents, causing testicular lesions, 190–195
   avitaminosis, 196–197
   chemical agents, 192–195
   heat, 191–192
   malnutrition, 196
   minerals, 197–198
   peripheral nervous system lesions, 198–199
   x-rays, 190–191
Pituitary gland, 178–180
Pluriglandular insufficiency, 187–188
Polyembryoma, 311
Popliteal web syndrome, 134
Prader-Labhart-Willi syndrome (HHHO syndrome), 173
Precocious puberty, 114–119
   causes, 114
   heterosexual pseudoprecocious puberty, 118
   idiopathic precocious puberty, 116
   isosexual pseudoprecocious puberty, 116–118
   juvenile hypothyroidism, 115–116
   McCune-Albright syndrome, 115
   neurogenic form, 114–115
   pseudoprecocious puberty, 116
Precocious testicular maturation, *see* Precocious puberty
Progressive muscular dystrophy, 162
Prune-belly syndrome, 134
Pyridoxine, 197

Regulatory cycles, 66–67
Reifenstein syndrome, 253
Rete testis, 52–54
   adenocarcinoma, 331–332
Retractile testes, 140–144
   diagnosis, 140
   germ cell hypoplasia, 143
   seminiferous tubule lesions, 140–142
   Sertoli cell atrophy, 143
   teratospermia, 143
Rhabdomyosarcoma, 344–345
Richards-Rundle syndrome, 176
Rosewater, Gwinup and Hamwi syndrome, 253
Rubinstein-Taybis syndrome, 133
Rudimentary testes syndrome, 164
Russell-Silver's syndrome, 135

Sanctis-Cacchione's xerodermic idiotia, 135
Sarcomas, 341

Seckel's syndrome, 133
Secondary hypogonadisms, 168–177
  ataxia, 174
  Biedmond syndrome, 175–176
  Borjeson syndrome, 176
  Carpenter syndrome, 175
  constitutional delay of puberty, 168
  dwarfism, 175
  ichthyosis, 174
  idiopathic hypogonadotrophic hypogonadism, 168–169
  Kraus-Ruppert syndrome, 174
  Laurence-Moon-Rozabal-Bardet Biedl (LMB) syndrome, 173–174
  Maestre de San Juan-Kallmann-de-Morsier syndrome, 169–171
  Pasqualini-Bure-McCullagh syndrome, 171–173
  Prader-Labhart-Willi syndrome (HHHO), 173
  Richards-Rundle syndrome, 176
Semen analysis, 227
Seminoma, 302–303
  anaplastic, 305–306
  classical or typical, 303
  cribiform and sclerosing, 305
  intratubular, 303–304
  scirrhous, 304–305
  spermatocytic, 306–307
  with trophoblastocarcinoma, 306
Sertoli cell tumor, 323–324
Sexual determination, sequence of, 6
Smith-Lemli-Opitz syndrome, 133
Sohval-Soffer syndrome, 164
Specialized gonad stroma tumors, 320–324
  Leydig cell tumor, 320–323
  Sertoli cell tumor, 323–324
Spermatic cord hematoma, 343–344
Spermatic cord torsion, 208–212
Spermatic cord tumors, 342–347
  benign tumors, 343–344
  dermoid cysts, 343
  fibrosarcoma, 345
  leiomyosarcoma, 345
  lipoma, 343
  liposarcoma, 345
  lymphangiomas, 343
  malignant fibrous histiocytoma, 345–347
  malignant tumors, 344–347
  pseudotumors, 347
  rhabdomyosarcoma, 344–345
  spermatic cord hematoma, 343–344
Spermatic duct ectasia, 278–280

Spermatic ducts, development of, 9–10
Spermatic ducts and epididymis, 52–62
  ductuli recti, 52
  efferent ducts, 54
  epididymal duct, 55–57
  rete testis, 52–54
  spermatic ducts, nerve supply, 59–61
  spermatic ducts, vascularization, 59
  straight ducts, 52
  vas deferens, 57–59
Spermatic duct obstructive lesions, 278–287
  brown patches, epididymis, 283–284
  spermatic duct ectasia, 278–280
  spermatocele, 282–283
  sperm granuloma, 280–281
  vasectomy, 284–286
Spermatic head and middle piece connection defect, 232–233
Spermatocele, 282–283
Spermatogenesis, 26, 32–36
  diakinesis, 34–35
  diplotene, 34
  leptotene stage, 33
  pachytene, 34
  spermiogenesis, 36
  telophase, 35
  zygotene, 33
Spermatogonia, 31–32
Spermatozoa morphological abnormalities, see Specific abnormalities
Sperm granuloma, 280–281
Spermiogenesis, 36–40
Spironolactones, 193–194
Steroidogenesis, 64–66
Syphilis, 268–269

Tail abnormalities, 234–238
  axoneme, 236–237
  coiled sperm tail, 236
  fibrous sheath, 237
  lack of sperm tail, 235
  mitochondrial sheath, 237
  morphology, 232
  multiple sperm tails, 236
  outer fibers, 237
  short or thick sperm tail, 235–236
  ultrastructural sperm tail, 236
Teratoma, 311–313
  organoid, 312
Testicular amyloidosis, 208
Testicular angiomas, 327–328
Testicular arteriolar hyalinosis, 205–208
Testicular artery occulsion, 201–202

Testicular biopsy, 94–113
  adult testis, 99–111
  basement membrane hyalinization, 102–103
  diffuse tubular hypoplasia, 100–101
  focal germinal hypoplasia, 108
  focal tubular hypoplasia, 101
  germ cell absence, 107
  germ cell hypoplasia, 103–105
  immature germ cell sloughing, 107
  Leydig cell alterations, 97–99
  maturation arrest, 105–107
  mean tubular diameter (MTD), 95–96
  peritubular fibrosis, 103
  prepubertal testis, 95–99
  seminiferous epithelial focal alterations, 108
  seminiferous epithelium, diffuse alterations, 103
  Sertoli cell athrocytosis, 108
  Sertoli cell index, 97
  Sertoli cell oncocytic transformation, 109
  Sertoli cell vacuolation, 108–109
  spermatic granuloma, 108
  spermatocele, 108
  spermatozoon maturation anomalies, 107
  techniques, 94–95
  testicular atrophy, 99
  tubular alterations, 95, 97
  tubular atrophic mosaicism, 107–108
  tubular development failure, 100
  tubular fertility index (TFI), 96–97
  tubular malformations, 97
  tubular maturation, 99
  tubulointerstitial maturation, 99
  tunica propri alterations, 101–102
Testicular carcinoid, 314
Testicular feminization syndrome, 249–252
Testicular fibromas, 328
Testicular functions, hormonal control, 63–71
  acetate transformed into cholesterol, 65
  adenohypophysis, 63–64
  clomiphene tests, 70
  estrogens, 68
  gonadotropins, 68
  hypothalamo-pituitary axis, 63–64
  hypothalamus, 64
  intrahypothalamic control, 67
  pituitary control of hypothalamus, 67
  regulatory cycles, 66–67
  response tests, 68–69
  seminal fluid examination, 68
  spermatogenesis and release of FSH, 66–67
  steroidogenesis, 64–66
  steroidogenesis and release of testosterone, 66
  stimulation tests, 69
Testicular function tests, 67–70
  clomiphene tests, 70
  gonadotropins, 68
  seminal fluid tests, 68
  stimulation tests, 69
  testosterone, 68
Testicular leiomyomas, 329
Testicular lymphoma, 329–331
Testicular neurofibromas, 328
Testicular tumors, 298–332
  germ cell tumors, 298–320
  gonadoblastoma, 324–327
  intratesticular spermatic duct tumors, 331–332
  nonspecialized gonad stroma tumors, 327–331
  primary tumors, 298–331
  rete testis adenocarcinoma, 331–332
  secondary testis, 331
  specialized gonad stroma tumors, 320–324
  See also Specific tumors
Testicular tumor markers, 316–318
Testicular tumor metastasis, 315–316
Testicular tumor treatment, 318–320
Testis
  descent of, 11–12
  development of, 6–9
  and epididymis, birth, 11
Testis development, birth to puberty, 14–25
  active growth phase, 21
  germ cells, infantile testis, 17
  histochemical features, 23–24
  maturation phase, 21–24
  newborn, 14–18
  resting phase, 18–21
Testosterone, 197
Thiamin, 197
Thyroid gland, 180–181
Traumatic testicular rupture, 293–294
Trisomy 13 syndrome, 133
Trisomy 18 syndrome, 133
True hermaphroditism, 242–245
  varieties, 242
Tuberculosis, 266–268
Tunica vaginalis, 288–297
  fibrous pseudotumor, 291
  glove-powder granuloma, 292–293

Tunica vaginalis (*continued*)
  hematocele, 294
  hydrocele, 288–289
  idiopathic fibromatosis, 291
  meconium vaginalitis, 291–292
  mesothelial hyperplasia, 289–290
  mesothelioma, 295–296
  nodular periorchitis, 291
  traumatic testicular rupture, 293–294
Turner's syndrome, 241

Undifferentiated external genitalia, 3–6
Undifferentiated gonad, evolution of, 1–2

Van Beuthrem's syndrome, 135
Varicocele, 214–224
  anatomical bases, 215–216
  clinical classification, 214–215
  contralateral testis, 221–222
  diagnosis and treatment, 223
  effect on pregnancy rate, 224
  etiology, 216
  hormonal regulation, 223
  incidence, 214
  intratesticular spermatic pathways, 218
  ipsilateral testis, 219–221
  kidney metabolites, 218–219
  physiopathology, 217
  reduced oxygen tension, 218
  seminiferous tubule lesions, 220–221
  spermiogram, 222–223, 224
  surgical results, 223
  testis, histopathology, 219
  thermoregulation alterations, 217–218
  tunica albuginea lesions, 220
  vascular lesions, 219–220
Vascular disorders, testis, 201–226
  aneurysm formation, 214
  arteriosclerosis, testicular lesions, 203–204
  arteritis, polyarteritis nodosa, 212–214
  contralateral testis, 202–203
  fibrinoid reaction, 213
  hypertension, 204–205
  inflammatory reaction, 213–214
  intravascular coagulation, 212
  spermatic cord torsion, 208–212
  testicular amyloidosis, 208
  testicular and epididymal appendix torsion, 212
  testicular arteriolar hyalinosis, 205–208
  testicular artery occlusion, 201–202
  thrombosis, 214
  varicocele, 214–224
Vas deferens, 57–59
Vasectomy, 284–286
  late complications, 285–286
  precocious complications, 284–285
  secondary complications, 285
Vasitis nodosa, 281
Virilizing adrenal hyperplasias, 181–182
Vitamin A, 197
Vitamin B_{12} deficiency, 197
Vitamin C, 197
Vitamin E, 196–197

Weinstein's syndrome, 164
Werner's syndrome, 162

XO gonadal dysgenesis, 241
XX gonadal dysgenesis, 241
XY gonadal dysgenesis, 241
46, XX males, 153–157
XXXXY syndrome, 133
XYY syndrome, 157–158

Yolk sac tumor, 309–311
Young's syndrome, 278

Zellweger's syndrome, 133
Zinc, 197–198